OCN Exam Study Guide

OCN Review + 600 Test Questions with In-Depth Answer Explanations for the ONCC Oncology Certified Nurse Exam

Jennifer L. Bradley
© 2023-2024
Printed in USA.

Disclaimer:

© Copyright 2023 by Jennifer L. Bradley . All rights reserved.

All rights reserved. It is illegal to distribute, reproduce or transmit any part of this book by any means or forms. Every effort has been made by the author and editor to ensure correct information in this book. This book is prepared with extreme care to give the best to its readers. However, the author and editor hereby disclaim any liability to any part for any loss, or damage caused by errors or omission. Recording, photocopying or any other mechanical or electronic transmission of the book without prior permission of the publisher is not permitted, except in the case of critical reviews and certain other non-commercial uses permitted by copyright law.

Printed in the United States of America.
OCN ®, ONCC ® are registered trademarks. They hold no affiliation with this product. We are not affiliated with or endorsed by any official testing organization.

Contents

1 Care Continuum

1.1 Health promotion and disease prevention (e.g., high-risk behaviors; preventive health practices:

1.2 Screening and early detection

1.3 Navigation and coordination of care

1.4 Advance care planning (e.g., advance directives)

1.5 Epidemiology

    1.5.1 Modifiable risk factors (e.g., smoking, diet, exercise, occupation)

    1.5.2 Non-modifiable risk factors (e.g., age, gender, genetics)

1.6 Survivorship

    1.6.1 Rehabilitation

    1.6.2 Recurrence concerns

    1.6.3 Family and social support concerns

    1.6.4 Sexuality concerns

    1.6.5 Discrimination concerns

1.7 Treatment-related considerations

    1.7.1 Delayed-onset side effects

    1.7.2 Chronic side effects

    1.7.3 Subsequent malignancies

    1.7.4 Follow-up car

1.8 End-of-Life Care

    1.8.1 Grief

    1.8.2 Bereavement

    1.8.3 Hospice care

    1.8.4 Caregiver support

    1.8.5 Interdisciplinary team

    1.8.6 Pharmacologic comfort measures

    1.8.7 Non-pharmacologic comfort measure

2 Oncology Nursing Practice

2.1 Scientific basis

    2.1.1 Carcinogenesis

    2.1.2 Immunology

    2.1.3 Clinical trials (e.g., research protocols)

    2.1.4 Molecular testing and genetics

2.2 Site-specific cancer considerations

    2.2.1 Pathophysiology

2.2.2 Common metastatic locations

   2.2.3 Diagnostic measures

   2.2.4 Prognosis

   2.2.5 Classification

   2.2.6 Staging and histological grading

 2.3 Scope and Standards of Practice

   2.3.1 Accreditation (e.g., The Joint Commission, QOPI, MAGNET)

   2.3.2 Collaboration

   2.3.3 Communication

   2.3.4 Culturally congruent care

   2.3.5 Environmental health (e.g., safety, personal protective equipment, safe handling)

   2.3.6 Ethics (e.g., patient advocacy)

   2.3.7 Evidence-based practice and research

   2.3.8 Leadership

   2.3.9 Legal, license, and protection of practice (including documentation)

   2.3.10 Professional practice evaluation

   2.3.11 Quality of practice

   2.3.12 Resource utilization

   2.3.13 Self-care (e.g., managing compassion fatigue)

   2.3.14 Standards of care (nursing process)

3 Treatment Modalities

 3.1 Surgical and procedural interventions

 3.2 Blood and marrow transplant

 3.3 Radiation therapy

 3.4 Chemotherapy

 3.5 Biotherapy

 3.6 Immunotherapy

 3.7 Vascular access devices (VADs) for treatment administration

 3.8 Targeted therapies

4 Symptom Management and Palliative Care

 4.1 Etiology and patterns of symptoms (acute, chronic, late)

 4.2 Anatomical and surgical alterations (e.g., lymphedema, ostomy, site-specific radiation)

 4.3 Pharmacologic interventions

 4.4 Complementary and integrative modalities (e.g., massage, acupuncture, herbal supplements)

 4.5 Palliative care considerations

 4.6 Alterations in functioning

   4.6.1 Hematologic

    4.6.2 Immune system
    4.6.3 Gastrointestinal
    4.6.4 Genitourinary
    4.6.5 Integumentary
    4.6.6 Respiratory
    4.6.7 Cardiovascular
    4.6.8 Neurological
    4.6.9 Musculoskeletal
    4.6.10 Nutrition
    4.6.11 Cognition
    4.6.12 Energy level (i.e., fatigue)
  4.7 Pain Management

5 Oncologic Emergencies
  5.1 Disseminated intravascular coagulation (DIC)
  5.2 Syndrome of inappropriate antidiuretic hormone secretion (SIADH)
  5.3 Sepsis (including septic shock)
  5.4 Tumor lysis syndrome
  5.5 Hypersensitivity
  5.6 Anaphylaxis
  5.7 Hypercalcemia
  5.8 Cardiac tamponade
  5.9 Spinal cord compression
  5.10 Superior vena cava syndrome
  5.11 Increased intracranial pressure
  5.12 Obstructions (bowel and urinary)
  5.13 Pneumonitis
  5.14 Extravasations
  5.15 Immune-related adverse events
  5.16 Venous thromboembolism

6 Psychosocial Dimensions of Care
  6.1 Cultural, spiritual, and religious diversity
  6.2 Financial concerns
    6.2.1 Employment
    6.2.2 Insurance
    6.2.3 Resources
  6.3 Altered Body Image
  6.4 Learning preferences and barriers to learning

6.5 Social relationships and family dynamics

6.6 Coping mechanisms and skills

6.7 Support

   6.7.1 Patient (i.e., individual and group)

   6.7.2 Caregiver (including family)

6.8 Psychosocial distress

   6.8.1 Anxiety

   6.8.2 Loss and grief

   6.8.3 Depression

   6.8.4 Loss of personal control

   6.8.5 Spiritual distress

   6.8.6 Caregiver fatigue

   6.8.7 Crisis management (e.g., domestic violence, suicidal ideation)

6.9 Sexuality

   6.9.1 Reproductive issues (e.g., contraception, fertility)

   6.9.2 Sexual dysfunction (e.g., physical and psychological effects)

   6.9.3 Intimacy

   6.9.4 Considerations for sexual and gender minorities

OCN Practice Test 1
Answers with Explanation for Practice Test 1
OCN Practice Test 2
Answers with Explanation for Practice Test 2
OCN Practice Test 3
Answers with Explanation for Practice Test 3
OCN Practice Test 4
Answers with Explanation for Practice Test 4

Why do you need to be OCN Certified?

1. Enhanced Knowledge and Skills: Obtaining OCN certification signifies that you possess a comprehensive understanding of the principles and practices in the field of oncology nursing. It demonstrates your ability to provide specialized care and support to patients diagnosed with cancer. The certification process helps you expand your knowledge base and acquire advanced skillsets required in this specialized area of nursing.

2. Professional Credibility: OCN certification adds professional credibility to your profile. It demonstrates your commitment to continuous learning and improvement in the field of oncology nursing. Employers, patients, and colleagues recognize OCN certification as a mark of excellence, which can enhance your reputation and standing within the healthcare community.

3. Career Advancement Opportunities: Being OCN certified can open doors to various career opportunities in oncology nursing. Many hospitals, clinics, and healthcare organizations prioritize hiring certified oncology nurses due to their specialized knowledge and skillset. OCN certification can increase your chances of securing a promotion, assuming leadership roles, or gaining access to advanced oncology nursing positions.

4. Personal and Financial Benefits: Professionally, OCN certification can bring personal satisfaction and fulfillment. It validates your expertise and dedication in caring for individuals with cancer, contributing to your overall job satisfaction. Additionally, many organizations offer financial incentives, such as salary increases or bonuses, to OCN certified nurses as a recognition of their specialized skills and expertise. This certification can also increase job security, as employers may prioritize certified nurses during downsizing or restructuring processes.

Overall, becoming OCN certified offers numerous benefits, including expanded knowledge and skills, professional credibility, career advancement opportunities, and personal and financial rewards. It can elevate your nursing career and allow you to make a significant impact in the lives of patients battling cancer.

Willing To Join Our Author Panel?

Dear Registered Nurses,

We would like to invite you to join our 'Panel Of Authors'.

First of all, Thank you for your hard work and dedication to your patients. We know that the hours are long and the workload is demanding, but you do it with grace and dignity. Your compassion is evident in the way you treat your patients, and we are grateful for all that you do.

We believe that your expertise and experience as nurses will be a valuable contribution to our books. Our goal is to provide valuable content that helps nurses to step forward in their career development. This is a unique opportunity to share your expertise with other nurses and help shape the future of nursing.

The requirements for joining our panel of authors are as follows:
- A minimum experience of 8 years in nursing
- Proper certification from a renowned organization
- Good writing and teaching skills
- Enthusiasm in sharing knowledge

If you meet these requirements and are interested in joining our panel, please send us your resume along with a writing sample for our review to propublisher@zohomail.com . We would be happy to have you on board!

We are happy that our panel of authors can provide the best content because they are experienced and passionate about nursing. We would love for you to join our panel of authors and help us continue to provide quality content for nurses. You will also be able to connect with other nurses from around the world and build a network of support. Undoubtedly, this will be a great opportunity for you to make a difference in the nursing profession.

Thank You.

Why is this book the right choice for you to clear the OCN Exam?

Latest Study Guide:

If you are looking for an up-to-date study guide for the OCN Exam, then look no further than this book. This book provides everything you need to know to ace the exam with tons of practice questions to help you prepare. This book is also constantly updated to ensure that it always covers the latest information on the exam as per the outline provided by the ONCC®.

OCN® EXAM CONTENT OUTLINE
1. Care Continuum
2. Oncology Nursing Practice
3. Treatment Modalities
4. Symptom Management and Palliative Care
5. Oncologic Emergencies
6. Psychosocial Dimensions of Care

Experienced Set of Authors:

There are many reasons to choose this book over others, but one of the most important is that it is written by experienced authors who are OCN Certified. The authors of this book have a wealth of experience in taking and passing exams, and we have used our knowledge to create a study guide that is comprehensive and easy to follow.

With our experienced authors and comprehensive coverage, our book is the best way to prepare for this important test.

Detailed rationale for the answer:

We provide an in-depth explanation for each question, so you can understand not only the correct answer but also why it is correct. This book also gives you an ample amount of practice to help you feel confident on exam day.

Similar Question Format as that in the actual exam:

One of the most important features of this book is that the questions and answers follow the same pattern as the actual exam. This is extremely important because you need to be familiar with the format of the exam to do well on it.

Fine Tunes your thinking:

Going through the questions, answers and explanations repeatedly will sharpen your thinking and understanding ability. This will help you to understand the root of the question in the OCN Exam and make the right selection of the answer.

Clear and Concise:

This OCN Prep is written in simple language and is not overly technical. This sets this book apart from other study materials because when you are studying for the OCN Exam, you need to be able to understand the material without getting bogged down in details. This book will help you do just that. This combination of easy-to-understand language and practical testing will help you be successful on the OCN exam.

Magical Steps to Pass the OCN Exam with Ease:

1. Belief: You must believe that you can pass the OCN exam with ease. This belief will help you stay focused and motivated throughout your studies. We help build your confidence by giving you the feel of attending virtual exams in our book, making you familiar with the type of questions that will be asked in the exam, and giving you a thorough idea about all the topics as specified by ONCC®.

2. Visualization: Visualize yourself passing the OCN exam with flying colors. This will help you stay positive and focused on your goal. Taking multiple tests and solving various questions will help improve your positivity and confidence. We try our best to improve your positivity.

3. Study: Make sure to study all the material thoroughly. Quality Learning is more important than Quantity Learning. Time yourself when you take tests and try to complete them within the stipulated time.

4. Practice: The more you practice the more is the chance of passing the exam. By doing this, you will get a feel for the types of questions that will be asked and how to best answer them. We have an abundant number of questions for you to practice.

5. Relax: On the day of the exam, make sure to relax and stay calm. This will help you think more clearly and perform at your best.

Smart Learning with Trust in Yourself will make Success knock at your door! All the Best!

OCN Guide

1 Care Continuum

1.1 Health promotion and disease prevention (e.g., high-rik behaviors; preventive health practices)

Health promotion and disease prevention are essential components of the care continuum for Oncology **Nurse**s. These practices aim to reduce the incidence of cancer and other diseases by addressing high-risk behaviors and promoting preventive health measures.

High-risk behaviors that contribute to the development of cancer include tobacco smoking, excessive alcohol consumption, poor dietary choices, and lack of physical activity. Oncology Nurses play a crucial role in identifying these behaviors and educating patients about their harmful effects. By promoting healthy lifestyle choices, such as smoking cessation, moderation in alcohol intake, and regular exercise, nurses can help reduce the risk of cancer and improve overall health.

Preventive health practices are equally important in the care continuum for Oncology **Nurse**s. These measures involve early detection of cancer and the implementation of interventions to prevent further progression. Screening tests, such as mammograms, colonoscopies, and Pap smears, are instrumental in detecting cancer at an early stage when treatment is more effective. Oncology **Nurse**s are responsible for educating individuals about the importance of these tests and ensuring their participation.

Vaccinations are another aspect of preventive health practices in oncology care. Certain viruses, such as human papillomavirus (HPV) and hepatitis B, can increase the risk of developing certain types of cancer. Oncology **Nurse**s educate patients and their families about the benefits of vaccinations, such as the HPV vaccine for cervical cancer prevention or the hepatitis B vaccine for liver cancer prevention.

Education on sun protection is crucial for preventing skin cancer. Oncology **Nurse**s advise patients about the consistent use of sunscreens, protective clothing, and avoiding excessive sun exposure, especially during peak hours. This information helps patients reduce their risk of developing skin cancer.

Psychological support and counseling also play a vital role in health promotion and disease prevention. Stress, anxiety, and depression can weaken the immune system and increase the risk of cancer and other diseases. Oncology **Nurse**s provide emotional support, coping strategies, and referral to mental health **professional**s when needed to help patients manage these psychological factors.

1.2 Screening and early detection

Screening and early detection are crucial components of the care continuum for oncology **nurse**s. These processes help identify cancer at its earliest stages, increasing the chances of successful treatment and improving patient outcomes.

The primary goal of screening is to detect cancer or precancerous conditions before they develop symptoms. It involves the use of various tests such as mammograms, colonoscopies, and Pap smears to identify abnormalities in the body. By detecting cancer early, healthcare providers can intervene promptly, potentially preventing or curing the disease.

Breast cancer screening, for example, plays a significant role in early detection. Mammograms are commonly used to screen for breast cancer in women, particularly those above the age of **40**. These tests help identify any signs of cancerous cells before they form a lump or cause symptoms. Early detection through mammograms increases the likelihood of successful treatment and reduces mortality rates.

Another crucial aspect of screening and early detection is educating individuals about the importance of regular screenings. Oncology **nurse**s play a vital role in raising awareness and promoting the adoption of screening practices among the general population. They provide information about the benefits of early detection, the available screening methods, and the recommended screening intervals based on individual risk factors.

In addition to screening, early detection involves recognizing potential signs and symptoms of cancer. Training oncology **nurse**s to identify early warning signs allows for timely intervention. This includes the knowledge of specific symptoms associated with different types of cancer, such as persistent coughing, unexplained weight loss, or changes in skin color or texture. Early detection through symptom recognition can lead to prompt diagnostic testing and subsequent treatment.

Furthermore, oncology **nurse**s collaborate closely with other healthcare **professional**s to ensure effective care coordination. They work with radiologists, pathologists, and other specialists to interpret screening results accurately. Oncology **nurse**s also provide emotional support and education to patients and their families regarding the next steps in the care continuum, such as further diagnostic tests, treatment options, and potential side effects.

1.3 Navigation and coordination of care

Navigation and coordination of care play a crucial role in the care continuum for Oncology **Nurse**s. It involves guiding patients through a complex healthcare system and ensuring seamless transitions between various healthcare providers and settings.

One important aspect of navigation and coordination of care is patient advocacy. Oncology **Nurse**s act as advocates for their patients, helping them navigate through the often overwhelming process of cancer treatment. They assist patients in making informed decisions regarding their care, ensuring that their preferences and values are respected.

Another aspect is coordinating appointments and services for patients. Oncology **Nurse**s work closely with other healthcare **professional**s to schedule and coordinate appointments for surgeries, chemotherapy sessions, radiation therapy, and other treatments. They ensure that these services are aligned and minimize the burden on the patient, reducing delays or unnecessary waiting times.

Furthermore, navigation and coordination of care involve managing medical records and information. Oncology **Nurse**s are responsible for organizing and updating patient records, ensuring that information is accurate and easily accessible to the healthcare team. They play a crucial role in facilitating communication between different healthcare providers, ensuring that everyone involved in the patient's care is aware of their medical history, treatment plan, and progress.

Education and support are also essential in navigation and coordination of care. Oncology **Nurse**s provide education to patients and their families, helping them understand their diagnosis, treatment options, and potential side effects. They offer emotional support, addressing the fears and concerns of patients, and connecting them with support groups or counseling services if needed.

In addition, navigation and coordination of care extend beyond the healthcare setting. Oncology **Nurse**s may assist patients in accessing community resources such as transportation services, financial assistance programs, and home care services. They help in coordinating the provision of these resources, ensuring that patients have the necessary support to navigate the challenges of their cancer journey.

1.4 Advance care planning (e.g., advance directives)

Advanced care planning, such as advance directives, is a crucial part of the care continuum in oncology nursing. It involves conversations and documentation regarding a patient's preferences for future healthcare decisions, especially in situations where the patient may become unable to make decisions due to their medical condition. This **topic** encompasses various aspects that are crucial for oncology **nurse**s to understand and implement effectively.

One important aspect of advance care planning is discussing and documenting the patient's values, goals, and preferences for their care. This includes exploring their thoughts on life-sustaining treatments, resuscitation, and interventions that may be necessary during their cancer journey. These discussions can be sensitive, requiring empathy, active listening, and providing emotional support to the patient and their families.

Another sub**topic** within advance care planning is the importance of advance directives. These legal documents, including living wills and healthcare proxies, allow patients to express their wishes in writing regarding their medical care. Living wills outline specific medical interventions the patient may or may not want, while healthcare proxies appoint a trusted person to make decisions on behalf of the patient if they are unable to do so. Oncology **nurse**s play a significant role in facilitating the completion, understanding, and regular review of these advance directives, ensuring they accurately represent the patient's current preferences.

Additionally, discussing potential future scenarios and outcomes is vital in advance care planning. This involves conversations about the progression of the patient's cancer, treatment options, and potential complications. Oncology **nurse**s should provide information and explanations in a clear and compassionate manner, allowing the patient and their families to make informed decisions about their care.

Furthermore, integrating advance care planning into interdisciplinary healthcare teams is essential. Collaboration with **physician**s, social workers, chaplains, and other healthcare **professional**s helps ensure that the patient's goals and preferences are incorporated into their overall treatment plan. This inter**professional** approach also promotes continuity of care as patients transition between different healthcare settings.

Lastly, ongoing reassessment and documentation of advance care planning discussions and decisions are necessary. Oncology **nurse**s should regularly review these documents and ensure they are up to date, reflecting the patient's current wishes. Furthermore, these conversations should be revisited regularly to address any changes in the patient's condition or goals of care.

1.5 Epidemiology

Epidemiology is a branch of public health that focuses on the study of diseases and their patterns within specific populations. In the context of oncology nursing, epidemiology plays a crucial role in understanding the incidence, prevalence, and distribution of cancer cases.

One important aspect of epidemiology is the identification of risk factors that contribute to the development of cancer. These risk factors can be genetic, environmental, behavioral, or related to certain occupational exposures. By studying these risk factors, oncology **nurse**s can better educate patients on prevention strategies and promote healthy lifestyle choices.

Another key aspect of epidemiology in oncology nursing is the surveillance of cancer cases. Epidemiologists analyze data from cancer registries to monitor trends in cancer incidence and mortality rates. This information helps in identifying high-risk populations and developing targeted interventions for cancer prevention and control.

Epidemiology also plays a role in evaluating the impact of cancer screening programs. Oncology **nurse**s work closely with epidemiologists to assess the effectiveness of early detection initiatives such as mammography, colonoscopy, and Pap smears. By analyzing screening data and following up with patients, healthcare **professional**s can assess the overall outcomes of these programs and make necessary improvements.

In addition, epidemiology contributes to the understanding of cancer disparities among different populations. By analyzing data on socioeconomic status, race, ethnicity, and access to healthcare, epidemiologists can identify disparities in cancer outcomes. This information helps oncology **nurse**s advocate for equal access to cancer prevention, screening, and treatment services.

Furthermore, epidemiology plays a critical role in research and clinical trials. Tracking and analyzing data from clinical trials is essential for determining the efficacy and safety of new cancer treatments. Oncology **nurse**s play a vital role in conducting these trials and collecting accurate data, which is then analyzed by epidemiologists for evidence-based practice.

1.5.1 Modifiable risk factors (e.g., smoking, diet, exercise, occupation)

Modifiable risk factors are key determinants of cancer that can be changed or controlled, and they play a significant role in the prevention and management of the disease. Some of the most common modifiable risk factors include smoking, diet, exercise, and occupation.

Smoking is one of the leading causes of cancer and is responsible for an alarming number of cases. It has been firmly established that tobacco smoke contains numerous carcinogens, which cause mutations in our DNA and ultimately lead to the development of cancer. As an oncology **nurse**, it is essential to educate patients about the dangers of smoking and assist them in cessation efforts.

Diet is another crucial modifiable risk factor. Certain dietary choices, such as excessive consumption of processed meats, sugary foods, and a lack of fruits and vegetables, can significantly increase the risk of developing cancer. Encouraging patients to adopt a healthy, balanced diet rich in nutrients and antioxidants can help reduce the incidence of cancer and improve overall well-being.

Regular exercise has been shown to have numerous health benefits, including reducing the risk of cancer. Physical activity hels maintain a healthy weight, strengthens the immune system, and improves overall cardiovascular health. As an oncology **nurse**, it is important to promote regular physical activity and encourage patients to engage in activities they enjoy.

Occupational factors can also contribute to the development of cancer. Some occupations involve exposure to harmful substances such as asbestos, benzene, or ionizing radiation, which can increase the risk of certain cancers. It is essential to assess patients' occupational history and identify any potential risks, advocating for appropriate protective measures in the workplace.

In addition to these modifiable risk factors, other lifestyle choices such as alcohol consumption and sun exposure can also influence cancer risk. Alcohol, when consumed in excess, can increase the risk of various cancers, including those of the breast, liver, and colon. Promoting moderate alcohol consumption or abstinence can greatly reduce this risk. Additionally, excessive sun exposure without protection can lead to skin cancer, emphasizing the importance of sun safety measures such as wearing sunscreen and protective clothing.

As an oncology **nurse**, understanding and addressing modifiable risk factors is crucial in the care continuum of cancer patients. By educating patients about the impact of smoking, diet, exercise, and occupation on cancer risk, and supporting them in making positive lifestyle changes, we can contribute to preventing cancer and improving outcomes for those already diagnosed. Remember, every small step towards modifying these risk factors can have a significant impact on overall health and well-being

1.5.2 Non-modifiable risk factors (e.g., age, gender, genetics)

Non-modifiable risk factors in oncology refer to the characteristics or variables that cannot be changed or modified, and yet play a significant role in an individual's susceptibility to developing cancer. These risk factors include age, gender, and genetics.

Age is considered a non-modifiable risk factor because as individuals grow older, their cells are more likely to accumulate genetic mutations that can potentially lead to cancer. Advanced age is associated with an increased risk of various types of cancer, such as breast, prostate, and colorectal cancer.

Gender is another non-modifiable risk factor, as certain types of cancer are more prevalent in one gender compared to the other. For instance, breast cancer is more common in females, while prostate cancer is predominantly seen in males. The differences in hormone levels and reproductive system structure contribute to these gender-based disparities in cancer risk.

Genetics, or an individual's inherited traits, can also influence their susceptibility to cancer. Some people may inherit specific gene mutations, such as BRCA1 and BRCA2, which significantly increase the risk of developing breast and ovarian cancer. Genetic factors can also affect the body's ability to metabolize carcinogens or repair damaged DNA, making certain individuals more vulnerable to developing cancer.

It is important for oncology **nurse**s to be aware of these non-modifiable risk factors, as they can help identify individuals who may be at higher risk of developing cancer. By understanding the influence of age, gender, and genetics on cancer risk, **nurse**s can provide targeted education, screening, and preventive measures to improve patient outcomes.

In addition to age, gender, and genetics, there are other non-modifiable risk factors in oncology that warrant attention. These include a family history of cancer, certain ethnicities or race, and previous personal history of cancer or certain benign conditions. By considering these non-modifiable risk factors, **nurse**s can develop individualized care plans and implement appropriate screening protocols to detect cancer at earlier stages or even prevent its occurrence.

1.6 Survivorship

Survivorship in the field of oncology refers to the period after a person has completed their cancer treatment and is living with or beyond the disease. This phase is an important part of the care continuum for oncology **nurse**s to address, as it focuses on the long-term physical, emotional, and psychosocial needs of cancer survivors. Survivorship encompasses a range of aspects that require attention in order to provide comprehensive care and support to cancer survivors.

One crucial aspect of survivorship care is the monitoring and management of late and long-term effects of cancer treatment. Oncology **nurse**s play a pivotal role in assessing and addressing these effects, such as fatigue, pain, cognitive changes, and emotional distress. Regular follow-up visits, symptom management, and referrals to specialists are all part of the survivorship care plan.

Another key element of survivorship care is providing education and counseling to survivors about healthy lifestyle choices. **Nurse**s can guide patients in adopting behaviors that promote overall well-being, such as proper nutrition, regular exercise, smoking cessation, and stress reduction techniques. By empowering survivors with knowledge and skills, **nurse**s can help improve their quality of life and reduce the risk of other chronic illnesses.

Additionally, psychosocial support is vital during survivorship. **Nurse**s must be attuned to the emotional and psychological needs of cancer survivors, as they may experience fear, anxiety, depression, or survivor's guilt. Providing a compassionate and supportive environment, connecting them with support groups, and facilitating access to counseling services are integral aspects of survivorship care.

Furthermore, survivorship care also involves addressing the financial, employment, and insurance-related issues faced by cancer survivors. Navigating through these challenges can be overwhelming, and oncology **nurse**s can assist survivors in accessing resources, understanding their rights, and advocating for their needs.

1.6.1 Rehabilitation

Rehabilitation plays a crucial role in the survivorship care continuum for oncology patients. It encompasses a wide range of interventions aimed at helping patients regain their physical, emotional, and social well-being after cancer treatment. The goal of rehabilitation is to optimize patients' functioning, improve their quality of life, and promote their overall recovery.

In the context of oncology, rehabilitation begins as soon as the patient is diagnosed with cancer. Before treatment even starts, healthcare **professional**s assess the patient's physical and functional status to establish a baseline for rehabilitation interventions. This evaluation helps identify potential impairments, such as pain, weakness, or reduced mobility, that may arise as a result of cancer or its treatment.

During active treatment, rehabilitation focuses on managing treatment-related side effects and minimizing their impact on the patient's daily life. For example, physical therapists may use exercise programs and manual techniques to address musculoskeletal issues caused by surgery, radiation, or chemotherapy. Occupational therapists help patients adapt to any physical or cognitive changes that affect their ability to perform daily activities, such as dressing or cooking.

After treatment, rehabilitation shifts towards supporting survivors in their transition back to normal life. This phase often involves helping patients manage the long-term effects of cancer and its treatments. Rehabilitation specialists provide education and guidance on strategies to cope with fatigue, neuropathy, lymphedema, or emotional distress. They also offer options for addressing sexual dysfunction, sleep disturbances, or cognitive difficulties that may persist post-treatment.

Psychosocial rehabilitation is another vital aspect of survivorship care. Oncology nurses often collaborate with psychologists or social workers to address patients' emotional and social needs. They may facilitate individual or group counseling sessions, offer support groups, or refer patients to community resources for additional assistance.

In addition to physical and emotional rehabilitation, optimizing nutrition is a vital part of the overall rehabilitation process. Dietitians help oncology patients develop healthy eating habits to support their recovery, manage treatment-related side effects, and reduce the risk of cancer recurrence.

To ensure the effectiveness of rehabilitation interventions, a multidisciplinary approach is essential. Oncology nurses collaborate with various healthcare **professional**s, including physical and occupational therapists, psychologists, dietitians, and social workers, to deliver comprehensive care. They communicate and coordinate with these team members to develop personalized rehabilitation plans that meet each patient's unique needs and goals.

1.6.2 Recurrence concerns

Recurrence concerns are a significant aspect of survivorship and care continuum in oncology nursing. Recurrence refers to the return or reappearance of cancer after a period of remission or successful treatment. It is a **topic** of great importance for oncology **nurse**s as it has a profound impact on the physical and emotional well-being of cancer survivors.

One of the key concerns related to recurrence is the detection and early diagnosis of recurring cancer. Oncology **nurse**s play a crucial role in educating patients about the signs and symptoms of recurrence and encouraging them to report any unusual changes in their health. Regular follow-up visits and surveillance are essential to monitor the patient's condition and detect any recurrence at the earliest stage possible.

Another aspect of recurrence concerns is the psychological impact it has on patients. The fear and anxiety associated with the possibility of cancer coming back can be overwhelming for survivors. As part of their role, oncology **nurse**s provide emotional support and counseling to help patients cope with this fear and manage their anxiety. They also collaborate with other healthcare **professional**s to develop survivorship care plans that address the unique needs of each individual.

Furthermore, recurrence concerns also involve the development of strategies for managing the physical and functional consequences of recurrent cancer. Oncology **nurse**s work closely with the healthcare team to address side effects of treatment, manage pain, and improve the patient's overall quality of life. They educate patients on self-care measures, such as proper nutrition, exercise, and medication adherence, which can help reduce the risk of recurrence and improve outcomes.

Within the broader **topic** of recurrence concerns, sub**topic**s can include risk factors for recurrence, such as tumor characteristics and individual patient factors. **Nurse**s need to be knowledgeable about these risk factors and tailor their care accordingly. Additionally, survivorship programs and support groups can aid in addressing the concerns related to recurrence by providing a platform for survivors to share experiences and seek advice from others who have gone through similar challenges.

1.6.3 Family and social support concerns

Family and social support concerns are significant aspects of survivorship and the care continuum in oncology. When individuals are diagnosed with cancer, it not only affects them but also their families and social networks. Understanding and addressing these concerns is essential for the holistic well-being of the patient.

One important family concern is the emotional impact of the cancer diagnosis. Family members may experience fear, anxiety, and uncertainty about the future. Providing emotional support to both the patient and their family is crucial in helping them cope with these feelings. Oncology **nurse**s play a vital role in facilitating open communication and providing resources for addressing these emotional concerns.

Another aspect of family support involves practical considerations. Cancer treatment often involves multiple appointments, medications, and lifestyle adjustments. Family members may need to provide assistance with transportation, childcare, or even financial support. Assessing the family's practical needs and coordinating resources can help alleviate some of the burdens associated with cancer treatment.

Additionally, the family dynamics may undergo changes after a cancer diagnosis. Roles within the family may shift, and new challenges may arise. It is important for **nurse**s to assess and address any potential disruptions in the family system and provide support as needed. This may involve providing education on coping strategies, facilitating family meetings, or referring to support groups.

Social support beyond the family unit is also crucial for the well-being of cancer survivors. Friends, coworkers, and community networks can provide valuable emotional support and help reduce feelings of isolation. **Nurse**s can encourage patients to maintain and strengthen their social connections and, if needed, refer them to support groups or counseling services.

Furthermore, cultural and religious beliefs can influence how individuals and their families cope with cancer. Understanding and respecting these beliefs is vital in providing culturally competent care. Oncology **nurse**s should assess the spiritual needs of patients and their families and collaborate with the healthcare team to provide appropriate support.

1.6.4 Sexuality concerns

Sexuality concerns are an important aspect of survivorship in oncology care. Cancer and its treatment can affect various aspects of an individual's sexual health, including desire, arousal, and satisfaction. It is crucial for oncology **nurse**s to address and support patients' sexuality concerns to improve their quality of life.

One of the primary concerns in this area is the impact of cancer treatment on fertility. Some cancer treatments, such as chemotherapy and radiation therapy, can significantly affect a person's reproductive organs and hormonal balance. Discussing fertility preservation options, such as sperm or egg freezing, before treatment is essential for patients who want to have children in the future.

Body image plays a vital role in an individual's sexuality, and cancer can have a significant impact on body image. Surgeries, scars, hair loss, weight changes, and mastectomies can all contribute to body image concerns in cancer survivors. Oncology **nurse**s can provide emotional support, refer patients to support groups or counseling services, and offer resources to help individuals cope with their changing body image.

Changes in sexual desire, functioning, and satisfaction are another common concern. Cancer treatments can lead to hormonal imbalances, fatigue, pain, and emotional distress, all of which can significantly impact a survivor's sexual well-being. Oncology **nurse**s can provide education on managing symptoms, recommend medications or therapies to address sexual dysfunction, and refer patients to sexual health specialists as needed.

Communication is crucial in addressing sexuality concerns. Many patients may feel uncomfortable discussing their sexual issues due to embarrassment or fear of judgment. Encouraging open and non-judgmental communication can help patients feel more comfortable discussing their concerns. Oncology **nurse**s can initiate conversations about sexuality, create a safe and supportive environment, and provide resources to help patients explore their sexual health concerns further.

It is important to acknowledge that sexuality concerns may extend beyond the individual survivor to include their partners. Providing resources and support for couples can help them navigate these changes together and maintain a healthy intimate relationship.

1.6.5 Discrimination concerns

Discrimination concerns are a significant issue in the field of oncology nursing, as they affect the overall survivorship and care continuum for cancer patients. Discrimination can occur in various forms and can have detrimental effects on both the patients and the healthcare **professional**s involved in their care.

One aspect of discrimination concerns in oncology nursing is the unequal treatment of patients based on their demographic characteristics such as race, ethnicity, age, or socioeconomic status. This can result in disparities in access to quality care, treatment options, and supportive services. It is crucial for oncology **nurse**s to be aware of these disparities and advocate for equal treatment and resources for all patients.

Another aspect of discrimination concerns is the stigmatization of certain types of cancer or patient populations. Patients with certain types of cancer, such as lung cancer or skin cancer, may face judgment or blame for their condition due to societal perceptions or stereotypes. Oncology **nurse**s must provide unbiased and non-judgmental care to all patients, regardless of the type of cancer or any associated stigma.

Discrimination can also occur within the healthcare system itself, where healthcare **professional**s may face discrimination based on their gender, race, or other factors. This can create a hostile work environment and affect the quality of care provided to patients. It is important for healthcare organizations to foster an inclusive and supportive work culture where discrimination is not tolerated.

To address discrimination concerns in oncology nursing, education and training programs should emphasize cultural competency, diversity, and inclusion. Oncology **nurse**s should be equipped with the knowledge and skills to provide culturally sensitive care to diverse populations. Additionally, healthcare organizations should implement policies and procedures that promote equality and discourage discrimination.

Furthermore, collaboration with community organizations and advocacy groups can help raise awareness about discrimination concerns and work towards eliminating them. These organizations can provide support and resources for both patients and healthcare **professional**s, ensuring that discrimination is addressed effectively.

1.7 Treatment-related considerations

Treatment-related considerations are an essential aspect of the care continuum for oncology **nurse**s. These considerations involve various factors that need to be taken into account during the treatment of cancer patients. It is crucial for **nurse**s to have a thorough understanding of these considerations to provide optimal care to their patients.

One important treatment-related consideration is the choice of treatment modalities. Oncology **nurse**s must be familiar with different treatment options such as surgery, radiation therapy, chemotherapy, immunotherapy, and targeted therapy. Each modality has its own benefits, risks, and side effects, which the **nurse** must explain to the patient and address any concerns or questions.

Another consideration is the timing and sequencing of treatments. Depending on the type and stage of cancer, patients may receive treatments in a specific order or combination. **Nurse**s must closely monitor treatment schedules and ensure patients understand the importance of adherence.

Managing side effects is also a critical consideration. Cancer treatments often have side effects, which can significantly impact a patient's quality of life. Oncology **nurse**s must be knowledgeable about common side effects and their management strategies. This includes educating patients about potential side effects, monitoring their symptoms, and providing appropriate interventions or referrals.

Supportive care is another significant aspect of treatment-related considerations. Oncology **nurse**s play a vital role in providing supportive care to patients. This may include assessing and managing symptoms such as pain, fatigue, nausea, and neuropathy, as well as addressing psychosocial and emotional needs. **Nurse**s may collaborate with other healthcare **professional**s, such as social workers or palliative care specialists, to ensure comprehensive support for patients.

Additionally, oncology **nurse**s must consider the patient's overall health and comorbidities when planning treatments. They need to assess patients' functional status and evaluate if any adjustments to treatment regimens are necessary to optimize outcomes and minimize risks.

Furthermore, treatment-related considerations extend beyond the hospital or clinic setting. **Nurse**s should educate patients about self-care practices, such as proper nutrition, physical activity, and medication management, to promote treatment effectiveness and overall well-being.

1.7.1 Delayed-onset side effects

Delayed-onset side effects are adverse reactions that occur after a certain time period following a specific treatment in oncology patients. It is crucial for oncology **nurse**s to be aware of these delayed-onset side effects as they can impact the patients' well-being and quality of life. One common delayed-onset side effect is peripheral neuropathy, which can occur after receiving chemotherapy or radiation therapy. This condition affects the nerves in the extremities, such as the hands and feet, causing symptoms like numbness, tingling, and pain. It is important for **nurse**s to educate patients about the potential for peripheral neuropathy and monitor their symptoms throughout treatment and beyond.

Another delayed-onset side effect is lymphedema, which can develop several months or even years after surgical removal of lymph nodes. This condition occurs when the lymphatic system becomes impaired, leading to swelling and fluid retention in the affected area. Oncology **nurse**s should educate patients about the risk factors for lymphedema, such as obesity or infection, and provide guidance on preventive measures, including proper skin care and exercise.

Oncology patients may also experience late-onset cardiac toxicity as a side effect of certain chemotherapy drugs or radiation therapy to the chest area. This can manifest as heart failure or arrhythmias and requires close monitoring by **nurse**s to detect any signs or symptoms early. It is essential for **nurse**s to educate patients on the importance of reporting any cardiovascular symptoms promptly.

Delayed-onset side effects can also include hormonal imbalances, such as hypothyroidism or infertility, which may arise months or even years after treatment completion. Oncology **nurse**s should educate patients about these potential long-term effects, monitor hormone levels, and collaborate with other healthcare providers to manage these conditions effectively.

Psychosocial side effects like depression, anxiety, or post-traumatic stress disorder (PTSD) can also manifest after cancer treatment. Oncology **nurse**s should provide emotional support, refer patients to appropriate mental health **professional**s if needed, and encourage patients to engage in support groups or counseling services.

1.7.2 Chronic side effects

Chronic side effects are important considerations in the treatment of cancer patients, as they can greatly impact their quality of life and overall well-being. These side effects can occur due to various treatment modalities such as chemotherapy, radiation therapy, hormonal therapy, targeted therapy, and immunotherapy. Understanding and managing these chronic side effects is crucial for oncology **nurse**s to provide optimal care to their patients.

One common chronic side effect is fatigue, which is characterized by extreme tiredness and lack of energy. It can persist long after the completion of treatment and may negatively affect a patient's ability to perform daily activities. Oncology **nurse**s can educate patients about energy conservation techniques and encourage them to engage in regular physical activity to help alleviate fatigue.

Another chronic side effect is peripheral neuropathy, which is a condition that causes numbness, tingling, and pain in the hands and feet. This side effect is commonly associated with certain chemotherapy drugs and can impact a patient's ability to perform fine motor tasks. **Nurse**s can assess and monitor patients for signs of neuropathy and collaborate with the healthcare team to adjust treatment regimens if necessary.

Lymphedema is a chronic side effect that can occur after surgery or radiation therapy for cancer. It is characterized by the accumulation of lymph fluid, leading to swelling and discomfort in the affected limb or body part. Oncology **nurse**s can educate patients about proper skincare, exercise, and self-management techniques to prevent or manage lymphedema.

Cardiotoxicity is a chronic side effect that can occur with certain cancer treatments, particularly some chemotherapy drugs. It can lead to heart damage and increase the risk of cardiovascular events. Oncology **nurse**s play a crucial role in monitoring patients' cardiac function and collaborating with the healthcare team to manage cardiotoxicity.

Gastrointestinal issues such as diarrhea, constipation, and nausea are also common chronic side effects in cancer patients. These can significantly impact a patient's quality of life and nutritional status. Oncology **nurse**s can provide education on diet modifications, medication management, and symptom control strategies to help patients manage these gastrointestinal side effects.

1.7.3 Subsequent malignancies

Subsequent malignancies, also known as second primary cancers, are new malignant tumors that develop in individuals who have previously been treated for cancer. These secondary malignancies are often related to the primary cancer treatment received, such as radiation therapy, chemotherapy, or certain targeted therapies. Understanding and managing subsequent malignancies is an important aspect of the care continuum for oncology **nurse**s.

One of the key factors contributing to the development of subsequent malignancies is the damage caused by cancer treatments. Radiation therapy, while effective in killing cancer cells, can also damage healthy cells and increase the risk of genetic mutations leading to new cancers. Similarly, chemotherapy drugs can affect DNA replication, potentially leading to the development of secondary tumors.

Different types of subsequent malignancies can arise depending on the type of primary cancer and the treatment received. For example, individuals treated with radiation therapy for breast cancer may have an increased risk of developing subsequent lung cancer. Those who have undergone chemotherapy for leukemia may be at risk for developing secondary solid tumors, such as lung or breast cancer.

Screening and early detection play a crucial role in managing subsequent malignancies. Oncology **nurse**s can assist in coordinating and educating patients about regular screenings for these secondary tumors. This may involve recommending mammograms, pap smears, colonoscopies, or other appropriate screening tests based on the patient's treatment history and risk factors.

Furthermore, oncology **nurse**s can educate patients about lifestyle modifications and strategies to reduce their risk of subsequent malignancies. This may include promoting smoking cessation programs, encouraging a healthy diet and exercise, and minimizing exposure to known carcinogens.

Collaboration with other healthcare **professional**s is vital in addressing subsequent malignancies. Oncology **nurse**s can work closely with radiation oncologists, medical oncologists, and surgical oncologists to ensure comprehensive care for patients at risk of developing secondary tumors. This collaboration involves monitoring and managing potential side effects of treatment, as well as coordinating multidisciplinary care.

1.7.4 Follow-up care

Follow-up care is a crucial component in the treatment journey of oncology patients. It refers to the ongoing monitoring and support provided to patients after they have completed their primary treatment for cancer. This stage is essential for evaluating the patient's progress, managing side effects, detecting recurrence or new cancer, and addressing the patient's overall well-being.

The primary goal of follow-up care is to ensure that patients remain in remission and maintain their quality of life. Regular check-ups and tests are conducted to assess the patient's physical and emotional health, as well as to detect any signs of cancer recurrence. These follow-up appointments typically involve a physical examination, reviewing the patient's medical history, and conducting various diagnostic tests such as blood work, imaging scans, and biopsies.

The frequency and duration of follow-up appointments vary depending on the type and stage of cancer, as well as the individual patient's condition. Generally, patients undergo more frequent follow-up visits during the first few years after treatment and less frequent visits as time goes on.

During these appointments, oncology **nurse**s play a crucial role in providing education and support to patients. They guide patients on self-monitoring for potential symptoms and side effects of treatment. Oncology **nurse**s also address any concerns or questions that arise, providing emotional support and counseling when needed.

Monitoring and managing treatment-related side effects are an integral part of follow-up care. Oncology **nurse**s assess the patient's overall well-being, physical functioning, and quality of life. They may provide interventions to manage symptoms such as pain, fatigue, nausea, or emotional distress. They also work closely with other healthcare **professional**s, such as oncologists and social workers, to ensure comprehensive care for the patient.

In addition to physical and emotional support, follow-up care also focuses on preventive measures and health promotion. Oncology **nurse**s educate patients about lifestyle modifications, such as adopting a healthy diet, engaging in regular exercise, and avoiding tobacco and excessive alcohol consumption. They also emphasize the importance of regular screenings and vaccinations to detect and prevent other health conditions.

1.8   End-of-Life Care

End-of-life care is a crucial aspect of the care continuum for oncology **nurse**s. This type of care involves providing holistic support to patients who are in the final stages of their life and are facing a terminal illness, such as cancer.

One important aspect of end-of-life care is symptom management. Oncology **nurse**s play a vital role in assessing and addressing the physical and emotional symptoms that arise as patients near the end of their life. This may include managing pain, nausea, fatigue, and other symptoms that can impact a patient's quality of life.

Another key component of end-of-life care is facilitating communication and decision-making. Oncology **nurse**s work closely with patients and their families to ensure that they have the information and support they need to make informed decisions about their care. This may involve discussing treatment options, exploring palliative care or hospice services, and assisting with advance care planning, such as creating a living will or designating a healthcare proxy.

Psychosocial support is also a crucial aspect of end-of-life care. Oncology **nurse**s provide emotional support to patients and their families, helping them navigate the complex emotions and challenges that arise during this difficult time. This may involve providing counseling, connecting patients and families with support groups or mental health services, and addressing spiritual or existential concerns.

Another important aspect of end-of-life care is ensuring that patients receive culturally sensitive and individualized care. Oncology **nurse**s strive to understand and respect the unique beliefs, values, and preferences of each patient and their family, tailoring their care accordingly. This may involve collaborating with interdisciplinary teams, such as social workers, chaplains, and translators, to address cultural, religious, or language barriers.

Lastly, bereavement support is a significant component of end-of-life care for oncology **nurse**s. They continue to offer support to the families and loved ones of patients even after their passing. This may involve providing grief counseling, connecting them with appropriate resources and support services, and assisting with memorial or funeral arrangements.

1.8.1   Grief

Grief is a complex emotional response that individuals experience following a significant loss or death. As an oncology **nurse**, it is crucial to understand and address the **topic** of grief in the context of end-of-life care and the care continuum for patients and their families.

Grief can be divided into different stages or phases, including shock and denial, anger, bargaining, depression, and acceptance. Each stage is unique and varies in duration and intensity for each individual. Understanding these stages can help oncology **nurse**s provide effective and empathetic support to patients and their families.

One aspect of grief is anticipatory grief, which occurs when individuals anticipate the impending loss of a loved one. This type of grief can begin before the actual death and can be equally challenging for patients and their families. Oncology **nurse**s should be prepared to address anticipatory grief by providing emotional support, facilitating open communication, and connecting families with appropriate resources such as counseling or support groups.

Additionally, grief can manifest in physical and psychological symptoms. Physical symptoms may include fatigue, sleep disturbances, loss of appetite, or physical pain. Oncology **nurse**s should monitor and address these symptoms to ensure the overall well-being of their patients. Psychological symptoms of grief may include sadness, guilt, anxiety, or difficulty concentrating. **Nurse**s should provide a safe space for patients and families to express these emotions and refer them to mental health **professional**s if necessary.

Supporting bereaved individuals is another essential aspect of grief in end-of-life care. Oncology **nurse**s should offer compassionate care to families and friends after the loss of a loved one. This can be done by providing information about grief support services, encouraging self-care practices, and conducting bereavement follow-up to assess the grieving process.

It is important for oncology **nurse**s to assess their own emotional well-being while supporting individuals experiencing grief. Self-care practices, such as debriefing sessions, counseling, and engaging in hobbies or self-reflection, can help **nurse**s cope with the emotional demands of their work

1.8.2   Bereavement

Bereavement refers to the period of adjustment and mourning that follows the loss of a loved one. In the context of end-of-life care and the care continuum for oncology **nurse**s, bereavement plays a crucial role in supporting both patients and their families.

When a patient passes away, the family members may experience a range of emotions such as sadness, anger, guilt, and even relief. It is vital for oncology **nurse**s to understand these complex emotions and provide compassionate support during this difficult time.

One important aspect of bereavement is the grieving process. Grief can manifest in various ways, including emotional, physical, cognitive, and social reactions. Emotional reactions may include feelings of sadness, loneliness, and despair. Physical reactions can manifest as fatigue, loss of appetite, or sleep disturbances. Cognitive reactions may involve difficulties in concentration or memory, while social reactions can lead to withdrawal from social activities or strained relationships.

Nurses can help individuals navigate through the grieving process by providing them with a safe space to express their emotions, validating their feelings, and offering empathy and active listening. It is crucial to respect cultural and religious beliefs surrounding grief and to provide necessary resources such as support groups or counseling services.

Supporting bereaved family members is equally important as they may also experience profound grief and struggle with adjusting to life without their loved one. **Nurse**s can provide emotional support, offer practical assistance, and encourage the use of community resources.

Another significant aspect of bereavement is anticipatory grief. This type of grief occurs when individuals and their families prepare for the impending loss of a loved one. Oncology **nurse**s can help patients and their families cope with anticipatory grief by providing information about the disease progression, treatment options, and available support services.

Furthermore, understanding the concept of complicated grief is crucial for oncology **nurse**s. Complicated grief refers to an intense and prolonged form of grief that may require **professional** intervention. **Nurse**s should be aware of the signs of complicated grief and refer individuals to appropriate mental health services when necessary.

1.8.3 Hospice care

Hospice care is a vital component of end-of-life care in the continuum of care for patients with terminal illnesses. Oncology **nurse**s play a crucial role in providing compassionate and holistic care during this stage of a patient's journey.

Hospice care focuses on enhancing the quality of life for patients with limited life expectancy, typically those with advanced cancer or other terminal illnesses. The aim is to provide physical, emotional, and spiritual support to both the patient and their loved ones.

One important aspect of hospice care is managing pain and symptoms. **Nurse**s work closely with the interdisciplinary team to develop personalized care plans that address the patient's specific needs. This may include administering medications, providing comfort measures, and promoting relaxation techniques.

Another key element is psychosocial support. Oncology **nurse**s offer counseling and support to patients and their families, helping them navigate through the emotional challenges that arise during the end-of-life stage. They provide a listening ear, facilitate open communication, and offer guidance in decision-making.

Communication and education are essential within the hospice setting. **Nurse**s help patients and their families understand the disease process, treatment options, and what to expect as the illness progresses. They empower patients to make informed choices and ensure their wishes are respected.

Collaboration with the interdisciplinary team is crucial in hospice care. **Nurse**s work closely with **physician**s, social workers, spiritual counselors, and other healthcare **professional**s to create a comprehensive care plan. This team approach ensures that all aspects of the patient's well-being are addressed.

Supporting the family is a significant part of oncology **nurse**s' role in hospice care. They provide emotional support, guidance in caregiving, and help with making end-of-life decisions. **Nurse**s also assist in facilitating family meetings to ensure effective communication and shared decision-making.

As part of their responsibilities, oncology **nurse**s play a pivotal role in advocating for patients and their families. They ensure that care is delivered with dignity and respect, while honoring the patient's cultural and religious beliefs. **Nurse**s also strive to provide a peaceful and comfortable environment for patients as they near the end of life.

Continuity of care is vital in hospice care. **Nurse**s work closely with the healthcare team to ensure a smooth transition between care settings, such as hospital to home or hospice facility. They provide education and support to the patient's caregivers, equipping them with the necessary skills to manage the patient's care at home.

1.8.4 Caregiver support

Caregiver support is a crucial aspect of end-of-life care in the oncology field. Oncology **nurse**s play a vital role in providing support and guidance to caregivers, who are often family members or close friends of the patient. Understanding and addressing the specific needs of caregivers can greatly enhance the quality of care provided to the patient.

One important aspect of caregiver support is education. Oncology **nurse**s can educate caregivers about the patient's condition, treatment options, and potential side effects. This knowledge empowers caregivers to make informed decisions and actively participate in the patient's care. **Nurse**s can also provide information about community resources, support groups, and counseling services available to caregivers.

Practical assistance is another crucial component of caregiver support. **Nurse**s can offer guidance on managing medications, providing personal care, and addressing the patient's emotional and psychological needs. They can also teach caregivers techniques for managing pain, reducing discomfort, and promoting a peaceful and comfortable environment for the patient.

Emotional support is equally important for caregivers. Oncology **nurse**s can provide a listening ear, offer empathy, and validate the caregiver's feelings and experiences. They can create a safe space for caregivers to express their concerns, fears, and grief. By acknowledging and addressing these emotions, **nurse**s can help caregivers maintain their own mental and emotional well-being while caring for their loved ones.

Respite care is a sub**topic** that should be addressed when discussing caregiver support. **Nurse**s can help identify and facilitate respite care options, where caregivers can take a short break from their caregiving responsibilities to rest and recharge. This respite can help prevent caregiver burnout and ensure they have the energy and emotional capacity to provide optimal care for the patient.

Collaboration with the interdisciplinary team is essential for effective caregiver support. Oncology **nurse**s can work closely with social workers, counselors, and other healthcare **professional**s to develop a comprehensive care plan that addresses the needs of both the patient and the caregiver. Regular communication and coordination with the team can ensure that caregivers receive the support they need throughout the end-of-life care continuum.

1.8.5 Interdisciplinary team

In end-of-life care within the oncology setting, the interdisciplinary team plays a crucial role in ensuring comprehensive and holistic patient care. The interdisciplinary team consists of healthcare **professional**s from various disciplines who collaborate to provide optimal care to patients at the end of their lives.

One of the primary goals of the interdisciplinary team is to manage symptoms and promote quality of life for patients. This team typically includes oncology **nurse**s, **physician**s, social workers, psychologists, nutritionists, and other specialists. Each member brings their unique **expert**ise to the team, allowing for a comprehensive approach to patient care.

The oncology **nurse**, as a vital member of the interdisciplinary team, plays a pivotal role in coordinating and delivering end-of-life care. They act as a liaison between patient and team, advocating for the patient's needs and ensuring their preferences are respected. The **nurse** closely monitors the patient's physical and emotional well-being, addressing any symptoms and providing comfort measures.

Collaboration and communication are key aspects of the interdisciplinary team's functioning. Regular meetings are held to discuss each patient's care plan, assess progress, and make necessary adjustments. This ensures that all team members are aware of the patient's condition and goals of care. Open lines of communication enable the team to work together seamlessly and make informed decisions.

The interdisciplinary team also focuses on providing psychosocial support to both patients and their families. Social workers and psychologists help patients cope with emotional distress, anxiety, and depression that may arise during this challenging time. They provide counseling, facilitate support groups, and guide families in making difficult decisions.

Additionally, the interdisciplinary team emphasizes the importance of spiritual care. Chaplains or spiritual counselors may be included to address the patient's spiritual needs and provide comfort through religious practices or rituals.

End-of-life care often involves complex decision-making, such as advance care planning and discussions regarding resuscitation, ventilation, and palliative sedation. The interdisciplinary team ensures that these conversations are guided by ethical principles and the patient's wishes are respected.

1.8.6 Pharmacologic comfort measures

End-of-life care in oncology nursing is a crucial aspect of providing comfort and support to patients during their final stage of life. Pharmacologic comfort measures play a significant role in managing symptoms and ensuring a peaceful experience for patients.

Pharmacologic comfort measures refer to the use of medications or drugs to alleviate pain, manage symptoms, and improve patients' quality of life. These measures are designed to address physical, emotional, and psychological distress that patients may encounter during end-of-life care.

One of the main objectives of pharmacologic comfort measures is pain management. Oncology **nurse**s work closely with healthcare teams to assess and evaluate the intensity of a patient's pain and prescribe appropriate medications. These medications may include opioids, nonsteroidal anti-inflammatory drugs (NSAIDs), or other analgesics, depending on the severity of the patient's pain.

In addition to pain management, pharmacologic comfort measures encompass various other symptoms that patients may experience. This includes addressing symptoms such as nausea, vomiting, dyspnea, anxiety, depression, and delirium. Medications such as antiemetics, benzodiazepines, antidepressants, and antipsychotics may be used to alleviate these symptoms.

Another important aspect of pharmacologic comfort measures is the consideration of individual patient preferences and goals of care. Oncology **nurse**s are responsible for engaging in meaningful conversations with patients and their families to understand their values, wishes, and treatment goals. These discussions help guide the selection of appropriate medications and dosages while aligning with the patient's overall care plan.

Oncology **nurse**s also play a vital role in educating patients and their families about the potential benefits and side effects of medications used for comfort measures. It is essential to provide clear instructions on administration, dosage, and potential adverse reactions. This empowers patients and their families to make informed decisions and actively participate in their care.

Continual reassessment and adjustment of pharmacologic comfort measures are crucial in end-of-life care. Oncology **nurse**s closely monitor patients' symptoms, assess the effectiveness of medications, and communicate any changes to the healthcare team. Regular evaluation ensures that optimal symptom management is achieved, and any necessary adjustments are made promptly.

1.8.7 Non-pharmacologic comfort measure

Non-pharmacologic comfort measures are an essential aspect of end-of-life care in oncology. These measures focus on providing comfort and alleviating symptoms without relying solely on medications. They play a crucial role in enhancing the quality of life for patients who may be experiencing physical, emotional, or spiritual distress.

One important aspect of non-pharmacologic comfort measures is the promotion of a soothing and calm environment. This can be achieved by ensuring that the patient's room is peaceful, with dimmed lighting and minimal noise. Creating a serene atmosphere can help reduce anxiety and promote relaxation.

Another key element is the provision of physical comfort. Oncology **nurse**s can assist patients by positioning them in a comfortable manner, using pillows and cushions to support their body and joints. Gentle massages or touch therapies, such as hand-holding or therapeutic touch, can also be beneficial in relieving pain and promoting a sense of well-being.

Emotional support is crucial for patients nearing the end of life. Oncology **nurse**s can provide active listening, empathy, and emotional validation to patients and their families. Encouraging open communication and creating a space for patients to express their fears, concerns, or wishes can help alleviate emotional distress.

Spiritual care is another vital component of non-pharmacologic comfort measures. Oncology **nurse**s can support patients' spiritual needs by facilitating access to chaplains, offering opportunities for prayer or meditation, and respecting patients' cultural or religious beliefs and practices. Spiritual care can provide comfort and a sense of purpose, helping patients find solace during this vulnerable time.

Promoting comfort also involves managing symptoms that may arise in end-of-life care. This can include techniques such as deep breathing exercises, relaxation techniques, and distraction methods, like music or guided imagery. These interventions can help patients cope with pain, dyspnea, or nausea, reducing reliance on pharmacologic interventions.

Education and support for caregivers are integral parts of non-pharmacologic comfort measures. Providing information on how to assist in pain management, administer non-pharmacologic interventions, and implement self-care strategies can empower caregivers and improve their ability to support their loved ones.

2 Oncology Nursing Practice

2.1 Scientific basis

Scientific basis forms a significant aspect of oncology nursing practice. It encompasses the knowledge and understanding of scientific principles that underpin the delivery of care to individuals with cancer. By focusing on evidence-based practice, oncology **nurse**s can provide the highest quality of care to their patients.

One essential component of the scientific basis in oncology nursing practice is understanding the biology of cancer. Knowledge of how cancer develops, grows, and spreads is crucial for **nurse**s in order to comprehend the disease process and effectively manage the care of patients. This includes understanding the different types of cancer, their risk factors, and their specific treatment options.

Another key aspect is the comprehension of the various treatment modalities available for cancer patients. This involves staying up-to-date with the latest advancements in oncology, including emerging therapies and clinical trials. By understanding the scientific basis behind different treatments, oncology **nurse**s can educate their patients about the potential benefits and risks, and support them in making informed decisions about their care.

Moreover, a solid foundation in research and evidence-based practice is essential for oncology **nurse**s. They need to be able to critically analyze scientific literature and research studies to ensure that their practice is based on the best available evidence. This involves staying abreast of current research findings, attending conferences, and engaging in continuous **professional** development opportunities.

In addition to understanding the scientific principles of cancer, oncology **nurse**s also need to have a comprehensive knowledge of symptom management and supportive care. This includes the management of side effects from treatments, such as chemotherapy-induced nausea and vomiting, fatigue, and pain. By utilizing evidence-based strategies, **nurse**s can help alleviate these symptoms and improve the quality of life for their patients.

Furthermore, the scientific basis in oncology nursing practice extends to the use of technology and informatics. **Nurse**s need to be proficient in utilizing electronic health records, medication administration systems, and other technological advancements to ensure accurate and efficient care delivery. This also includes understanding the ethical considerations and privacy issues related to the use of technology in healthcare.

2.1.1 Carcinogenesis

Carcinogenesis is the process of the development of cancer in the body. It involves the transformation of normal cells into cancerous cells through a series of genetic mutations. Carcinogenesis can be divided into several stages: initiation, promotion, and progression. Each stage plays a crucial role in the development and progression of cancer.

In the initiation stage, exposure to certain carcinogens, such as chemicals, radiation, or viruses, damages the DNA of normal cells. This DNA damage can result in mutations, which can disrupt the normal functions of the cells and lead to the development of cancer. These mutations can be inherited or acquired during a person's lifetime.

During the promotion stage, the mutated cells undergo further changes that allow them to divide and proliferate. This can be triggered by various factors, including hormonal changes, chronic inflammation, or exposure to certain chemicals. The promotion stage can last for years and increases the likelihood of cancer development.

In the progression stage, the cancer cells continue to grow and invade nearby tissues. They can also spread to other parts of the body through the bloodstream or lymphatic system, a process known as metastasis. The progression of cancer is influenced by various factors, including the type of cancer, the aggressiveness of the tumor, and the individual's immune system.

Understanding the mechanisms of carcinogenesis is essential in the field of oncology nursing practice. Oncology **nurse**s play a vital role in educating patients about the risk factors for cancer and promoting healthy behaviors to prevent its development. They also provide support and care for patients undergoing cancer treatment, including chemotherapy, radiation therapy, and surgery.

Early detection of cancer is another crucial aspect of oncology nursing. **Nurse**s are often involved in screening programs and can help identify individuals who may be at higher risk for developing cancer. By detecting cancer at an early stage, treatment outcomes can be improved, and the chances of survival can be increased.

2.1.2 Immunology

Immunology is a branch of science that focuses on the study of the immune system, which plays a crucial role in protecting the body from foreign substances such as viruses, bacteria, and cancer cells. It is an important **topic** for oncology **nurse**s as it helps them understand the complexities of the immune system and its role in cancer development and treatment.

One of the key concepts in immunology is the distinction between the innate and adaptive immune responses. The innate immune system provides the first line of defense against pathogens and is composed of physical barriers, such as the skin, as well as cells and molecules that can quickly recognize and eliminate foreign substances. On the other hand, the adaptive immune system is more specific and involves the production of antibodies and activation of specialized immune cells, such as T and B lymphocytes, which work together to recognize and eliminate specific pathogens.

Understanding the immune system's response to cancer is essential for oncology **nurse**s. Cancer cells can evade immune surveillance by developing mechanisms to avoid detection and destruction by the immune system. Immunotherapy, a rapidly advancing field in cancer treatment, aims to harness the power of the immune system to target and eliminate cancer cells. Several types of immunotherapy, such as immune checkpoint inhibitors and CAR-T cell therapy, have shown promising results in various types of cancers.

Oncology **nurse**s need to be familiar with the various immunotherapeutic agents used in cancer treatment, their mechanisms of action, potential side effects, and monitoring requirements. They play a vital role in educating and counseling patients about immunotherapy, managing treatment-related adverse events, and assessing treatment response.

Furthermore, immunology also encompasses the study of immune deficiencies, autoimmune diseases, and hypersensitivity reactions, which are relevant **topic**s for oncology **nurse**s caring for patients with cancer. Understanding these conditions can help **nurse**s identify and manage potential complications and provide appropriate supportive care.

2.1.3 Clinical trials (e.g., research protocols)

Clinical trials, specifically research protocols, play a critical role in the scientific basis of oncology nursing practice. These trials are conducted to evaluate new treatments, therapies, and interventions for various types of cancer. They are designed to test the safety and efficacy of these interventions in order to improve patient outcomes and advance medical knowledge.

In a clinical trial, a group of patients who share similar characteristics and have a specific type of cancer are enrolled and assigned to different treatment groups. The treatments being studied can range from new drugs or combination therapies to surgical procedures or radiation techniques. Each treatment group is closely monitored and compared to determine its effectiveness and potential side effects.

The research protocols of clinical trials are meticulously planned and regulated. Before a trial can begin, it must be approved by an institutional review board (IRB) to ensure that it meets ethical standards and protects the rights and welfare of the participants. These protocols outline the study objectives, inclusion and exclusion criteria for participation, treatment schedules, data collection methods, and statistical analyses.

One important aspect of clinical trials is informed consent. Oncology **nurse**s play a vital role in educating and supporting patients and their families about the trial, its potential risks and benefits, and their rights as participants. They help individuals make informed decisions by providing understandable and accurate information.

During the clinical trial, oncology **nurse**s serve as integral members of the research team. They actively participate in patient recruitment, data collection, and adverse event reporting. They closely monitor patients for any changes in their condition and ensure that they receive proper care and follow-up.

The results of clinical trials are crucial in shaping oncology nursing practice. They provide evidence for evidence-based practice, guide treatment decision-making, and contribute to the development of clinical guidelines. **Nurse**s who are actively involved in clinical trials gain valuable knowledge and experience that they can apply in their everyday practice to deliver high-quality care to cancer patients.

2.1.4 Molecular testing and genetics

Molecular testing and genetics play a crucial role in the scientific basis of oncology nursing practice. These fields of study help healthcare **professional**s better understand the genetic makeup of cancer cells and how they interact with various treatments. By analyzing the molecular characteristics of tumors, oncology **nurse**s can provide personalized and targeted care to their patients.

One important aspect of molecular testing is the identification of genetic mutations within cancer cells. These mutations can provide valuable information about the specific type of cancer a patient has and its potential response to different treatments. By understanding the genetic profile of a tumor, oncology **nurse**s can recommend personalized therapies that target these specific mutations, leading to more effective treatment outcomes.

In addition to identifying genetic mutations, molecular testing also allows for the monitoring of treatment response and disease progression. By analyzing the levels of specific biomarkers in a patient's blood or tissue samples, oncology **nurse**s can determine whether a treatment is working or if the cancer is becoming resistant to the therapy. This information is vital in adapting the treatment plan and making informed decisions about patient care.

Genetics also plays a crucial role in determining an individual's susceptibility to certain types of cancer. Some people may inherit gene mutations that increase their risk of developing specific cancers, such as breast or colorectal cancer. Oncology **nurse**s can help identify individuals at higher risk through genetic counseling and testing. This information allows for early detection, preventive measures, and tailored screening protocols.

Furthermore, molecular testing and genetics aid in the identification and monitoring of minimal residual disease (MRD). MRD refers to the small number of cancer cells that remain in a patient's body after treatment. By utilizing sensitive molecular tests, oncology **nurse**s can detect and monitor these residual cells to assess the effectiveness of treatment and determine if further interventions are necessary.

Molecular testing and genetics also have a significant impact on the field of targeted therapies. These therapies specifically target the underlying molecular alterations in cancer cells. Oncology **nurse**s play a crucial role in educating patients about the benefits and potential side effects of these treatments. They also closely monitor patients for any adverse reactions or treatment-related complications.

2.2 Site-specific cancer considerations

Site-specific cancer considerations in oncology nursing practice refer to the identification and management of unique factors associated with cancers that occur in specific locations or organs in the body. These considerations are essential for **nurse**s to effectively provide comprehensive and individualized care to cancer patients.

One important aspect of site-specific cancer considerations is understanding the distinct risk factors associated with different types of cancers. For example, lung cancer is strongly linked to smoking, while skin cancer can be caused by overexposure to sunlight. By recognizing these risk factors, oncology **nurse**s can educate patients on prevention strategies and early detection.

Additionally, **nurse**s must be knowledgeable about the signs and symptoms specific to various types of cancers. Breast cancer, for instance, may present with a breast lump or change in breast shape, while colon cancer can cause abdominal pain and changes in bowel habits. Recognizing these symptoms allows **nurse**s to promptly refer patients for further evaluation and potential diagnosis.

Furthermore, site-specific cancer considerations involve understanding the diagnostic procedures and treatment modalities used for each cancer type. **Nurse**s must be familiar with imaging techniques such as mammography for breast cancer or colonoscopy for colon cancer. They should also be aware of the various treatment options available, including surgery, chemotherapy, radiation therapy, and targeted therapies.

Nurses should also be well-versed in the potential complications and side effects associated with specific cancer treatments. For example, radiation therapy to the head and neck region may result in oral mucositis or dysphagia, while chemotherapy can cause nausea, vomiting, and hair loss. By anticipating and managing these complications, **nurses** can improve patients' quality of life during and after treatment.
In addition to medical aspects, site-specific cancer considerations extend to the psychosocial and emotional needs of patients. **Nurse**s should provide emotional support and guidance to help patients and their families cope with the challenges of cancer. They should also facilitate access to support groups, counseling services, and community resources.
Finally, site-specific cancer considerations may involve coordinating care across multiple healthcare disciplines. **Nurse**s collaborate with surgeons, oncologists, radiologists, and other healthcare **professional**s to ensure comprehensive and coordinated care. This collaboration includes the effective communication of patient information, facilitating referrals, and advocating for the best interests of the patient.

2.2.1 Pathophysiology

Pathophysiology is a branch of medical science that focuses on the study of the functional changes that occur as a result of a disease or injury within the body. In the context of site-specific cancer considerations in the field of oncology nursing, understanding the pathophysiology of different types of cancer is crucial for providing effective care and treatment to patients.
One important aspect of studying the pathophysiology of cancer is understanding the cellular changes that lead to its development. Cancer is characterized by the uncontrolled growth and division of abnormal cells, which can form tumors and invade surrounding tissues. Genetic mutations play a key role in initiating and promoting this abnormal cell growth, and they can occur as a result of various factors such as exposure to carcinogens, family history, or underlying genetic abnormalities.
Furthermore, the pathophysiology of cancer involves the interaction between malignant cells and the body's immune system. Cancer cells can evade immune surveillance and suppression mechanisms, allowing them to proliferate and spread throughout the body. This interaction between cancer cells and the immune system also plays a significant role in the effectiveness of cancer treatment options such as immunotherapy.
Different types of cancer present unique pathophysiological features that impact patient care. For example, breast cancer pathophysiology involves the proliferation of abnormal cells within the breast tissue, leading to the formation of tumors. Understanding the specific molecular markers and genetic mutations associated with breast cancer helps guide treatment decisions, such as targeted therapy or hormone therapy.
Similarly, lung cancer pathophysiology is influenced by various factors, including exposure to tobacco smoke and genetic predisposition. The understanding of lung cancer subtypes, such as non-small cell lung cancer and small cell lung cancer, allows for tailored treatment approaches including surgery, radiation, or chemotherapy.

2.2.2 Common metastatic locations

Common metastatic locations refer to the areas where cancer cells often spread from the primary site. Metastasis occurs when cancer cells break away from the tumor and travel through the bloodstream or lymphatic system to other parts of the body. Identifying the common sites of metastasis is crucial for oncology **nurses** to provide effective care and support to cancer patients.
One of the most common sites of metastasis is the bones. Cancer cells have a tendency to spread to the bones, especially the spine, hips, and long bones. This can cause severe pain, fractures, and other complications. Oncology **nurse**s need to be vigilant in assessing for bone metastasis and providing appropriate pain management and supportive care.
Another common location for metastasis is the liver. Many types of cancer, such as colon, breast, lung, and pancreatic cancer, have a high likelihood of spreading to the liver. Liver metastases can cause symptoms like abdominal pain, jaundice, and liver dysfunction. Oncology **nurse**s play a crucial role in monitoring liver function and managing symptoms in patients with liver metastasis.
The lungs are also frequently affected by metastatic cancer. Cancers of the breast, colon, kidney, and bladder often spread to the lungs. Lung metastases can lead to respiratory symptoms like cough, shortness of breath, and chest pain. Oncology **nurse**s need to assess respiratory function regularly and provide interventions to alleviate symptoms and improve quality of life.
Brain metastasis is another significant concern in cancer patients. Breast, lung, and melanoma cancers are commonly associated with metastases to the brain. Metastatic brain tumors can cause neurological symptoms such as headaches, seizures, and changes in cognitive function. Oncology **nurse**s should be knowledgeable about the signs and symptoms of brain metastasis and collaborate with the healthcare team to provide appropriate care and support to patients.
Other common sites of metastasis include the lymph nodes, adrenal glands, and distant organs such as the ovaries, abdominal organs, and skin. Each of these sites presents unique challenges and requires specific assessments and interventions from oncology **nurse**s.

2.2.3 Diagnostic measures

Diagnostic measures play a crucial role in the field of oncology nursing when considering site-specific cancer. These measures involve various tests and procedures that help in the identification and assessment of cancer in specific areas of the body. By employing these diagnostic measures, oncology **nurse**s can gather important information that guides the overall management and treatment of cancer.
One of the common diagnostic measures utilized in oncology nursing practice is imaging tests. These tests include X-rays, computed tomography (CT) scans, magnetic resonance imaging (MRI), and positron emission tomography (PET) scans. They help in visualizing organs and tissues, allowing **nurses** and doctors to detect any abnormalities or tumors in the specific site of concern.
In addition to imaging tests, biopsies are essential diagnostic measures used by oncology **nurse**s. Through this procedure, a small sample of tissue or cells is taken from the suspected area and examined under a microscope. This helps in confirming the presence of cancer cells and determining the stage and type of cancer. There are various types of biopsies, such as needle biopsies, endoscopic biopsies, and surgical biopsies, each having its own advantages and considerations.
Moreover, blood tests play a crucial role in the diagnostic process. Oncology **nurse**s may collect blood samples to assess tumor markers or specific biomarkers associated with certain types of cancer. These tests aid in monitoring the response to treatment, detecting recurrence, and assessing the overall health status of the patient.

Diagnostic measures in oncology nursing also extend to genetic testing. Genetic tests analyze an individual's DNA to identify any inherited gene mutations that may increase the risk of developing certain types of cancer. By identifying these genetic variations, oncology **nurse**s can provide patients and their families with appropriate counseling and guidance regarding preventive measures or surveillance strategies. Another important aspect of diagnostic measures in oncology nursing is staging and grading. Staging determines the extent and spread of cancer, while grading evaluates the aggressiveness and characteristics of the cancer cells. These assessments help oncology **nurse**s and other healthcare **professional**s in devising personalized treatment plans and predicting the prognosis for the patient.

2.2.4 Prognosis

Prognosis is an essential aspect of oncology nursing practice, specifically when considering site-specific cancers. It refers to the predicted outcome or course of a disease, particularly cancer, based on various factors such as the stage of the cancer, the patient's overall health, and the response to treatment.

Understanding the prognosis of a site-specific cancer plays a crucial role in planning and providing effective nursing care. The prognosis can help **nurse**s communicate effectively with patients and their families, provide emotional support, and assist in making informed decisions about treatment options.

When discussing the prognosis of a site-specific cancer, it is important to consider factors such as the stage of the cancer. The staging system helps determine the extent and spread of the cancer, aiding in predicting the disease's course. **Nurse**s need to have a comprehensive understanding of the staging system specific to each cancer type to effectively assess the prognosis.

Another aspect to consider when discussing prognosis is the patient's overall health. Pre-existing conditions, comorbidities, and overall physical and mental well-being can significantly impact the prognosis. **Nurse**s need to assess these factors thoroughly and collaborate with other healthcare providers to provide comprehensive care.

Response to treatment is also a crucial factor in determining prognosis. Some cancers respond well to specific therapies, while others may be more resistant. **Nurse**s play a vital role in monitoring treatment response, managing side effects, and educating patients about the signs and symptoms of treatment effectiveness or failure.

Additionally, **nurse**s need to provide ongoing support and education to patients and their families regarding prognosis. This can involve explaining medical terminologies, discussing treatment options, and addressing any concerns or anxieties they may have. **Nurse**s should encourage patients and families to ask questions and actively participate in decision-making processes.

Furthermore, it is essential for **nurse**s to stay updated with the latest research and advancements in cancer treatment to accurately discuss prognosis with patients and families. Evidence-based practice ensures that **nurse**s provide accurate information and stay informed about emerging treatment options that may improve prognosis.

2.2.5 Classification

Classification is a crucial aspect of oncology nursing practice when considering site-specific cancers. It involves categorizing malignancies based on their anatomical location, histological characteristics, and molecular profiles. This classification allows healthcare **professional**s, including oncology **nurse**s, to develop targeted treatment and care plans for patients.

One primary aspect of classification is the anatomical location of the cancer. Site-specific cancers, such as breast, lung, colorectal, or prostate cancer, are named after the organ or tissue in which they originate. Understanding the site of the cancer helps oncology **nurse**s in identifying potential symptoms and planning appropriate interventions.

Histological classification is another essential component of cancer classification. It involves examining the microscopic characteristics of cancer cells and assigning them to specific subtypes. For example, breast cancer can be classified into subtypes like invasive ductal carcinoma or lobular carcinoma based on the appearance of cells under a microscope. By categorizing cancers histologically, oncology **nurse**s can better understand the disease process and predict its behavior.

The advancement of molecular profiling has significantly influenced cancer classification. Molecular classification involves analyzing the genetic and molecular alterations present in cancer cells. This information helps in identifying specific biomarkers, such as mutations or gene expression patterns, that can guide treatment decisions. Oncology **nurse**s play a vital role in understanding and interpreting the results of molecular tests, enabling personalized care for patients.

Sub**topic**s related to classification in oncology nursing practice include staging and grading systems. Staging is the process of determining the extent of cancer spread, while grading assesses the aggressiveness of tumor cells. These systems provide valuable information for treatment planning and prognosis assessment.

Furthermore, classification in oncology nursing practice also involves recognizing and understanding cancer subtypes that may have unique clinical characteristics and treatment options. For example, within lung cancer, there are different subtypes such as non-small cell lung cancer and small cell lung cancer, each requiring tailored approaches to care.

2.2.6 Staging and histological grading

Staging and histological grading are essential components in the field of oncology nursing practice, specifically when considering site-specific cancers. These tools allow oncology **nurse**s to accurately assess and classify tumors, enabling them to provide appropriate treatment and care for patients.

Staging refers to the process of determining the extent and spread of cancer within the body. It involves gathering information from various sources such as physical exams, imaging tests, and biopsies. The primary goal of staging is to determine the size of the tumor, whether it has spread to nearby tissues or lymph nodes, and if it has metastasized to distant organs. This information is crucial for developing an effective treatment plan and predicting the patient's prognosis.

Histological grading, on the other hand, focuses on the characteristics of cancer cells under a microscope. Pathologists analyze tissue samples obtained through biopsies or surgical procedures to determine the grade of the tumor. This grading system classifies tumors into different grades based on their degree of differentiation and cellular abnormalities. Higher-grade tumors tend to be more aggressive and have a poorer prognosis compared to lower-grade tumors.

When considering site-specific cancers, staging and histological grading become even more vital. Different cancers have specific staging systems tailored to their unique characteristics. For example, breast cancer uses the TNM system, which evaluates tumor size, lymph node involvement, and metastasis. Staging allows oncology **nurse**s to accurately communicate the disease stage to other healthcare **professional**s, facilitate treatment decisions, and provide patients with information about their prognosis and potential treatment outcomes. Histological grading provides valuable insights into the aggressiveness and behavior of site-specific cancers. **Nurse**s can use this information to educate patients about their disease, potential treatment options, and the importance of early detection. It also helps **nurse**s assess the response to treatment and monitor for disease recurrence. By understanding the specific grading system for a particular cancer, oncology **nurse**s can provide appropriate support and guidance to patients and their families throughout the cancer journey.

2.3 Scope and Standards of Practice

Scope and Standards of Practice in oncology nursing encompass the range of responsibilities and tasks that an oncology **nurse** is expected to carry out. These standards are set by **professional** nursing organizations and serve as a guide for the practice of oncology nursing. The scope of practice defines the boundaries within which an oncology **nurse** can function. It encompasses the knowledge, skills, and abilities that an oncology **nurse** must possess to provide quality care to patients with cancer. This includes assessing and diagnosing patients, developing and implementing care plans, administering medications and treatments, and providing emotional support to patients and their families.

The standards of practice outline the level of care that is expected from an oncology **nurse**. These standards cover a wide range of areas such as assessment and screening of patients, prevention and management of complications, coordination of care with other healthcare **professional**s, education and guidance for patients and their families, and participation in research and quality improvement initiatives.

Within the scope of practice, oncology **nurse**s are responsible for assessing the physical, emotional, and psychosocial needs of patients with cancer. They monitor patients for signs and symptoms of complications, administer medications and treatments, and provide education and counseling to patients and their families regarding the disease and its management. They also coordinate care with other members of the healthcare team to ensure continuity and effectiveness of treatment.

Oncology **nurse**s play a crucial role in supporting patients and their families throughout the cancer journey. They offer emotional support, provide information about treatment options and their potential side effects, and assist in decision-making processes. They also advocate for patients' rights and preferences, ensuring that their individual needs are met.

Furthermore, oncology **nurse**s contribute to the advancement of cancer care through their involvement in research and quality improvement initiatives. They participate in clinical trials, contribute to evidence-based practice, and strive to improve the quality of care provided to patients with cancer.

2.3.1 Accreditation (e.g., The Joint Commission, QOPI, MAGNET)

Accreditation plays a crucial role in ensuring the delivery of high-quality healthcare services, including oncology nursing practice. Several organizations are responsible for accrediting healthcare facilities and recognizing excellence in the field of oncology nursing. The most prominent accrediting bodies include The Joint Commission, QOPI (Quality Oncology Practice Initiative), and MAGNET (The Magnet Recognition Program).

The Joint Commission is a well-known organization that accredits and certifies healthcare organizations in the United States. It sets rigorous standards and conducts comprehensive evaluations to ensure that healthcare facilities meet or exceed the criteria for quality and safety. The accreditation process involves an on-site survey conducted by trained **professional**s who assess various aspects of patient care, including oncology nursing practices. The Joint Commission's accreditation is highly regarded and demonstrates a commitment to exceptional patient care.

QOPI, on the other hand, is a robust quality improvement program specifically designed for oncology practices. It focuses on measuring and improving the quality of cancer care provided by healthcare **professional**s. QOPI certification requires participating oncology practices to undergo a rigorous evaluation process, including documentation review and on-site visits. This accreditation signifies a dedication to delivering evidence-based, high-quality cancer care.

MAGNET accreditation recognizes nursing excellence in healthcare organizations. To achieve this prestigious designation, healthcare facilities must demonstrate exceptional nursing leadership, **professional** development opportunities, and a positive work environment. MAGNET-accredited hospitals have highly skilled and empowered oncology nursing staff, who provide excellent patient-centered care. This recognition enhances the reputation and credibility of nursing **professional**s within the organization and the broader healthcare community.

Accreditation by these organizations provides numerous benefits to oncology **nurse**s and their patients. It assures patients that they are receiving care from healthcare facilities that meet stringent quality and safety standards. For oncology **nurse**s, it represents **professional** growth opportunities, as maintaining accreditation often necessitates continuous learning and improvement. Accreditation also fosters a culture of accountability and encourages the adoption of best practices in oncology nursing.

2.3.2 Collaboration

Collaboration plays a crucial role in the scope and standards of practice for oncology nursing. It refers to the process of working together with other healthcare **professional**s, patients, and their families to provide comprehensive and holistic care to individuals affected by cancer.

One important aspect of collaboration in oncology nursing is interdisciplinary teamwork. Oncology **nurse**s often work alongside **physician**s, surgeons, radiologists, and other specialists to develop and implement individualized treatment plans for cancer patients. By collaborating with these **professional**s, oncology **nurse**s can contribute their specialized knowledge and skills to ensure the best possible outcomes for their patients.

Effective communication is another essential component of collaboration in oncology nursing practice. Nurses must communicate information about the patient's condition, treatment options, and any potential side effects or complications to the interdisciplinary team. In turn, they also gather feedback and recommendations from other team members to provide a comprehensive care plan for the patient. Collaboration also extends beyond healthcare professionals to include patients and their families. Oncology nurses work collaboratively with patients to educate them about their diagnosis, treatment options, and self-care strategies. By involving patients in the decision-making process, nurses empower them to take an active role in managing their disease and improving their quality of life.

Furthermore, collaboration with patients and their families helps in addressing their emotional and psychosocial needs. Oncology nurses provide support, counseling, and resources to help patients cope with the challenges that cancer brings. By collaborating with patients and their families, nurses can develop individualized care plans that consider their preferences, values, and goals.

In addition to interdisciplinary teamwork and patient/family collaboration, oncology nurses also collaborate with community resources and organizations. They establish partnerships with cancer support groups, rehabilitation centers, and palliative care services to provide a continuum of care for patients beyond the hospital setting. These partnerships ensure that patients have access to comprehensive and integrated services that address their physical, emotional, and spiritual needs.

2.3.3 Communication

Communication is a vital aspect of oncology nursing practice. Effective communication is essential for providing comprehensive care to oncology patients. It involves the exchange of information, thoughts, and feelings between the oncology nurse and the patient, as well as with other healthcare professionals.

One important aspect of communication in oncology nursing practice is establishing rapport and building trust with patients. This involves active listening, empathizing with their concerns, and showing genuine care and compassion. By doing so, the oncology nurse can create a supportive and therapeutic environment for the patient.

Clear and concise communication is crucial in conveying important medical information to patients. Oncology nurses must be able to explain complex medical concepts in a way that patients and their families can understand. This requires using simple language, avoiding medical jargon, and providing visual aids or written materials when necessary.

In addition to verbal communication, non-verbal cues such as body language and facial expressions also play a significant role in effective communication. Oncology nurses need to be aware of their own non-verbal communication as well as accurately interpreting the non-verbal cues of their patients. This can facilitate a better understanding of emotions and needs.

Another subtopic related to communication is the importance of interdisciplinary collaboration. Oncology nurses must communicate effectively with other members of the healthcare team, including physicians, pharmacists, and social workers. This ensures that everyone is working together to provide the best possible care for the patient.

Communication also encompasses the documentation of patient information. Oncology nurses must accurately and comprehensively record patient assessments, interventions, and outcomes. This documentation serves as a communication tool for other healthcare professionals involved in the patient's care and helps ensure continuity of care.

Furthermore, communication extends beyond the patient and healthcare team to include the patient's family and support system. Oncology nurses need to effectively communicate with family members, providing emotional support, answering their questions, and involving them in care decisions when appropriate

2.3.4 Culturally congruent care

Culturally congruent care is an essential aspect of oncology nursing practice that focuses on providing care that is sensitive and responsive to the cultural beliefs, values, and practices of patients from diverse backgrounds.

One important aspect of culturally congruent care is cultural awareness. Oncology nurses need to be aware of their own cultural biases and beliefs in order to deliver care that is unbiased and respectful of the patient's cultural identity. This involves recognizing and understanding the impact of culture on health beliefs, attitudes towards illness, and treatment preferences.

Cultural knowledge is also crucial in providing culturally congruent care. Oncology nurses should seek to understand the cultural practices, traditions, and healthcare beliefs of their patients. This includes knowledge about cultural norms related to communication, decision-making, and end-of-life care. By having a deeper understanding of their patients' cultural backgrounds, oncology nurses can provide care that is appropriate and respectful.

Another important aspect of culturally congruent care is communication. Clear and effective communication is essential in building trust and understanding with patients from different cultures. It is important for oncology nurses to be aware of language barriers, use interpreters when necessary, and employ culturally appropriate communication techniques, such as using visual aids or gestures. Good communication also involves active listening and seeking clarification to ensure accurate understanding.

Respecting cultural preferences and beliefs is another key component of culturally congruent care. Oncology nurses should be sensitive to the values and preferences of patients, such as religious or spiritual beliefs, dietary restrictions, and preferences for gender-specific care providers. Respecting these preferences helps to foster a trusting and collaborative relationship with patients and can positively impact their overall satisfaction and outcomes.

Culturally congruent care also involves advocating for patients by addressing any cultural barriers that may affect their access to care or treatment. This may include collaborating with interdisciplinary teams to develop culturally appropriate care plans, connecting patients with community resources, or advocating for translation services.

2.3.5 Environmental health (e.g., safety, personal protective equipment, safe handling)

Environmental health is a crucial aspect of oncology nursing practice as it encompasses various elements such as safety, personal protective equipment (PPE), and safe handling. By prioritizing environmental health, oncology nurses can create a safe and secure environment for both patients and themselves.

Safety is of utmost importance in oncology nursing practice. **Nurse**s must adhere to strict safety protocols to prevent accidents, injuries, and the spread of infections. This includes maintaining a clean and clutter-free workspace, ensuring proper disposal of hazardous waste, and regularly sanitizing equipment and surfaces.

Personal protective equipment plays a vital role in shielding **nurse**s from potential health hazards. Oncology **nurse**s commonly use PPE such as gloves, masks, gowns, and goggles to protect themselves and prevent the transmission of infectious agents. It is crucial to utilize appropriate PPE and ensure its proper usage, including correct donning and doffing techniques.

Safe handling practices are essential to minimize occupational hazards in oncology nursing. This involves correctly handling and disposing of hazardous substances, such as chemotherapy drugs, which can pose risks to both **nurse**s and the environment if mishandled. **Nurse**s should receive thorough training on safe handling procedures and be knowledgeable about local regulations regarding the disposal of hazardous materials.

Additionally, environmental health extends beyond the physical work environment. Oncology **nurse**s also need to educate patients and their families about the importance of maintaining a safe home environment. This may include providing guidance on storing medications securely, minimizing exposure to environmental toxins, and promoting practices that enhance overall well-being.

Sub**topic**s that fall under environmental health include:
1. Safety protocols in oncology nursing practice.
2. Importance of personal protective equipment (PPE) for oncology **nurse**s.
3. Proper usage and disposal of PPE.
4. Safe handling of hazardous substances, such as chemotherapy drugs.
5. Training on safe handling procedures and compliance with regulations.
6. Educating patients and families about creating a safe home environment.

2.3.6 Ethics (e.g., patient advocacy)

Ethics, specifically patient advocacy, is a critical aspect of the scope and standards of practice in oncology nursing. Patient advocacy refers to the ethical responsibility of the oncology **nurse** to advocate for the best interests and well-being of their patients throughout their cancer journey. This involves promoting autonomy, respect for patient choices, and ensuring the provision of high-quality care.

One important aspect of patient advocacy is respecting the autonomy and decision-making capacity of the patient. Oncology **nurse**s must empower their patients by providing them with accurate and comprehensive information about their condition, treatment options, and potential outcomes. This allows patients to make informed decisions about their care, taking into account their values and preferences.

Another crucial aspect of patient advocacy is ensuring that the patient's rights are protected and their needs are met. Oncology **nurse**s have a responsibility to address any concerns or complaints their patients may have and to advocate for fair and equitable healthcare practices. This may involve collaborating with other healthcare **professional**s to establish effective communication channels, ensuring the patient's access to appropriate resources, and addressing any barriers they may face in receiving optimal care.

In addition to individual patient advocacy, oncology **nurse**s also play a role in advocating for broader systemic changes that improve the overall quality of cancer care. This may involve participating in policy development, research initiatives, and quality improvement projects. By actively engaging in these activities, oncology **nurse**s can contribute to the enhancement of patient care and the advancement of ethical standards within the field.

Ethics in patient advocacy also encompasses the principles of beneficence and nonmaleficence. Oncology **nurse**s have a duty to act in the best interests of their patients and to avoid causing harm. This involves regularly assessing the patient's physical, emotional, and psychosocial well-being, and intervening appropriately to alleviate their suffering.

2.3.7 Evidence-based practice and research

Evidence-based practice and research is an integral component of oncology nursing practice. It involves using the best available evidence to inform clinical decision-making and improve patient outcomes.

Oncology **nurse**s who practice evidence-based care utilize scientific research, clinical **expert**ise, and patient preferences to guide their interventions. By integrating these three components, **nurse**s are able to provide the highest quality of care that is individualized to meet each patient's unique needs.

One important aspect of evidence-based practice is the use of research findings. **Nurse**s critically appraise peer-reviewed articles, clinical practice guidelines, and systematic reviews to identify the most current and relevant evidence. Research studies help **nurse**s understand the efficacy of various treatments and interventions, allowing them to make informed decisions about patient care.

Another aspect of evidence-based practice is the integration of clinical **expert**ise. **Nurse**s draw upon their own knowledge and experience to assess patient needs, develop nursing diagnoses, and plan appropriate interventions. This **expert**ise is essential in understanding the unique complexities and challenges of oncology patients.

Patient preferences also play a significant role in evidence-based practice. Oncology **nurse**s consider individual patient values, beliefs, and priorities when making care decisions. By involving patients in their own care, **nurse**s ensure that treatment plans are aligned with individual goals and preferences.

The implementation of evidence-based practice involves a systematic approach. **Nurse**s engage in a process that includes asking clinical questions, searching for and appraising evidence, integrating the evidence into practice, and evaluating the outcomes. This cyclic process allows **nurse**s to continually improve the quality of care they provide.

The ultimate goal of evidence-based practice and research in oncology nursing is to enhance patient outcomes. By integrating the best available evidence, clinical **expert**ise, and patient preferences, **nurse**s can optimize treatment plans, improve symptom management, and enhance overall quality of life for patients with cancer.

2.3.8 Leadership

Leadership is a crucial aspect of oncology nursing practice, falling under the broad **topic** of Scope and Standards of Practice. As an oncology **nurse**, developing strong leadership skills is vital for providing high-quality patient care and ensuring positive outcomes.

At its core, leadership in oncology nursing involves guiding and inspiring individuals and teams towards achieving common goals. It requires the ability to effectively communicate, collaborate, and make critical decisions in a dynamic healthcare environment. Leading by example and being a role model for others is also an essential component of effective leadership.

Within the realm of oncology nursing, there are several key aspects that encompass leadership. Firstly, oncology **nurse** leaders must possess clinical **expert**ise and stay updated on the latest evidence-based practices and advancements in the field. This knowledge enables them to provide competent and comprehensive care to cancer patients.

Furthermore, leadership in oncology nursing involves advocating for patients and their families. This includes ensuring their rights are protected, actively involving them in decision-making processes, and providing emotional support throughout their cancer journey. Oncology **nurse** leaders also collaborate with other healthcare **professional**s to develop and implement interdisciplinary care plans that address the physical, emotional, and psychosocial needs of patients.

In addition, effective leadership in oncology nursing involves fostering a positive and inclusive work environment. This includes promoting a culture of respect, open communication, and teamwork. By empowering and supporting their colleagues, **nurse** leaders enable them to provide the best possible care to patients. They also play a pivotal role in mentoring and developing other **nurse**s, helping them grow both **professional**ly and personally.

In order to become effective leaders, oncology **nurse**s can benefit from specialized leadership training and education. This may include courses on communication skills, conflict resolution, critical thinking, and decision-making. Developing leadership skills can also involve seeking opportunities for additional certifications and involvement in **professional** organizations related to oncology nursing.

2.3.9 Legal, license, and protection of practice (including documentation)

Legal, license, and protection of practice are crucial aspects of the scope and standards of practice in oncology nursing. It is essential for oncology **nurse**s to adhere to the legal and regulatory requirements in order to ensure patient safety and maintain **professional** integrity. One of the key components in the legal aspect is obtaining and maintaining a valid nursing license. **Nurse**s must have a current and unrestricted license to practice oncology nursing in their respective state or jurisdiction. This license serves as a legal document that validates an individual's qualifications and competence to provide safe and effective care to oncology patients.

In addition to holding a nursing license, oncology **nurse**s must also comply with various laws, regulations, and policies related to the practice of nursing. These regulations are designed to protect patients and promote high-quality care. **Nurse**s should have a thorough understanding of these laws and ensure compliance with documentation, confidentiality, and consent requirements.

Documentation plays a crucial role in nursing practice, including oncology nursing. Accurate and comprehensive documentation is essential for communication, continuity of care, legal protection, and reimbursement purposes. Oncology **nurse**s must maintain detailed records of assessments, interventions, medication administration, patient education, and any adverse events or complications.

Furthermore, **nurse**s should be aware of the legal and ethical considerations regarding patient confidentiality. Protecting patient privacy and maintaining confidentiality of medical information is of utmost importance. Oncology **nurse**s must adhere to HIPAA regulations and other applicable laws to safeguard patient information and only share necessary information with relevant healthcare providers.

Oncology **nurse**s must also be aware of their responsibility to report any incidents, errors, or near misses that may compromise patient safety. Reporting such occurrences can help identify systemic issues and improve patient care outcomes. Whistleblower protection laws exist to safeguard **nurse**s who report violations and protect them from retaliation.

Continuous **professional** development and ongoing education are vital for oncology **nurse**s to stay current with legal and regulatory changes in their practice. **Nurse**s should actively seek opportunities for learning and **professional** growth to ensure they are providing safe and ethical care to oncology patients.

2.3.10 Professional practice evaluation

Professional practice evaluation is a crucial aspect of oncology nursing practice. It involves a comprehensive assessment of an oncology **nurse**'s clinical skills, knowledge, and overall performance in providing care to oncology patients. This evaluation helps ensure that the **nurse** is delivering the highest quality care and meeting the established standards of practice.

One important component of **professional** practice evaluation is the assessment of clinical competence. This includes evaluating the **nurse**'s ability to perform various nursing procedures and interventions specific to oncology care. It assesses their knowledge of the disease process, treatment modalities, symptom management, and evidence-based practices in oncology nursing.

Another aspect of **professional** practice evaluation is the evaluation of critical thinking and problem-solving skills. Oncology **nurse**s must be able to analyze complex situations, prioritize patient needs, and make sound clinical judgments. They should demonstrate the ability to assess, plan, implement, and evaluate patient care effectively.

Continuing education and **professional** development are essential in oncology nursing. Therefore, **professional** practice evaluation also focuses on assessing a **nurse**'s commitment to ongoing learning and growth. This may involve reviewing the **nurse**'s participation in workshops, conferences, certifications, and other educational activities that enhance their knowledge and skills.

Furthermore, **professional** practice evaluation considers the **nurse**'s adherence to ethical and legal standards. Oncology **nurse**s must uphold a high level of integrity, confidentiality, and respect for patient autonomy. Compliance with institutional policies, standards, and regulatory requirements is also assessed during the evaluation process.

Effective communication and collaboration are vital skills for oncology **nurse**s. Hence, **professional** practice evaluation may involve assessing the **nurse**'s ability to communicate effectively with patients, families, and inter**professional** teams. This includes conveying complex medical information, providing emotional support, and facilitating shared decision-making.

Self-reflection and self-assessment play a crucial role in **professional** growth. Thus, **professional** practice evaluation may encourage oncology **nurse**s to engage in self-evaluation, identifying their strengths and areas for improvement. Self-assessment promotes personal and **professional** development, leading to enhanced patient outcomes.

2.3.11 Quality of practice

The quality of practice in oncology nursing is of utmost importance in providing optimal care to patients. It encompasses various aspects that contribute to the overall effectiveness and excellence of nursing practice in the field of oncology.

One crucial aspect of quality practice is the utilization of evidence-based practice. This involves using the best available evidence from research studies, clinical **expert**ise, and patient preferences to guide decision-making and nursing interventions. By incorporating evidence-based practice, oncology **nurse**s can ensure that their care is based on the most up-to-date and effective interventions, leading to improved patient outcomes.

Another important element is the establishment of clear standards and guidelines for oncology nursing practice. These standards outline the expectations and responsibilities of oncology **nurse**s and provide a framework for consistent and high-quality care. They cover various aspects, such as assessment, communication, symptom management, end-of-life care, and patient education. Adhering to these standards ensures that oncology **nurse**s are providing safe, effective, and patient-centered care.

Continuing education and **professional** development also contribute to the quality of practice in oncology nursing. As the field of oncology constantly evolves, it is crucial for **nurse**s to stay updated with the latest advancements, treatment modalities, and research findings. By participating in educational programs, attending conferences, and obtaining certifications, oncology **nurse**s can enhance their knowledge and skills, ultimately leading to improved patient care.

Collaboration and interdisciplinary teamwork are additional components of quality practice in oncology nursing. Oncology **nurse**s work closely with other healthcare **professional**s, such as **physician**s, pharmacists, social workers, and nutritionists, to develop comprehensive care plans and ensure coordinated and holistic care for their patients. Effective communication, mutual respect, and shared decision-making among the healthcare team are vital in delivering high-quality care and optimizing patient outcomes.

Patient advocacy is a fundamental aspect of quality practice in oncology nursing. Oncology **nurse**s serve as advocates for their patients, ensuring their rights are respected, and their needs are met. This involves empowering patients to make informed decisions about their care, promoting their autonomy, and addressing their concerns and preferences. By advocating for their patients, oncology **nurse**s can help improve patient satisfaction and contribute to their overall well-being.

2.3.12 Resource utilization

Resource utilization in oncology nursing practice refers to the efficient and effective management of various resources, including time, personnel, equipment, and supplies, to deliver quality care to individuals with cancer. This **topic** covers several important aspects that help oncology **nurse**s optimize resource utilization and enhance patient outcomes.

One essential aspect of resource utilization is time management. Oncology **nurse**s must prioritize their tasks, plan their schedules, and allocate their time efficiently to provide timely and comprehensive care to their patients. They need to ensure that they have ample time for assessments, treatments, medication administration, and patient education, while also considering factors such as emergencies or unexpected events.

Another crucial aspect is personnel management. Oncology **nurse**s work as part of an interdisciplinary team, which includes **physician**s, **nurse** practitioners, pharmacists, social workers, and other healthcare **professional**s. Effective resource utilization involves coordinating with team members, delegating tasks appropriately, and collaborating to provide comprehensive care. This includes utilizing the **expert**ise and skills of each team member to their fullest potential and promoting teamwork and communication.

Equipment and supplies management is also vital in resource utilization. Oncology **nurse**s must ensure that they have the necessary equipment and supplies readily available for various procedures and treatments. This involves proper inventory management, regular maintenance, and effective communication with supply chains to prevent delays or shortages. It is important to have protocols in place for equipment handling, storage, and replacement to optimize resource utilization and minimize waste.

In addition to managing these resources, oncology **nurse**s also play a role in cost-effective practice. They need to consider the cost implications of different interventions or treatments and work towards minimizing unnecessary expenditures without compromising patient care. This can be achieved through evidence-based practice, standardization of protocols, and collaboration with financial advisors and administrators.

Furthermore, education and training are essential for resource utilization in oncology nursing practice. **Nurse**s should stay updated with the latest advancements, guidelines, and protocols in cancer care to ensure efficient and effective resource utilization. Continuous **professional** development and training programs can enhance their knowledge and skills, allowing them to provide comprehensive care while making the best use of available resources.

2.3.13 Self-care (e.g., managing compassion fatigue)

Self-care, specifically managing compassion fatigue, is a crucial aspect of oncology nursing practice that **nurse**s need to prioritize for their own well-being. Compassion fatigue refers to the emotional and physical exhaustion experienced by healthcare **professional**s who are constantly exposed to the suffering of others. It can be particularly prevalent in the field of oncology nursing, which deals with patients facing serious illnesses, pain, and the potential for loss.

To effectively manage compassion fatigue, oncology **nurse**s should engage in self-care practices that address their physical, emotional, and spiritual needs. This includes practicing regular exercise, maintaining a balanced diet, and getting enough restorative sleep. **Nurse**s should also make time for activities they enjoy and find fulfilling outside of work. Engaging in hobbies, spending time with loved ones, and participating in support groups can help alleviate stress and promote overall well-being.

Another important aspect of self-care for oncology **nurse**s is developing healthy coping strategies. This involves recognizing and acknowledging their own emotions and seeking support when needed. **Nurse**s can benefit from talking to trusted colleagues, seeking **professional** counseling services, or participating in debriefing sessions with their team. Engaging in mindfulness or relaxation exercises, such as deep breathing or meditation, can also help reduce stress levels and promote emotional resilience.

Building and maintaining supportive relationships is essential for managing compassion fatigue. **Nurse**s can benefit from connecting with a network of colleagues who understand the unique challenges they face, as well as seeking guidance from mentors or supervisors. Balancing personal and **professional** relationships helps prevent isolation and provides a support system that understands the demands of the oncology nursing profession.

Additionally, setting boundaries and practicing self-compassion are crucial components of self-care. **Nurse**s need to recognize their limitations and learn to say no when necessary. Prioritizing their own well-being allows them to provide the best possible care to their patients. **Nurse**s should also practice self-compassion by acknowledging their efforts and achievements, and not being too hard on themselves when faced with challenges or setbacks

2.3.14 Standards of care (nursing process)

Standards of care in the nursing process are essential in oncology nursing practice. These standards serve as guidelines and protocols to ensure high-quality patient care. They encompass various aspects, including assessment, diagnosis, planning, implementation, and evaluation.
1. Assessment: The first step in the nursing process is to assess the patient's physical, emotional, and psychosocial condition. Oncology **nurse**s gather relevant information about the patient's medical history, perform thorough physical examinations, and assess the impact of cancer and its treatment on the patient's overall well-being. They also evaluate the patient's support system and identify potential barriers to care.
2. Diagnosis: After assessing the patient, oncology **nurse**s identify actual or potential nursing diagnoses. These diagnoses help **nurse**s understand the patient's specific needs, concerns, and goals. Common nursing diagnoses in oncology nursing may include pain, nausea, altered body image, impaired mobility, or anxiety.
3. Planning: Oncology **nurse**s collaborate with the patient, their family, and the healthcare team to develop an individualized plan of care. This plan includes setting realistic and measurable goals, establishing appropriate interventions, and coordinating supportive care services. The plan also addresses strategies for symptom management, psychosocial support, and patient education.
4. Implementation: Oncology **nurse**s play a vital role in implementing the plan of care. They provide direct patient care, administer medications, monitor vital signs, manage symptoms, and coordinate treatments. They advocate for patients' needs, offer emotional support, and facilitate referrals to supportive care resources such as nutritionists, social workers, or palliative care specialists.
5. Evaluation: The final step in the nursing process is the evaluation of the patient's response to interventions. Oncology **nurse**s assess the effectiveness of the care provided, modify the plan as needed, and promote continuity of care. They monitor treatment outcomes, evaluate symptom control, and assess the patient's overall well-being. Regular evaluation helps identify areas for improvement and ensures optimal patient outcomes.
The standards of care in the nursing process require oncology **nurse**s to stay updated with current evidence-based practices and participate in continuing education. They should maintain clear and concise documentation, adhere to ethical principles, and promote patient advocacy. Collaboration and effective communication within the healthcare team are also essential for comprehensive and coordinated oncology nursing care.

3 Treatment Modalities

3.1 Surgical and procedural interventions

Surgical and procedural interventions are important treatment modalities in oncology care. These interventions involve various surgical techniques and procedures aimed at diagnosing, treating, and managing cancer.
One common surgical intervention is a biopsy, which involves the removal of a small sample of tissue for examination and diagnosis. This procedure helps determine the type and stage of cancer, guiding further treatment decisions. Another common intervention is the removal of tumors through surgery, also known as tumor resection. This can be done through open surgery or minimally invasive techniques, such as laparoscopy or robotic-assisted surgery.
In some cases, surgical interventions are curative, aiming to completely remove the cancerous tissues. This is often the case for localized tumors that haven't spread to other parts of the body. Surgical resections can help eliminate tumors in organs like the breast, colon, lung, or prostate. In cases where complete removal is not feasible, surgery can still be used to debulk the tumor, reducing its size and relieving symptoms.
Surgical interventions can also be used to create access points for other treatments. For instance, the insertion of a port or catheter allows for the administration of chemotherapy or other medications directly into the bloodstream. This helps minimize the need for repeated needle sticks and can make treatments more comfortable for the patient.
Additionally, surgical procedures can be performed to alleviate cancer-related symptoms and improve quality of life. These interventions can include the removal of obstructions caused by a tumor, such as relieving bowel or urinary blockages. Palliative surgeries can also be done to manage pain or improve mobility.
It is important for oncology **nurse**s to have a comprehensive understanding of surgical and procedural interventions. They play a crucial role in preoperative and postoperative care, working closely with surgical teams to ensure patient safety and optimal outcomes. **Nurse**s provide education and support to patients and their families, explaining the purpose and expectations of surgical interventions, as well as potential complications and recovery processes.

3.2 Blood and marrow transplant

Blood and marrow transplant, also known as hematopoietic stem cell transplant, is a treatment modality used in oncology to treat various types of cancers and blood disorders. It involves replacing the damaged or diseased bone marrow with healthy stem cells to restore the body's ability to produce healthy blood cells.

There are two main types of blood and marrow transplant: autologous transplant and allogeneic transplant. In autologous transplant, the patient's own stem cells are collected and stored before undergoing high-dose chemotherapy or radiation. After the treatment, the stored stem cells are infused back into the patient's body to replenish the depleted bone marrow. This type of transplant is commonly used to treat some lymphomas, multiple myeloma, and certain solid tumors.

On the other hand, allogeneic transplant involves using stem cells from a donor, typically a sibling or unrelated matched donor. The donor's stem cells are collected and infused into the patient's body after undergoing a conditioning regimen of chemotherapy and/or radiation. The donor stem cells then take over the function of the patient's damaged bone marrow and start producing healthy blood cells. Allogeneic transplant is used to treat various types of leukemia, myelodysplastic syndromes, and other blood disorders.

Before the transplant, patients undergo a thorough evaluation to determine their eligibility and assess any potential risks or complications. This evaluation includes a series of tests to evaluate the patient's overall health, heart and lung function, and the presence of any infections or other diseases. The patient's mental and emotional well-being is also assessed, as the transplant process can be physically and emotionally challenging.

During the transplant, the patient receives high-dose chemotherapy and radiation to destroy the cancer cells or diseased bone marrow. This conditioning regimen also helps suppress the patient's immune system to prevent rejection of the donor stem cells. After the infusion of stem cells, the patient is closely monitored for any complications, such as infections, graft versus host disease, and organ damage. Supportive care, including medications, blood transfusions, and nutritional support, is provided to help manage these potential complications.

Recovery after a blood and marrow transplant can be a long and challenging process. Patients require special care to support their immune system, prevent infections, and manage any side effects or complications. They may need ongoing medical follow-up, including regular blood tests, imaging studies, and check-ups to monitor their progress and detect any signs of relapse or complications.

3.3 Radiation therapy

Radiation therapy is a common treatment modality used in oncology to fight cancer. It involves using high-energy radiation beams to target and destroy cancer cells. This therapy can be delivered externally or internally, depending on the type and location of the tumor.

External radiation therapy, also known as external beam radiation, is the most common form of radiation therapy. It involves directing a focused beam of radiation from an external machine towards the tumor. This beam of radiation damages the DNA of cancer cells, preventing their ability to divide and grow. The treatment is painless and typically delivered on an outpatient basis over several weeks.

Internal radiation therapy, also called brachytherapy, involves placing a radiation source directly into or near the tumor. This allows for a higher concentration of radiation to be delivered to the cancer cells while minimizing damage to surrounding healthy tissues. This method is often used for cancers in the cervix, prostate, and breast.

Radiation therapy can be used with the goal of cure, control, or palliation. In curative intent, the radiation is usually delivered with the intent of eradicating the tumor completely. In control intent, the goal is to shrink or slow down the growth of the tumor. Palliative radiation aims to relieve symptoms and improve the quality of life by reducing pain or pressure caused by the tumor.

Before initiating radiation therapy, thorough planning is essential. This includes obtaining accurate imaging, such as CT scans or MRI, to precisely map the tumor and surrounding structures. The radiation oncologist then determines the appropriate dose and technique for treatment.

During treatment, the radiation therapist uses specialized equipment to deliver the radiation accurately and safely. Patients are positioned on a treatment table, and the radiation beams are directed precisely to the tumor site while sparing healthy tissues. Advanced technologies such as intensity-modulated radiation therapy (IMRT) and stereotactic body radiation therapy (SBRT) allow for even more precise targeting of the tumor.

Radiation therapy is generally well-tolerated, but it can cause side effects. Common acute side effects include fatigue, skin irritation, and temporary hair loss in the treatment area. Long-term side effects may include organ dysfunction, lymphedema, or secondary malignancies. To ensure the safety and effectiveness of radiation therapy, the oncology **nurse** plays a crucial role in educating patients about the treatment, managing side effects, and providing emotional support. The **nurse** also monitors the patient's progress and collaborates with the radiation oncologist and other healthcare providers to ensure comprehensive care.

3.4 Chemotherapy

Chemotherapy is a treatment modality commonly used in the field of oncology. It involves the use of drugs to kill cancer cells or to prevent them from multiplying further. This method is often recommended for patients with different types and stages of cancer, and can be used as the primary treatment or in combination with other therapies.

The goal of chemotherapy is to target cancer cells that may have spread throughout the body, not just in the primary tumor site. This treatment can be administered in various ways, including intravenously, orally, **topic**ally, or by injection into a specific body cavity. The choice of administration depends on factors such as the type and stage of cancer, the drugs being used, and the patient's overall health.

Chemotherapy drugs work by interfering with the cell division process of cancer cells. They can either kill the cells directly or slow down their growth. However, normal cells that divide rapidly, such as those in the hair follicles, bone marrow, and digestive tract, can also be affected by these drugs, leading to side effects.

The side effects of chemotherapy can vary depending on the specific drugs used and the individual patient. Some common side effects include nausea, vomiting, hair loss, fatigue, and increased risk of infection. Oncology **nurse**s have a crucial role in managing these side effects and providing support to patients throughout their treatment.

Before starting chemotherapy, patients undergo a thorough evaluation, including blood tests, imaging studies, and other diagnostic procedures. This helps determine the most appropriate drugs and dosage for each patient. During treatment, regular monitoring is essential to assess the effectiveness of chemotherapy, manage side effects, and adjust the treatment plan as needed.

Chemotherapy is often given in cycles, with rest periods in between to allow the body to recover. The length and number of cycles depend on various factors, including the type and stage of cancer, the drugs used, and the response to treatment. In some cases, chemotherapy may be used before surgery or radiation therapy to shrink tumors, making them easier to remove or treat.

3.5 Biotherapy

Biotherapy is a treatment modality used in oncology to combat different types of cancer. It involves the use of biological substances and techniques to boost the body's natural defenses against cancer cells. The goal of biotherapy is to stimulate the immune system or directly target cancer cells, either killing them or preventing their growth.
There are various forms of biotherapy, each targeting different aspects of the immune system or cancer cells. One form is immunotherapy, which uses substances such as antibodies to strengthen the immune system's ability to recognize and destroy cancer cells. Another form is gene therapy, where genetic material is introduced into the body to correct genetic defects or enhance the body's ability to fight cancer.
One sub**topic** within biotherapy is monoclonal antibody therapy. Monoclonal antibodies specifically target certain proteins on the surface of cancer cells, blocking their growth or stimulating the immune system to attack them. These antibodies can be used alone or in combination with other treatments like chemotherapy.
Another sub**topic** is adoptive cell transfer therapy, which involves collecting and modifying a patient's own immune cells to enhance their cancer-fighting abilities. These modified cells are then reintroduced into the patient's body to target and eliminate cancer cells.
Biological response modifiers (BRMs) are another important aspect of biotherapy. These substances, such as interferons and interleukins, can directly affect the growth and activity of cancer cells. They can also enhance the immune system's response to cancer cells.
Biotherapy can be administered through different routes, including intravenous infusions, subcutaneous injections, or **topic**al applications. The specific route and dosage depend on the type of biotherapy being used and the patient's individual needs.
Like other cancer treatments, biotherapy can have side effects. Common side effects include fatigue, flu-like symptoms, and skin reactions at the injection site. However, these side effects are often temporary and can be managed with medications or supportive care.
It is important for oncology **nurse**s to stay updated on the latest advancements in biotherapy and to be familiar with its benefits, risks, and side effects. They play a crucial role in educating patients about their treatment options, monitoring their progress during therapy, and providing them with necessary support and guidance throughout the treatment process.

3.6 Immunotherapy

Immunotherapy is a type of treatment modality that harnesses the power of the immune system to fight against cancer. It uses substances made by the body or in a laboratory to boost, direct, or restore the body's natural defenses against cancer cells. This innovative approach has shown promising results in the field of oncology.
One major sub**topic** within immunotherapy is immune checkpoint inhibitors. These drugs target specific proteins on immune cells or cancer cells to unleash an immune response against the cancer. By blocking certain inhibitory pathways, immune checkpoint inhibitors can enhance the immune system's ability to recognize and attack cancer cells.
Another sub**topic** is adoptive cell transfer therapy. This involves removing immune cells, such as T cells, from a patient's body and modifying them in the laboratory to increase their cancer-fighting abilities. These enhanced cells are then reintroduced into the patient to attack and destroy the cancer.
Cancer vaccines also fall under the umbrella of immunotherapy. These vaccines stimulate an immune response against specific cancer antigens, helping the immune system recognize and attack cancer cells with greater precision. They can be used to prevent certain cancers or to treat existing tumors.
Additionally, monoclonal antibodies are another important aspect of immunotherapy. These laboratory-made antibodies can be designed to bind to specific proteins on cancer cells, flagging them for destruction by the immune system. Monoclonal antibodies can also deliver drugs directly to cancer cells, minimizing damage to healthy cells and reducing side effects.
Immunotherapy has transformed the treatment landscape for many types of cancer, offering new hope to patients who may not respond well to conventional therapies. It has been particularly successful in the treatment of melanoma, lung cancer, kidney cancer, and bladder cancer. Clinical trials are underway to explore its efficacy in a wide range of other cancers as well.
While immunotherapy has shown great promise, it does come with some potential side effects. These can include inflammation, fatigue, skin rashes, and autoimmune reactions. It is crucial for oncology **nurse**s to closely monitor patients undergoing immunotherapy and promptly address any adverse effects.

3.7 Vascular access devices (VADs) for treatment administration

Vascular access devices (VADs) play a crucial role in the administration of treatment to cancer patients. These devices are used to provide a reliable and safe route for delivering medications and fluids directly into the bloodstream. They eliminate the need for repeated invasive procedures, such as needle sticks, which can cause discomfort and increase the risk of complications.
One commonly used type of VAD is a central venous catheter (CVC). A CVC is typically inserted into a large vein near the heart, such as the subclavian or jugular vein. This type of access is commonly used for long-term treatment administration, as it provides a stable and durable option. Another type of VAD is a peripherally inserted central catheter (PICC), which is inserted into a peripheral vein, usually in the arm. PICCs are often used when treatment duration is shorter or when patients do not have suitable central veins for a CVC.
VADs offer several advantages in the administration of cancer therapy. Firstly, they allow for the administration of highly potent medications, such as chemotherapy drugs, that can cause irritation and damage to peripheral veins. Additionally, VADs provide a means for reliable and repeated blood sampling for laboratory testing, without the need for repeated needle sticks. This is especially important in oncology, as frequent blood tests are necessary to monitor treatment efficacy and detect any adverse effects.
The care and maintenance of VADs are essential to ensure their long-term functionality and prevent complications. After device insertion, healthcare providers must carefully monitor the insertion site for signs of infection or inflammation. Regular flushing of the device with a saline solution and heparin helps to prevent blockages and maintain patency. Sterile techniques should be followed during all interventions involving the VAD to minimize the risk of infection. Additionally, patients and caregivers should receive education on proper care and management of the device to promote its longevity.

Complications can arise with VADs, although they are relatively rare when proper care is taken. Some potential complications include infection, blood clots, catheter malfunction, and catheter-related bloodstream infections. These complications can lead to delays in treatment, extended hospital stays, and increased healthcare costs. Therefore, close surveillance and prompt management of any concerning signs or symptoms are crucial in the oncology setting.

3.8 Targeted therapies

Targeted therapies are a type of treatment modality used in oncology to specifically target and attack cancer cells while minimizing damage to normal, healthy cells. Unlike traditional chemotherapy, which can affect both cancerous and non-cancerous cells, targeted therapies are designed to interfere with the specific molecules and pathways involved in the growth and survival of cancer cells.

One sub**topic** of targeted therapies is monoclonal antibodies. Monoclonal antibodies are laboratory-produced molecules that can target specific proteins on the surface of cancer cells. By binding to these proteins, monoclonal antibodies can block signals that promote cell division and growth, or they can mark the cancer cells for destruction by the immune system.

Another sub**topic** of targeted therapies is small molecule inhibitors. Small molecule inhibitors are drugs that interfere with the signals inside cancer cells that promote their growth and survival. They work by inhibiting specific enzymes or proteins involved in these pathways, preventing the cancer cells from proliferating or inducing cell death.

Additionally, targeted therapies can also involve targeted drug delivery systems. These systems use nanoparticles or other carriers to deliver chemotherapy drugs directly to the tumor site, minimizing exposure to healthy tissues. This approach allows for higher drug concentrations at the tumor site, increasing their effectiveness while reducing side effects.

Furthermore, targeted therapies may be personalized based on the specific tumor characteristics of each patient. Molecular profiling of the tumor can identify specific genetic mutations or alterations that drive its growth. Based on this information, targeted therapies can be selected to match the specific molecular profile of the tumor, increasing the chances of a successful treatment outcome.

Targeted therapies have shown great promise in the treatment of various types of cancer, including breast, lung, colorectal, and prostate cancer, among others. They have proven to be effective in shrinking tumors, delaying disease progression, and improving overall survival rates. However, it's important to note that not all patients will respond to targeted therapies, as the effectiveness of these treatments can vary depending on individual characteristics and tumor heterogeneity.

4 Symptom Management and Palliative Care

4.1 Etiology and patterns of symptoms (acute, chronic, late)

Etiology and patterns of symptoms (acute, chronic, late) are important aspects of symptom management and palliative care in oncology nursing. Understanding the underlying causes and the different patterns of symptoms is crucial for effective symptom management and improved quality of life for cancer patients.

Etiology refers to the study of the causes or origins of a disease or symptoms. In oncology, symptoms can arise from various factors such as the underlying cancer itself, cancer treatments, or the side effects of medications. For example, pain may be caused by the tumor pressing on surrounding structures or by the side effects of chemotherapy or radiation therapy. By identifying the specific etiology of symptoms, **nurse**s can tailor interventions to address the root cause and provide targeted relief.

Symptoms can be classified into three main patterns: acute, chronic, and late. Acute symptoms are those that occur suddenly and have a short duration. These symptoms are often related to the immediate effects of cancer treatments such as nausea, vomiting, fatigue, and pain. Acute symptoms require prompt assessment and intervention to alleviate distress and enhance patient comfort.

Chronic symptoms, on the other hand, persist over an extended period. These symptoms may result from the ongoing cancer or its treatment, and they can significantly impact a patient's quality of life. Common chronic symptoms in oncology include persistent pain, fatigue, insomnia, and depression. **Nurse**s play a vital role in the ongoing management of chronic symptoms by monitoring their severity, providing education and support, and implementing appropriate interventions to relieve symptoms and improve patients' overall well-being.

Late symptoms are those that emerge or worsen as the disease progresses or after treatment completion. These symptoms can have a significant impact on patients and may require specialized interventions. Examples of late symptoms in oncology include lymphedema, cognitive impairment (commonly referred to as "chemo brain"), neuropathy, and long-term psychological distress. Oncology **nurse**s should be knowledgeable about late symptoms and their management to provide comprehensive care to patients throughout the disease trajectory.

4.2 Anatomical and surgical alterations (e.g., lymphedema, ostomy, site-specific radiation)

Anatomical and surgical alterations are important considerations in symptom management and palliative care for patients with cancer. These alterations can have a significant impact on their quality of life and require specialized care from oncology **nurse**s.

One common anatomical alteration is lymphedema, which is the swelling of tissues due to a build-up of lymph fluid. It often occurs in patients who have undergone surgery or radiation therapy, particularly in the lymph nodes. The role of an oncology **nurse** in managing lymphedema includes educating patients about risk reduction strategies, such as avoiding trauma to the affected area, maintaining good hygiene, and wearing compression garments. They may also provide lymphatic drainage massage and refer patients to physical therapy for exercises to reduce swelling.

Another surgical alteration that oncology **nurse**s may encounter is an ostomy. An ostomy is a surgical procedure that creates an opening in the body to divert waste products. This can be challenging for patients as it may affect their body image and cause physical discomfort.

Nurses play a crucial role in teaching patients how to care for their ostomy, including proper hygiene, skin protection, and appliance management. They also provide emotional support, helping patients adjust to the changes and address any concerns they may have. Site-specific radiation is another important aspect of anatomical and surgical alterations in cancer care. Radiation therapy is a common treatment modality that targets cancer cells while minimizing damage to surrounding healthy tissues. Oncology nurses play a key role in educating patients about the potential side effects of radiation therapy, such as skin changes, fatigue, and nausea. They offer strategies to manage these side effects, such as using gentle skincare products, practicing healthy sleep habits, and maintaining a balanced diet. **Nurse**s also closely monitor patients during treatment, assessing for any complications and providing appropriate interventions.

4.3 Pharmacologic interventions

Pharmacologic interventions play a crucial role in symptom management and palliative care for patients under the care of an oncology **nurse**. These interventions involve the use of medications to alleviate symptoms and improve the quality of life for patients with cancer. There are various important aspects that need to be considered when discussing pharmacologic interventions in this context.
One key aspect is pain management. Cancer patients often experience pain due to the disease itself or as a side effect of treatments such as surgery, chemotherapy, or radiation therapy. Pharmacologic interventions for pain management can include the use of analgesics such as opioids, nonsteroidal anti-inflammatory drugs (NSAIDs), and adjuvant medications. The selection of the appropriate medication depends on the intensity and type of pain, as well as the patient's medical history and individual needs.
Another aspect of pharmacologic interventions is nausea and vomiting control. Many cancer patients undergoing treatment experience these distressing symptoms, which can significantly impact their well-being and ability to tolerate anti-cancer therapies. Antiemetic medications, such as serotonin receptor antagonists, dopamine antagonists, and corticosteroids, are commonly used to manage nausea and vomiting in oncology patients.
Pharmacologic interventions also extend to managing other common symptoms related to cancer and its treatment. These may include fatigue, constipation, neuropathy, insomnia, anxiety, and depression. Medications like stimulants, laxatives, antidepressants, anxiolytics, and sedatives can be prescribed to address these symptoms and improve the patient's overall comfort and quality of life.
It is important for the oncology **nurse** to have a comprehensive understanding of the potential side effects and interactions of these medications. This knowledge enables them to educate the patient about the benefits and possible risks of pharmacologic interventions, as well as to monitor the patient closely for any adverse effects. The **nurse** should also be knowledgeable about dosage adjustments, potential drug interactions, and non-pharmacologic interventions that can complement pharmacologic interventions.

In addition to the appropriate selection and administration of medications, the **nurse** plays a crucial role in assessing the effectiveness of pharmacologic interventions and ensuring the patient's adherence to the prescribed regimen. Regular evaluation of symptom relief and close communication with the healthcare team are vital to make necessary adjustments in the treatment plan and optimize the patient's comfort.

4.4 Complementary and integrative modalities (e.g., massage, acupuncture, herbal supplements)

Complementary and integrative modalities are alternative approaches to symptom management and palliative care in oncology nursing. They include practices such as massage, acupuncture, and herbal supplements. These modalities are often used alongside conventional medical treatments to enhance patient well-being and provide relief from various symptoms associated with cancer and its treatments.
Massage therapy is a common complementary modality used in oncology care. It involves manipulating the body's soft tissues to reduce pain, promote relaxation, and improve circulation. Massage can alleviate muscle tension, decrease anxiety, and improve overall mood in oncology patients. It may be particularly beneficial for managing chemotherapy-induced peripheral neuropathy and lymphedema.
Acupuncture, an ancient Chinese practice, involves inserting thin needles into specific points on the body to stimulate energy flow. Oncology **nurse**s may refer patients to qualified acupuncturists to alleviate pain, nausea, and other treatment-related side effects. Acupuncture has been shown to have a positive impact on cancer-related fatigue, hot flashes, and chemotherapy-induced nausea and vomiting.
Herbal supplements, also known as botanicals, are derived from plants and may be taken orally or applied **topic**ally. Many oncology patients turn to herbal medicine for various reasons, such as managing symptoms, boosting the immune system, or reducing treatment side effects. However, it is essential for oncology **nurse**s to be cautious with herbal supplements due to potential drug interactions and lack of regulation in the industry. Patients should always consult their healthcare provider before starting any herbal treatment.
When integrating these modalities into patient care, oncology **nurse**s must prioritize safety, effectiveness, and evidence-based practice. Adhering to **professional** guidelines and standards is crucial in providing holistic care to patients. Communication and collaboration with the interdisciplinary healthcare team are also essential for incorporating complementary modalities into the overall treatment plan.
Furthermore, oncology **nurse**s should educate themselves on the latest research and evidence regarding complementary and integrative modalities. This knowledge will enable them to inform patients about the potential benefits and risks associated with these practices. **Nurse**s can help patients make informed decisions and ensure they receive appropriate care within a supportive and well-rounded approach.

4.5 Palliative care considerations

Palliative care considerations in the field of oncology nursing play a crucial role in managing symptoms and improving the quality of life for patients. These considerations revolve around addressing physical, emotional, and spiritual aspects of care to provide holistic support to patients and their families.
One important aspect of palliative care is pain management. Oncology **nurse**s should assess pain levels regularly and collaborate with the interdisciplinary team to develop a tailored pain management plan for each patient. This may include administering appropriate medications, such as opioids, and providing non-pharmacological interventions like relaxation techniques or massage therapy.

Symptom control is another key consideration in palliative care. **Nurse**s need to address symptoms such as nausea, fatigue, dyspnea, and constipation. They should closely monitor these symptoms, assess their impact on patients' daily lives, and work with the healthcare team to find suitable interventions. This may involve adjusting medications, recommending lifestyle modifications, or providing emotional support and counseling.

Psychosocial support forms an essential component of palliative care. Oncology **nurse**s should be vigilant for signs of distress, anxiety, depression, or spiritual distress in patients and their families. They should provide a listening ear, offer reassurance, and connect them with appropriate resources. Additionally, involving social workers, psychologists, or chaplains can further enhance the psychosocial support offered.

Communication is vital in palliative care, both with patients and their families. Oncology **nurse**s should ensure effective communication, including open and honest discussions about prognosis, treatment options, and goals of care. They should address patients' fears and concerns, facilitate advanced care planning, and help navigate difficult decisions. Regularly assessing and documenting patients' preferences and goals of care can guide future care decisions.

Ethical considerations also play a crucial role in palliative care. **Nurse**s should respect patients' autonomy, confidentiality, and cultural beliefs. They should be knowledgeable about ethical frameworks and guidelines to make informed decisions in complex situations, such as end-of-life care.

Lastly, facilitating a peaceful and comfortable environment is essential in palliative care. **Nurse**s should advocate for patient-centered care, ensure symptom control, maintain cleanliness, and offer emotional support. They should also involve patients' families in care planning and provide guidance on caregiving techniques and support services.

4.6 Alterations in functioning

Alterations in functioning refer to the changes that occur in an individual's physical, emotional, or cognitive abilities due to a disease or condition. In the context of palliative care for oncology patients, these alterations in functioning can have a significant impact on the patient's quality of life and overall well-being.

One of the key areas that alterations in functioning can affect is physical functioning. This refers to the ability of the patient to perform their daily activities, such as eating, bathing, or walking. Cancer and its treatments can cause various physical symptoms and side effects, such as pain, fatigue, nausea, and weakness, which can greatly limit the patient's ability to carry out these activities. It is important for oncology **nurse**s to assess and address these physical symptoms in order to enhance the patient's functioning and improve their quality of life.

Another aspect of alterations in functioning is emotional functioning. Dealing with a cancer diagnosis and its treatment can be emotionally challenging for patients. They may experience feelings of fear, anxiety, depression, or sadness. All of these emotions can have a significant impact on their overall functioning. Oncology **nurse**s can provide emotional support, counseling, and assistance in coping with these emotional changes to help patients optimize their emotional well-being.

Cognitive functioning can also be affected by cancer and its treatment. Patients may experience difficulty with memory, attention, concentration, and decision-making. These cognitive changes, often referred to as "chemo brain," can significantly impact a patient's ability to perform cognitive tasks, such as work or managing their daily activities. Oncology **nurse**s can work with patients to develop strategies to manage and cope with these cognitive changes, such as using memory aids or scheduling activities during times when cognitive functioning is at its best.

In addition to these specific areas of functioning, alterations in functioning can also have a broader impact on the patient's social and occupational roles. For example, a patient may be unable to work or fulfill their family responsibilities due to physical or cognitive limitations. This can lead to financial stress, strain on relationships, and feelings of loss and frustration. Oncology **nurse**s can provide support and resources to help patients navigate these challenges and maintain a sense of identity and purpose.

4.6.1 Hematologic

Hematologic refers to any condition or disease related to blood and blood-forming organs. In the context of oncology nursing, hematologic alterations in functioning, symptom management, and palliative care play a crucial role in the overall well-being and quality of life of patients with hematologic cancers.

One important aspect of hematologic alterations is understanding the various types of cancers that affect the blood and blood-forming organs. This includes leukemia, lymphoma, multiple myeloma, and myelodysplastic syndromes. Each of these cancers originates from different cells within the bone marrow and presents unique challenges in terms of diagnosis, treatment, and management.

It is vital for oncology **nurse**s to be knowledgeable about the signs and symptoms of hematologic cancers, which may include fatigue, unexplained weight loss, recurrent infections, easy bruising or bleeding, and enlarged lymph nodes. Early detection and prompt initiation of appropriate treatment can significantly impact patient outcomes.

When it comes to symptom management, hematologic cancers often present with various side effects related to treatment. These may include anemia, thrombocytopenia (low platelet count), neutropenia (low white blood cell count), and immunosuppression. Oncology **nurse**s should be skilled in assessing and managing these symptoms to optimize patient comfort and minimize potential complications.

Supportive care and palliative care are integral components of the comprehensive management of hematologic cancers. Oncology **nurse**s play a crucial role in providing physical, emotional, and psychosocial support to patients and their families throughout the trajectory of illness. They assist in pain and symptom management, assess and address psychosocial distress, facilitate discussions about end-of-life care, and ensure a dignified and peaceful transition.

Additionally, oncology **nurse**s must be well-versed in the administration and management of blood products, such as packed red blood cells, platelets, and fresh frozen plasma. They collaborate closely with the healthcare team to ensure appropriate blood product transfusions and monitor patients for potential transfusion reactions.

4.6.2 Immune system

The immune system plays a crucial role in the body's defense against diseases and infections. It is a complex network of organs, cells, and molecules that work together to recognize and destroy harmful substances. Understanding the immune system is vital for oncology **nurse**s as they must be able to recognize and manage alterations in its functioning, as well as provide symptom management and palliative care for patients.

The immune system can be divided into two main parts: the innate immune system and the adaptive immune system. The innate immune system is the body's first line of defense and includes physical barriers like the skin and mucous membranes, as well as white blood cells called phagocytes and natural killer cells. These cells act quickly to neutralize and destroy foreign invaders.

The adaptive immune system, on the other hand, is more specific and takes time to develop. It involves the activation of specialized immune cells called lymphocytes, which are made up of B cells and T cells. B cells produce antibodies that can recognize and neutralize specific pathogens, while T cells help in killing infected cells directly.

Alterations in the immune system's functioning can occur in various ways. Immunodeficiency disorders, such as HIV/AIDS, weaken the immune system, making individuals more susceptible to infections. Autoimmune disorders, such as rheumatoid arthritis and lupus, cause the immune system to mistakenly attack healthy cells and tissues. Oncology **nurse**s need to be aware of these alterations and provide appropriate care and support to patients.

Symptom management in relation to the immune system involves addressing the side effects of treatments like chemotherapy, which can weaken the immune system and lead to increased susceptibility to infections. **Nurses** must educate patients about the importance of hand hygiene, vaccinations, and avoiding exposure to people with contagious illnesses. They also play a crucial role in recognizing early signs of infection and facilitating timely medical intervention.

Palliative care in relation to the immune system focuses on maintaining patients' quality of life in the presence of advanced diseases. This involves managing symptoms like pain, fatigue, and infections that can arise due to a compromised immune system. It also entails providing emotional support, counseling, and facilitating open communication between patients, families, and the healthcare team.

4.6.3 Gastrointestinal

Gastrointestinal (GI) alterations are common in patients undergoing cancer treatment and can significantly impact their overall well-being. As an oncology **nurse**, it is important to understand the various aspects of GI alterations, symptom management, and palliative care in order to provide optimal care to patients.

The GI system refers to the organs involved in digestion, including the esophagus, stomach, small intestine, large intestine, and rectum. Patients with cancer may experience a range of GI alterations, such as nausea, vomiting, diarrhea, constipation, abdominal pain, and loss of appetite.

Nausea and vomiting are common side effects of chemotherapy and radiation therapy. It is crucial to assess the severity and frequency of these symptoms, as they can lead to dehydration and malnutrition. Antiemetic medications and lifestyle modifications, such as eating small, frequent meals and avoiding trigger foods, can help manage these symptoms.

Diarrhea can be caused by cancer treatments, infections, or medications. Monitoring stool frequency and consistency is essential in assessing the severity of diarrhea. Treatment strategies may include antidiarrheal medications, dietary modifications, fluid and electrolyte replacement, and addressing the underlying cause.

On the other hand, constipation can result from cancer treatments, decreased physical activity, inadequate fluid intake, and certain medications. Adequate hydration, dietary fiber, and routine bowel habits can help prevent and manage constipation. Laxatives and stool softeners may also be used to alleviate symptoms.

Abdominal pain is a complex symptom that can have various causes, such as tumor progression, inflammation, or treatment-related complications. Accurate assessment and management of pain are crucial to improving patients' quality of life. This may involve analgesic medications, non-pharmacological interventions, and addressing the underlying cause.

Loss of appetite and malnutrition are common among cancer patients and can be influenced by GI alterations. Nutritional support, such as dietary counseling, oral supplementation, or enteral feeding, may be necessary to ensure patients receive adequate nourishment.

Palliative care plays a significant role in managing GI alterations and improving symptom control. Effective communication with patients and their families is crucial to understanding their goals and tailoring care accordingly. Palliative care can involve pain management, optimizing nutrition, psychological support, and addressing any spiritual or emotional needs.

4.6.4 Genitourinary

Genitourinary issues are common among cancer patients and can significantly affect their quality of life. As an oncology **nurse**, it is important to have a thorough understanding of the genitourinary system and the alterations that can occur in its functioning, as well as strategies for symptom management and palliative care.

The genitourinary system encompasses the organs and structures involved in reproduction and waste elimination. It includes the kidneys, bladder, ureters, urethra, prostate, testes, and female reproductive organs. Cancer can affect any of these organs, leading to various alterations in their functioning.

One common genitourinary alteration in cancer patients is renal impairment. This can be caused by the cancer itself, as tumors can directly impact kidney function, or it can be a result of treatments such as chemotherapy or radiation therapy. Renal impairment can manifest as decreased urine output, changes in urine color or odor, and electrolyte imbalances. Close monitoring of kidney function and the implementation of appropriate interventions are crucial in managing this condition.

Another genitourinary issue in cancer patients is urinary incontinence. This can occur due to the tumor's direct involvement with the bladder or as a side effect of treatments like surgery or radiation therapy. **Nurses** should assess the severity and type of incontinence (stress, urge, or overflow) to guide appropriate interventions, which may include bladder training exercises, pelvic floor exercises, or the use of incontinence aids.

Sexual dysfunction is also common among cancer patients, particularly those with genitourinary cancers. Treatments like surgery, radiation therapy, or hormone therapy can cause erectile dysfunction in men and vaginal dryness or loss of libido in women. Open communication, emotional support, and the referral to counseling or support groups can help address these concerns and enhance patients' overall well-being.

Palliative care plays a crucial role in managing genitourinary symptoms in advanced cancer. This may involve the use of pharmacological interventions to alleviate pain, discomfort, or urinary symptoms. Additionally, **nurse**s can provide education and support on self-care practices such as maintaining good hydration, proper nutrition, and personal hygiene.

4.6.5 Integumentary

The integumentary system is the organ system that encompasses the skin, hair, nails, and associated glands. In the context of oncology nursing, alterations in the functioning of the integumentary system can occur as a result of cancer or its treatments. As an oncology **nurse**, it is vital to understand the various aspects of integumentary alterations, as well as symptom management and palliative care strategies.

One important aspect of integumentary alterations is skin changes. Cancer treatments such as chemotherapy and radiation therapy can cause skin reactions such as rashes, dryness, itching, and even blistering. These changes can be distressing for patients and may adversely affect their quality of life. It is crucial for oncology **nurse**s to be able to assess and document these alterations accurately.

Another significant aspect is hair loss. Cancer treatments often cause hair loss or alopecia. Understanding the emotional impact of hair loss on patients is essential. Providing emotional support, education regarding wig options, and scalp care can make the experience more manageable for patients.

Nail changes are also a common issue. Chemotherapy can cause nail discoloration, brittleness, and even nail loss. Oncology **nurse**s should educate patients on proper nail care, monitor for signs of infection, and recommend appropriate interventions to manage these changes.

Managing symptoms related to integumentary alterations is an integral part of an oncology **nurse**'s role. The use of **topic**al treatments, such as moisturizers and emollients, can help alleviate dryness and itching. For more severe skin reactions, **nurse**s may collaborate with dermatologists to prescribe specialized creams or ointments.

Pain management is crucial for patients experiencing integumentary alterations. Topical analgesics or systemic pain medications may be necessary. Emotional support and counseling can also play a significant role in helping patients cope with the physical and emotional side effects.

Palliative care strategies should also be considered when addressing integumentary alterations. Comfort measures, such as using soft fabrics, maintaining a comfortable room temperature, and gentle cleansing techniques, can provide relief. Additionally, interventions such as massage, relaxation techniques, and aromatherapy can help enhance patients' well-being.

4.6.6 Respiratory

Respiratory alterations are common among oncology patients and can significantly impact their overall functioning, quality of life, symptom management, and palliative care. In the oncology setting, it is essential for **nurse**s to have a comprehensive understanding of respiratory health and the various alterations that can occur.

Respiratory alterations encompass a range of conditions, such as dyspnea (shortness of breath), cough, wheezing, and increased respiratory rate. These alterations can arise from various factors, including the primary tumor's location, metastases to the lungs, radiation therapy, chemotherapy-induced lung toxicity, and non-neoplastic lung diseases.

One important aspect of respiratory management in oncology is the early identification and assessment of alterations. This involves vigilant monitoring of patients' respiratory status, including the assessment of respiratory rate, depth, and effort, as well as the presence of any abnormal breath sounds. Additionally, obtaining a detailed history and conducting a physical examination can provide valuable insights into the underlying cause of the respiratory alteration.

Depending on the identified alterations and their severity, various interventions can be employed to manage respiratory symptoms effectively. Pharmacological interventions, such as bronchodilators, corticosteroids, and opioids, may be initiated to alleviate symptoms and improve breathing. Non-pharmacological approaches, including oxygen therapy, respiratory exercises, relaxation techniques, and positioning, can also be utilized to enhance respiratory function and provide relief.

Furthermore, palliative care plays a vital role in addressing respiratory alterations in oncology patients. Palliative interventions aim to improve the patient's overall comfort and quality of life by focusing on symptom management, psychosocial support, and the enhancement of overall well-being. This may involve a multidisciplinary approach that includes collaboration with respiratory therapists, physiotherapists, social workers, and psychologists.

Educating patients and their families about respiratory alterations and their management is crucial for empowering them to actively participate in their care. This includes providing information about specific alterations, their causes, treatment options, and self-care strategies. **Nurse**s should ensure that patients understand the importance of reporting any changes in respiratory symptoms promptly and seeking timely medical attention.

4.6.7 Cardiovascular

Cardiovascular alterations are common among oncology patients and can significantly impact their overall health and quality of life. Understanding these alterations is essential for oncology **nurse**s to provide appropriate care and symptom management.

Cardiovascular alterations in oncology patients can occur due to multiple factors, including the tumor itself, cancer treatments, and the individual's pre-existing cardiovascular conditions. Tumors can directly invade blood vessels or release substances that affect blood flow and cardiac function. Cancer treatments, such as chemotherapy and radiation therapy, can also have toxic effects on the heart and blood vessels.

When managing cardiovascular alterations in oncology patients, it is crucial to assess and monitor for symptoms and changes in cardiac function. Common symptoms may include shortness of breath, chest pain, palpitations, edema, and fatigue. Regular monitoring of vital signs, such as blood pressure, heart rate, and oxygen saturation, helps identify any changes that might require intervention.

There are several sub**topic**s related to cardiovascular alterations in oncology patients that **nurse**s should be aware of. These include ischemic heart disease, heart failure, arrhythmias, and venous thromboembolism. Ischemic heart disease occurs when there is an inadequate blood supply to the heart muscle, leading to angina (chest pain) or myocardial infarction (heart attack). Heart failure refers to the heart's inability to pump blood effectively, causing fluid accumulation and symptoms such as shortness of breath and fatigue. Arrhythmias are abnormal heart rhythms that can be life-threatening in certain situations. Venous thromboembolism involves the formation of blood clots in veins, which can lead to dangerous complications if not treated promptly.

Palliative care plays a crucial role in managing cardiovascular alterations in oncology patients. It focuses on providing relief from symptoms, improving patients' quality of life, and supporting their emotional and psychological well-being. Symptom management strategies may include medications to control pain and discomfort, lifestyle modifications, and supportive therapies such as physical therapy and nutrition counseling.

Oncology **nurse**s should collaborate with a multidisciplinary team, including cardiologists, oncologists, and palliative care specialists, to provide comprehensive care for patients with cardiovascular alterations. Regular communication and coordination among team members ensure that patients receive appropriate interventions and follow-up care

4.6.8 Neurological

Neurological alterations are common in patients receiving palliative care for cancer. These alterations can arise as a result of the cancer itself or due to the side effects of cancer treatments. It is crucial for oncology **nurse**s to be knowledgeable about neurological symptoms and their management in order to provide effective care for their patients.

One important aspect of neurological alterations is the presence of neurological symptoms such as pain, numbness, tingling, weakness, or difficulty in movement. These symptoms may occur as a result of tumor growth or nerve damage caused by cancer treatments. Oncology **nurse**s need to assess these symptoms carefully and work with the healthcare team to develop a comprehensive treatment plan.

Pain that radiates along a specific nerve pathway can indicate nerve involvement by the tumor, known as neuropathic pain. This type of pain is often challenging to manage and requires a multimodal approach using medications such as gabapentin or pregabalin. Oncology **nurse**s should closely monitor the effectiveness of pain management strategies and promptly address any changes in symptoms.

In addition to pain, oncology **nurse**s should also be vigilant for signs of neurological deficits such as weakness, changes in coordination or balance, difficulty in swallowing or speaking, or changes in cognition. These symptoms may indicate the spread of cancer to the brain or spinal cord, known as metastatic disease. Prompt recognition of these symptoms is crucial for timely intervention and appropriate referral for further diagnostic testing or treatment.

Managing neurological symptoms also involves providing supportive care to alleviate distress and improve quality of life. This can include techniques such as relaxation exercises, massage, or physical therapy to address muscle weakness or loss of function. Additionally, oncology **nurse**s play a vital role in educating patients and their families about self-care techniques and coping strategies to manage the impact of neurological alterations on daily activities.

Furthermore, oncology **nurse**s may need to collaborate with other healthcare **professional**s such as neurologists or palliative care specialists to optimize symptom management. This interdisciplinary approach ensures that patients receive the most comprehensive care and support.

4.6.9 Musculoskeletal

The musculoskeletal system refers to the combination of muscles, bones, joints, ligaments, and tendons that provide the body with support, stability, and movement. In the context of oncology nursing, musculoskeletal alterations can arise from various factors such as cancer itself, its treatments, or other related conditions. These alterations can significantly impact a patient's functioning and overall quality of life.

One common musculoskeletal alteration in cancer patients is bone metastasis, which occurs when cancer cells spread to the bones. This can lead to bone pain, fractures, and spinal cord compression, resulting in decreased mobility and functional impairment. Oncology **nurse**s play a crucial role in assessing and managing these symptoms, ensuring appropriate pain management, and collaborating with the healthcare team to develop a comprehensive care plan.

Another aspect of musculoskeletal alterations in cancer patients is treatment-induced bone loss, commonly associated with therapies such as hormone therapy or chemotherapy. These treatments can disrupt the balance between bone formation and resorption, leading to osteoporosis or osteopenia. Oncology **nurse**s can educate patients about the importance of maintaining bone health, encourage lifestyle modifications, and facilitate appropriate screening and preventive measures.

Lymphedema is another musculoskeletal alteration that can occur as a result of cancer treatment, particularly in patients with breast cancer or gynecological malignancies. It is characterized by the accumulation of lymph fluid, leading to swelling, discomfort, and reduced mobility in the affected limb. Oncology **nurse**s play a pivotal role in educating patients about lymphedema prevention, monitoring for early signs, and implementing appropriate interventions such as compression garments and therapeutic exercises.

Musculoskeletal complications can also arise from cancer-related surgeries, such as limb amputations or reconstructive procedures. These alterations can have a profound impact on a patient's body image, psychological well-being, and functional abilities. Oncology **nurse**s provide support and counseling to patients undergoing these procedures, helping them adapt to their new physical changes and facilitating their rehabilitation process.

To effectively manage musculoskeletal alterations in cancer patients, oncology **nurse**s collaborate closely with other healthcare **professional**s, including physical therapists, occupational therapists, and pain specialists. They also stay updated on evidence-based practices and nursing interventions to optimize patient outcomes.

4.6.10 Nutrition

Nutrition plays a crucial role in the overall well-being of individuals, especially those undergoing oncology treatment. It is essential for oncology **nurse**s to have a comprehensive understanding of nutrition to support their patients effectively.

Firstly, a balanced diet rich in nutrients is vital for cancer patients. This includes consuming a variety of foods from all food groups, such as fruits, vegetables, whole grains, lean proteins, and dairy products. These provide essential vitamins, minerals, carbohydrates, proteins, and fats necessary for optimal health and energy levels.

One significant aspect of nutrition in oncology care is managing side effects and symptoms related to treatment. Certain treatments like chemotherapy and radiation therapy can cause nausea, vomiting, and taste changes, which can lead to weight loss and malnutrition. In these cases, oncology **nurse**s should recommend consuming small, frequent meals, avoiding strong-smelling foods, and trying different cooking methods to enhance taste. They may also suggest the use of anti-nausea medications prescribed by the medical team.

Hydration is another vital component of nutrition. Patients should be encouraged to drink an adequate amount of fluids to prevent dehydration, especially during treatment. Water, herbal teas, and fruit juices can be included to maintain hydration levels.

Specific diets, such as the neutropenic diet, may also be recommended for individuals with compromised immune systems. This diet restricts foods that may harbor bacteria or fungi, reducing the risk of infection. Oncology **nurse**s should educate patients on safe food handling practices and encourage them to avoid raw or undercooked foods.

In some cases, patients may require enteral or parenteral nutrition. Enteral nutrition involves a feeding tube that delivers nutrients directly into the stomach or small intestine, while parenteral nutrition is administered through a vein. Oncology **nurse**s should monitor the effectiveness of these feeding methods and provide education and support to patients and their families.

Furthermore, maintaining a healthy body weight is essential for cancer patients. Being underweight or overweight can impact treatment outcomes and overall wellness. Oncology **nurse**s can work closely with registered dietitians to develop personalized meal plans and provide recommendations for physical activity and exercise.

4.6.11 Cognition

Cognition is a crucial aspect of functioning that can be affected in individuals receiving oncology care. It refers to the mental processes involved in acquiring, processing, and understanding information, including perception, memory, attention, language, and problem-solving. Alterations in cognition can significantly impact a person's quality of life and their ability to manage symptoms and make informed decisions regarding their care.

One important aspect of cognition that oncology **nurse**s should be aware of is cognitive impairment, which can range from mild to severe. This impairment can be caused by various factors, including cancer itself, the side effects of cancer treatments such as chemotherapy or radiation therapy, and comorbidities like depression or anxiety. It can manifest as memory loss, difficulty concentrating, decreased attention span, confusion, or language problems.

Understanding the potential causes of cognitive impairment in cancer patients is crucial for symptom management and providing appropriate palliative care. Oncology **nurse**s should evaluate patients for any underlying medical conditions that might contribute to cognitive changes, provide education and support to patients and their families, and collaborate with the healthcare team to implement strategies that optimize cognitive function.

Sub**topic**s to consider when discussing cognition in oncology care include assessing cognitive function using various screening tools, implementing interventions like cognitive rehabilitation, providing education on strategies to manage cognitive changes, and addressing any emotional or psychological aspects associated with cognitive impairment.

When assessing cognitive function, **nurse**s can use tools such as the Mini-Mental State Examination (MMSE) or the Montreal Cognitive Assessment (MoCA). These tests provide a baseline assessment and can help identify any areas of cognitive impairment that require intervention.

Interventions for managing cognitive changes may include cognitive rehabilitation programs, which involve structured exercises and activities to enhance cognitive skills. Additionally, providing education on strategies such as maintaining a healthy lifestyle, engaging in mentally stimulating activities, and using memory aids can empower patients to manage their cognitive impairment more effectively.

Furthermore, it is essential to address the emotional and psychological aspects associated with cognitive impairment. Patients may experience frustration, anxiety, or depression due to their cognitive changes. Oncology **nurse**s can offer emotional support, encourage patients to share their concerns, and collaborate with the healthcare team to provide appropriate psychosocial interventions when needed.

4.6.12 Energy level (i.e., fatigue)

Energy level, or fatigue, is a common symptom experienced by individuals with cancer and can have a significant impact on their quality of life. Fatigue is characterized by a persistent lack of energy, tiredness, and exhaustion that is not relieved by rest or sleep. It can be both physical and mental, affecting a person's ability to perform everyday tasks and participate in activities they once enjoyed.

There are several factors that contribute to fatigue in individuals with cancer. One of the primary causes is the cancer itself, as the body expends a significant amount of energy in fighting the disease. Additionally, cancer treatments such as chemotherapy, radiation therapy, and surgery can also contribute to fatigue. These treatments can damage healthy cells, disrupt hormone levels, and cause inflammation, all of which can lead to increased fatigue.

Managing and alleviating fatigue is an important aspect of the care provided by oncology **nurse**s. There are several strategies that can be implemented to help patients cope with fatigue. One approach is to educate patients about the importance of conserving energy and prioritizing activities. By pacing themselves and taking regular breaks, patients can reduce the impact of fatigue on their daily lives.

Another aspect of managing fatigue is addressing any underlying causes or contributing factors. This may involve adjusting medication dosages, managing side effects, addressing sleep disturbances, and providing pain management. Additionally, oncology **nurse**s can assist patients in developing strategies for managing their daily routine, such as organizing activities and delegating tasks to conserve energy.

Promoting physical activity and exercise can also help reduce fatigue in cancer patients. While it may seem counterintuitive, regular exercise has been shown to improve energy levels and reduce fatigue. **Nurse**s can work with patients to develop safe and appropriate exercise plans that take into consideration their individual abilities and limitations.

Supportive care interventions, such as relaxation techniques, massage therapy, and counseling, can also be beneficial in managing fatigue. These interventions can help patients relax, reduce stress, and improve their overall sense of well-being, which can reduce the impact of fatigue.

4.7 Pain Management

Pain management is a critical aspect of symptom management and palliative care for oncology nurses. It involves the assessment, intervention, and ongoing evaluation of pain experienced by cancer patients. The goal of pain management is to provide relief, improve quality of life, and enhance physical and psychological well-being.

Assessment plays a crucial role in pain management. Oncology nurses should use various tools and techniques to assess the intensity, location, duration, and quality of pain experienced by patients. This helps in understanding the underlying cause of pain and guides the selection of appropriate interventions. Subtopics under assessment can include pain scales, pain diaries, and patient interviews.

Interventions for pain management encompass pharmacological and non-pharmacological approaches. Pharmacological interventions include the administration of analgesic medications such as opioids, non-opioids, and adjuvant drugs. It is important for oncology nurses to have a thorough understanding of these medications, their side effects, and potential interactions. They should also monitor patients closely for any adverse effects and adjust medications as necessary.

Non-pharmacological interventions are equally important in pain management. These can include relaxation techniques, breathing exercises, heat or cold therapy, massage, acupuncture, and guided imagery. These interventions can be used alone or in combination with pharmacological interventions to promote pain relief and improve overall well-being.

Education and counseling are vital components of pain management for oncology nurses. They should educate patients and their families about the nature of pain, its management, and the importance of adhering to the prescribed treatment plan. Effective communication and counseling can help alleviate fears and anxieties related to pain, foster trust, and improve patient outcomes.

Ongoing evaluation is essential to ensure the effectiveness of pain management interventions. Oncology nurses should regularly assess pain levels, monitor the response to treatment, and make modifications as needed. This includes adjusting medication dosage, timing, or route of administration, as well as exploring alternative interventions if necessary.

Collaboration with a multidisciplinary team is crucial in pain management. Oncology nurses should work closely with physicians, pharmacists, physical therapists, psychologists, and social workers to develop comprehensive and individualized pain management plans for each patient. This interdisciplinary approach ensures holistic care and enhances the overall outcomes.

5 Oncologic Emergencies

5.1 Disseminated intravascular coagulation (DIC)

Disseminated intravascular coagulation (DIC) is a serious condition that can occur as an oncologic emergency in cancer patients. DIC is a complex disorder characterized by the widespread activation of clotting factors, resulting in the formation of blood clots throughout the body's small blood vessels. This excessive clotting can lead to organ damage and even organ failure.

DIC often develops as a complication of other medical conditions, such as sepsis, trauma, or cancer. In cancer patients, DIC can be triggered by the release of cancer cells or cancer-related substances into the bloodstream, causing a systemic activation of the clotting system. The exact mechanisms underlying DIC in cancer are not fully understood, but it is believed that factors secreted by tumors can disrupt the normal balance between clotting and anticoagulant pathways.

The clinical presentation of DIC can vary depending on the underlying cause and the extent of clotting. Patients may experience symptoms such as excessive bleeding, bruising, and petechiae (small red or purple spots caused by bleeding into the skin). They may also develop signs of organ dysfunction, such as shortness of breath, confusion, or decreased urine output.

Diagnosis of DIC is based on a combination of clinical findings and laboratory tests. Common laboratory abnormalities include low platelet count, prolonged prothrombin time (PT) and activated partial thromboplastin time (aPTT), elevated levels of fibrin degradation products (FDPs), and decreased levels of fibrinogen. Imaging studies, such as ultrasound or computed tomography (CT) scan, may be performed to evaluate for the presence of blood clots in major organs.

The management of DIC in cancer patients is challenging, as it requires both treating the underlying cause and correcting the abnormal clotting. Treatment strategies may include addressing the underlying cancer, providing supportive care, and administering anticoagulant medications to prevent further clot formation. Blood transfusions may be necessary to replace depleted clotting factors or platelets.

Prognosis for patients with DIC depends on the underlying cause and the extent of organ damage. Prompt recognition and treatment are crucial to improve outcomes. Close monitoring of vital signs, laboratory values, and organ function is essential in managing DIC. Collaboration with a multidisciplinary team, including hematologists, oncologists, and critical care specialists, is often necessary to provide optimal care for patients with DIC.

5.2 Syndrome of inappropriate antidiuretic hormone secretion (SIADH)

The Syndrome of Inappropriate Antidiuretic Hormone Secretion (SIADH) is a condition that can occur in oncology patients as an oncologic emergency. It is characterized by excessive secretion of antidiuretic hormone (ADH), also known as vasopressin, by the pituitary gland or other sources. This hormone is responsible for regulating the amount of water excreted by the kidneys.

In patients with SIADH, there is a continuous release of ADH, which leads to the reabsorption of water by the kidneys and dilution of electrolytes in the body. This can result in hyponatremia, or low sodium levels, which can be extremely dangerous and even life-threatening.

There are several causes of SIADH in oncology patients. One common cause is the production of ADH by certain types of cancer cells, such as small cell lung cancer. Other causes include brain tumors, infections, medications, or a combination of factors.

The symptoms of SIADH can vary depending on the severity of hyponatremia, but they generally include nausea, vomiting, headache, confusion, seizures, and in severe cases, coma. It is important for oncology nurses to recognize these symptoms and initiate prompt treatment.

Diagnosis of SIADH involves measuring sodium levels in the blood and urine, as well as other electrolyte and hormone levels. Imaging studies, such as brain MRI, may be necessary to identify the underlying cause of SIADH.

The treatment of SIADH focuses on correcting the hyponatremia and addressing the underlying cause. This may involve restricting fluid intake and administering intravenous saline solutions to increase sodium levels. In some cases, medications called vasopressin receptor antagonists may be used to block the effects of ADH and promote water excretion.

Oncology **nurse**s play a crucial role in monitoring patients with SIADH and managing complications. They should closely monitor fluid intake and output, as well as electrolyte levels. Education and support for patients and their families are also essential in ensuring compliance with treatment and preventing recurrence.

5.3 Sepsis (including septic shock)

Sepsis is a potentially life-threatening condition that can occur when the body's response to infection causes damage to its own tissues and organs. It is a critical oncologic emergency that oncology **nurse**s need to be aware of and prepared to manage.

Sepsis can develop when an infection in the body, such as a urinary tract infection or pneumonia, spreads to the bloodstream. The immune system responds to the infection by releasing chemicals into the bloodstream, triggering widespread inflammation. This inflammation can lead to a cascade of events that can damage organs and impair their function.

One of the complications of sepsis is septic shock, which is characterized by a severe drop in blood pressure. In septic shock, the body is no longer able to maintain adequate blood flow to vital organs, such as the brain, heart, and kidneys. This can result in organ failure and, if not promptly treated, can be fatal.

The signs and symptoms of sepsis and septic shock can vary, but they often include fever, chills, rapid heart rate, rapid breathing, confusion, and decreased urine output. Early recognition and prompt treatment are essential to improve patient outcomes.

As an oncology **nurse**, it is important to closely monitor patients for signs of sepsis, especially those who are undergoing cancer treatment, as they may have a weakened immune system and be at higher risk of developing infections. Promptly assessing and identifying infections in these patients can help prevent the progression to sepsis.

When managing sepsis and septic shock, the **nurse**'s role includes administering intravenous fluids to restore blood pressure, initiating broad-spectrum antibiotics to target the infection, and closely monitoring the patient's vital signs and organ function. In some cases, the patient may require interventions such as vasopressor medications to support blood pressure or mechanical ventilation to assist with breathing.

Furthermore, the **nurse** plays a crucial role in educating patients and their families about the signs and symptoms of infection and when to seek medical attention. Implementing preventive measures, such as good hand hygiene, proper wound care, and adherence to infection control protocols, can also help reduce the risk of sepsis in oncology patients.

5.4 Tumor lysis syndrome

Tumor lysis syndrome (TLS) is an oncologic emergency that can occur when cancer cells are destroyed at a rapid rate, leading to the release of large amounts of cellular contents into the bloodstream. This condition is most commonly seen in patients with rapidly dividing, highly sensitive tumors, such as hematological malignancies, but can also occur in solid tumors.

TLS is characterized by several metabolic abnormalities, including hyperuricemia, hyperkalemia, hyperphosphatemia, and hypocalcemia. These imbalances can lead to serious complications, such as acute kidney injury, cardiac arrhythmias, seizures, and even death if not promptly managed.

The primary cause of TLS is the release of intracellular contents, such as nucleic acids and potassium, into the bloodstream following chemotherapy or radiation therapy. This sudden release overwhelms the body's normal mechanisms for processing and excreting these waste products, leading to metabolic disturbances.

TLS can be classified into two types: laboratory TLS and clinical TLS. Laboratory TLS is diagnosed when there are metabolic abnormalities without any clinical symptoms, while clinical TLS occurs when these abnormalities are accompanied by clinical manifestations. These manifestations may include renal impairment, cardiac arrhythmias, muscle cramps, seizures, and even sudden death in severe cases.

Early identification and prompt management of TLS are crucial to prevent serious complications. Treatment strategies focus on correcting metabolic imbalances and providing supportive care. This may involve measures such as aggressive hydration, alkalinization of the urine, administration of medications to lower uric acid levels, and monitoring of electrolyte levels.

Prevention plays a vital role in managing TLS. Risk stratification, based on factors such as tumor type, tumor burden, renal function, and previous episodes of TLS, can help identify patients who are at a higher risk. Prophylactic measures, such as the use of medications to reduce uric acid levels or increase uric acid excretion, may be considered in high-risk patients prior to initiating chemotherapy or radiation therapy.

5.5 Hypersensitivity

Hypersensitivity reactions are a common occurrence in oncologic emergencies. These reactions are an overreaction of the immune system to certain substances, such as medications given during cancer treatment. Hypersensitivity reactions can range from mild to severe, with potentially life-threatening consequences if not promptly managed.

There are four types of hypersensitivity reactions: type I, type II, type III, and type IV. Each type involves a different immune response mechanism and can present with varying symptoms.

Type I hypersensitivity reactions, also known as immediate hypersensitivity reactions, occur rapidly after exposure to an allergen. This can include symptoms such as itching, hives, swelling, wheezing, and difficulty breathing. Anaphylaxis, a severe and potentially life-threatening allergic reaction, can also occur in type I hypersensitivity reactions.

Type II hypersensitivity reactions involve the destruction of cells or tissues by antibodies. These reactions can result in complications such as autoimmune hemolytic anemia or immune thrombocytopenia, where the immune system attacks red blood cells or platelets, respectively.

Type III hypersensitivity reactions occur due to the formation of immune complexes in tissues or blood vessels. This can lead to inflammation and tissue damage, presenting as symptoms like joint pain, fever, and skin rashes. Conditions such as serum sickness or systemic lupus erythematosus can result from type III hypersensitivity reactions.

Type IV hypersensitivity reactions are delayed hypersensitivity reactions that typically occur hours to days after exposure to an allergen. These reactions involve the activation of immune cells such as T-cells, leading to inflammation and tissue damage. Contact dermatitis, such as poison ivy rashes, is a common example of a type IV hypersensitivity reaction.

Managing hypersensitivity reactions in oncology patients requires quick identification and prompt intervention. This includes stopping the suspected medication or substance triggering the reaction and administering appropriate medications to alleviate symptoms. Epinephrine is commonly used in the treatment of severe allergic reactions, while antihistamines and corticosteroids may be used for milder reactions.

Oncology **nurse**s play a crucial role in recognizing and managing hypersensitivity reactions in cancer patients. They must closely monitor patients during treatments and respond quickly to any signs or symptoms of a reaction. Education and awareness about potential allergens and hypersensitivity reactions are also essential in preventing and managing these emergencies.

5.6 Anaphylaxis

Anaphylaxis is a severe and potentially life-threatening allergic reaction that can occur in oncologic emergencies. It is a medical emergency that requires immediate attention and intervention. Anaphylaxis can be caused by a variety of triggers, such as medications, foods, insect stings, or latex.

When an oncology **nurse** encounters a patient experiencing anaphylaxis, it is crucial to recognize the signs and symptoms promptly. These can include difficulty breathing, wheezing, hives, swelling, rapid heartbeat, low blood pressure, and gastrointestinal symptoms. Timely identification of anaphylaxis can help in taking immediate action to prevent further complications.

The first step in managing anaphylaxis is to remove the trigger, if possible. For example, if the reaction is caused by a medication, discontinuing its administration is essential. Additionally, it is vital to call for emergency medical assistance immediately to ensure appropriate care and treatment.

Intramuscular epinephrine is the first-line treatment for anaphylaxis. It works by opening up the airways and reducing swelling, helping to improve breathing and blood pressure. Oncology **nurse**s should be familiar with the correct administration technique and dosage of epinephrine. It is important to note that individuals with a history of anaphylaxis may carry an epinephrine auto-injector for self-administration.

Supportive care is also crucial in managing anaphylaxis. This may involve administering oxygen to improve breathing and providing intravenous fluids to stabilize blood pressure. Antihistamines and corticosteroids can be used to help relieve symptoms and prevent a future reaction.

It is essential for oncology **nurse**s to educate patients about anaphylaxis and potential triggers related to their treatment. This includes learning about their medical history, allergies, and previous reactions. Patients should be educated on how to recognize early signs of an allergic reaction and when to seek immediate medical attention.

Prevention and preparedness are key to reducing the risk of anaphylaxis in oncologic emergencies. This involves comprehensive allergy assessments, proper documentation, and clear communication within the healthcare team. Oncology **nurse**s should be vigilant in monitoring patients for potential allergic reactions and have a readily available anaphylaxis emergency kit that includes epinephrine.

5.7 Hypercalcemia

Hypercalcemia is a condition characterized by high levels of calcium in the blood. It is one of the oncologic emergencies that oncology **nurse**s should be aware of and prepared to manage.

In cancer patients, hypercalcemia is often associated with malignancies, particularly those that have spread to the bone or produce hormones that affect calcium regulation. Some common cancers that can lead to hypercalcemia include breast cancer, lung cancer, multiple myeloma, and certain types of leukemia.

The main cause of hypercalcemia in cancer patients is bone metastases. When cancer cells invade the bone, they cause destruction, releasing calcium into the bloodstream. Additionally, some cancer cells can produce substances that imitate parathyroid hormone, leading to increased calcium levels.

The signs and symptoms of hypercalcemia can vary and may be subtle in some cases. Patients may experience fatigue, weakness, nausea, vomiting, constipation, increased thirst, frequent urination, confusion, and even coma in severe cases. It is important for oncology **nurse**s to monitor patients closely for these symptoms, as early intervention is crucial for preventing complications.

To diagnose hypercalcemia, blood tests are performed to measure calcium levels. Additionally, it is important to assess the patient's medical history, conduct a physical examination, and order imaging studies to determine the underlying cause.

Treatment of hypercalcemia aims to reduce calcium levels, alleviate symptoms, and address the underlying cause. Fluid hydration is typically the first-line treatment, as it helps to flush out excess calcium. Intravenous bisphosphonates, such as zoledronic acid and pamidronate, may also be administered to inhibit bone breakdown and lower calcium levels. Other treatment options include calcitonin, corticosteroids, and denosumab.

Oncology **nurse**s play a crucial role in the management of hypercalcemia. They should closely monitor patients for symptoms, assess calcium levels regularly, and assist in administering treatments. It is also important to educate patients and their families about the signs and symptoms of hypercalcemia and when to seek medical attention.

5.8 Cardiac tamponade

Cardiac tamponade is a potentially life-threatening oncologic emergency that requires prompt recognition and intervention. It occurs when fluid, such as blood or fluid from a tumor, accumulates in the pericardial sac, leading to compression of the heart. This compression restricts the heart's ability to fill and pump blood effectively, causing hemodynamic instability.

The most common cause of cardiac tamponade in oncology patients is the spread of cancer to the pericardium, the sac surrounding the heart. Other causes include radiation therapy to the chest, infection, or trauma. It can also occur as a consequence of complications from invasive procedures, such as placement of central venous catheters or cardiac surgery.

Patients with cardiac tamponade may present with symptoms such as shortness of breath, chest pain, low blood pressure, tachycardia, and signs of poor perfusion. Physical examination findings may include distant heart sounds, muffled heart sounds, jugular venous distention, and pulsus paradoxus (an exaggerated drop in blood pressure during inspiration).

Diagnosis of cardiac tamponade is typically made based on clinical suspicion and confirmed with various imaging modalities such as echocardiography or computed tomography (CT) scan. Echocardiography is particularly valuable as it can demonstrate the presence of pericardial effusion and signs of hemodynamic compromise.

The management of cardiac tamponade involves addressing the underlying cause and relieving the compression on the heart. Pericardiocentesis, a procedure in which a needle or catheter is inserted into the pericardial sac to drain the fluid, is often performed as an emergency intervention. A pericardial drain may be left in place to ensure continuous fluid drainage and prevent re-accumulation.

In some cases, surgical intervention may be necessary to treat the underlying cause of cardiac tamponade, such as resection of a tumor or repair of cardiac injuries. Supportive measures, including intravenous fluids and inotropic medications, may be required to stabilize the patient's hemodynamics during the acute phase.

The prognosis of cardiac tamponade depends on various factors, including the underlying cause, the degree of hemodynamic compromise at presentation, and the promptness of intervention. Early recognition and prompt intervention are crucial for improving outcomes in patients with this condition.

5.9 Spinal cord compression

Spinal cord compression is a serious condition that can occur in patients with cancer. It is considered an oncologic emergency because it requires prompt diagnosis and intervention to prevent permanent damage to the spinal cord.

Spinal cord compression happens when a tumor grows in or around the spinal cord, putting pressure on it. This pressure can cause a range of symptoms, including pain, weakness, numbness, and problems with bowel or bladder control.

The most common cause of spinal cord compression in cancer patients is the spread of cancer cells from the original tumor to the spine. Other causes include the growth of a new tumor in the spine or the collapse of a vertebra due to cancer-related bone loss.

Early recognition of spinal cord compression is crucial. Oncology **nurses** should be vigilant in assessing patients for signs and symptoms, such as back pain that worsens over time, weakness or numbness in the extremities, difficulty walking, or changes in bowel or bladder function.

Once spinal cord compression is suspected, appropriate diagnostic tests should be ordered to confirm the diagnosis. These may include imaging studies such as X-rays, computed tomography (CT) scans, or magnetic resonance imaging (MRI). The results of these tests can help determine the location and extent of the compression.

Treatment options for spinal cord compression depend on several factors, including the underlying cause, the location and extent of the compression, and the patient's overall health. In some cases, surgery may be necessary to remove the tumor or relieve the pressure on the spinal cord. Other treatment options may include radiation therapy to shrink the tumor, chemotherapy to slow its growth, or corticosteroids to reduce inflammation and swelling in the area.

In addition to medical interventions, oncology **nurses** play a crucial role in managing the symptoms and providing supportive care for patients with spinal cord compression. This may involve administering pain medication, assisting with mobility and positioning, providing education and emotional support to patients and their families, and coordinating care with other healthcare **professional**s.

5.10 Superior vena cava syndrome

Superior vena cava syndrome (SVCS) is a condition that occurs when there is a blockage or compression of the superior vena cava, a large vein that carries deoxygenated blood from the upper body to the heart. In the context of oncologic emergencies, SVCS is most often caused by a malignancy in the mediastinum, such as lung cancer or lymphoma.

The symptoms of SVCS can vary depending on the severity and location of the blockage. Common symptoms include swelling of the face, neck, and upper chest, difficulty breathing, coughing, and a feeling of fullness or tightness in the head or neck. Other symptoms may include hoarseness, difficulty swallowing, and dilated veins in the upper body.

The diagnosis of SVCS usually involves a combination of clinical evaluation and imaging studies, such as chest X-ray, computed tomography (CT) scan, or magnetic resonance imaging (MRI). These tests help determine the location and cause of the blockage, allowing for appropriate treatment planning.

The management of SVCS aims to relieve the obstruction and improve symptoms. The choice of treatment depends on the underlying cause, the patient's overall health, and the urgency of the situation. In some cases, urgent interventions may be necessary if there is respiratory compromise or other life-threatening complications.

One common approach to manage SVCS is the use of radiation therapy, which can help shrink the tumor causing the obstruction. Chemotherapy may also be employed to treat the underlying malignancy. In some cases, surgical intervention may be required to bypass or remove the blockage. Additionally, supportive measures such as diuretics, steroids, and pain management may be used to alleviate symptoms and improve the patient's comfort.

The care of patients with SVCS requires close collaboration between **nurses**, oncologists, radiation oncologists, and other healthcare **professional**s. It is crucial for oncology **nurses** to closely monitor patients for any changes in symptoms, vital signs, or clinical condition. They play a vital role in educating patients and their families about the condition, its treatment, and preventive measures to reduce the risk of complications.

5.11 Increased intracranial pressure

Increased intracranial pressure (ICP) refers to the buildup of pressure inside the skull, specifically in the brain. This can occur due to various reasons in patients with cancer, making it an important **topic** for oncology **nurse**s to be familiar with.

One common cause of increased intracranial pressure in cancer patients is brain metastases. When cancer spreads to the brain, it can cause the growth of tumors, resulting in increased pressure. This can lead to symptoms such as headaches, nausea, vomiting, changes in behavior, seizures, and even loss of consciousness.

Another cause can be the presence of a brain tumor itself, either primary or secondary. As the tumor grows, it occupies space inside the skull, leading to increased pressure. This can have detrimental effects on the brain and its functions.

In addition to brain tumors, other contributing factors to increased intracranial pressure in cancer patients include cerebral edema (swelling of the brain), hydrocephalus (accumulation of cerebrospinal fluid in the brain), and hemorrhage (bleeding) within the brain.

Recognizing the signs and symptoms of increased intracranial pressure is crucial for oncology **nurse**s. Prompt identification allows for early intervention and management, which can significantly improve patient outcomes. **Nurse**s should assess patients for symptoms like severe headaches, changes in mental status, altered consciousness, vomiting, vision changes, and seizures.

Diagnosing increased intracranial pressure requires a thorough evaluation by a healthcare provider, which may include a neurological exam, imaging studies such as CT scans or MRIs, and measuring the pressure directly through intracranial pressure monitoring.

Treatment for increased intracranial pressure aims to reduce the pressure and manage symptoms. This may involve medications to decrease brain swelling, such as corticosteroids, diuretics, and antiepileptic drugs. In some cases, surgical intervention, such as tumor removal or shunt placement, may be necessary.

Nurses play a crucial role in the management of patients with increased intracranial pressure. They provide education to patients and families, administer prescribed medications, monitor the patient's neurological status, and communicate any changes or concerns to the healthcare team.

5.12 Obstructions (bowel and urinary)

Obstructions of the bowel and urinary system can be potential oncologic emergencies that oncology **nurse**s should be aware of. Bowel obstruction refers to a blockage in the intestines that can occur due to tumors, adhesions, or inflammation. On the other hand, urinary obstruction refers to a blockage in the urinary tract caused by tumors or other obstructions. These obstructions can lead to various complications and require prompt intervention.

Bowel obstruction can present with symptoms such as abdominal pain, nausea, vomiting, bloating, and constipation. The oncology **nurse** should assess the patient's vital signs, perform a physical examination, and review their medical history. Diagnostic tests, such as X-rays, CT scans, or sigmoidoscopy, may be ordered to confirm the obstruction. Treatment options include bowel rest, intravenous fluids, pain management, and decompression through the use of a nasogastric tube. Surgery may be necessary in severe cases to remove the obstruction.

Urinary obstruction can manifest as urinary retention, flank pain, urinary frequency, or hematuria. The **nurse** should assess the patient's urinary output, perform a bladder scan, and assess for signs of infection. Depending on the severity of the obstruction, interventions may include the placement of a urinary catheter, administration of pain medication, or surgical intervention to remove the obstruction. It is important for the **nurse** to monitor the patient's urine output, assess for signs of infection, and provide appropriate education regarding catheter care.

Complications of bowel and urinary obstructions can include dehydration, electrolyte imbalances, infection, and tissue necrosis. **Nurse**s should closely monitor the patient's vital signs, fluid intake and output, and provide appropriate interventions to prevent complications. Additionally, close collaboration with the healthcare team, including surgeons and oncologists, is crucial to ensure timely and effective management of obstructions.

5.13 Pneumonitis

Pneumonitis is a condition that is commonly encountered in oncology patients. It refers to the inflammation of the lung tissue, which can be caused by various factors. This condition can be challenging to diagnose and manage, hence it is important for oncology **nurse**s to have a comprehensive understanding of pneumonitis.

One of the main causes of pneumonitis in oncology patients is radiation therapy. When radiation is used to treat tumors in the thoracic area, it can inadvertently damage the surrounding lung tissue, leading to inflammation. This type of pneumonitis is known as radiation-induced pneumonitis.

Chemotherapy can also contribute to the development of pneumonitis. Certain drugs used in the treatment of cancer, such as immunotherapy agents and targeted therapies, can cause inflammation in the lungs. This is known as drug-induced pneumonitis.

The symptoms of pneumonitis can vary depending on the severity of the inflammation. Patients may experience shortness of breath, cough, chest pain, fever, and fatigue. It is important for oncology **nurse**s to be vigilant in monitoring these symptoms, as early detection and intervention can improve patient outcomes.

Diagnosing pneumonitis involves a thorough evaluation of the patient's medical history, physical examination, and imaging studies such as chest X-rays or CT scans. In some cases, a lung biopsy may be necessary to confirm the diagnosis.

Once pneumonitis is diagnosed, the management approach will depend on the underlying cause and the severity of the symptoms. Treatment may involve discontinuing or adjusting the dose of the offending medication, providing supportive care such as supplemental oxygen or bronchodilators, and administering corticosteroids to reduce inflammation.

Oncology **nurse**s play a crucial role in the management of pneumonitis. They are responsible for closely monitoring patients for the development of symptoms, educating patients about potential risks and symptoms to watch out for, and providing emotional support to help patients cope with the challenges of managing this condition

5.14 Extravasations

Extravasations are a common oncologic emergency that oncology **nurse**s need to be aware of. It refers to the leakage of chemotherapy drugs or other irritant substances from the blood vessels into the surrounding tissues, resulting in local tissue damage.

One important aspect of extravasations is the identification of early signs and symptoms. It is crucial for oncology **nurse**s to closely monitor their patients for any signs of extravasation, such as pain, swelling, redness, or blistering at the infusion site. Prompt recognition of these signs can lead to early intervention and prevention of further complications.

Once extravasation is suspected, the **nurse** should stop the infusion and alert the healthcare team immediately. The next step is to assess the extent of the extravasation by carefully examining the affected area. This assessment includes determining the type of infiltrated substance, the volume of leakage, and the patient's symptoms.

The management of extravasations involves different interventions depending on the severity and type of infiltrated substance. For mild cases, the **nurse** may apply warm or cold compresses and elevate the affected limb to reduce swelling and discomfort. In more severe cases, specific antidotes or neutralizing agents may be needed to counteract the effects of the infiltrated substance.

Another important aspect of extravasations is prevention. Oncology **nurse**s should adhere to best practices, including proper insertion and securement of vascular access devices, adequate patient education on the signs of extravasation, and regular monitoring during infusion.

It is also essential for oncology **nurse**s to have a thorough understanding of the chemotherapy drugs they administer, including their vesicant properties and potential for extravasation. They should be knowledgeable about the appropriate management protocols for different types of drugs.

5.15 Immune-related adverse events

Immune-related adverse events (irAEs) are a significant concern in the field of oncology, particularly in the context of immunotherapy. As an oncology **nurse**, it is crucial to have a comprehensive understanding of irAEs and their management.

IrAEs are adverse events that occur as a result of the immune system's response to cancer treatment. They can affect various organs and systems in the body, leading to a wide range of symptoms and complications. Common irAEs include dermatologic reactions, gastrointestinal disturbances, hepatotoxicity, pneumonitis, endocrine dysfunction, and musculoskeletal disorders.

Dermatologic reactions are among the most frequently reported irAEs. These can manifest as rash, pruritus, or even severe blistering conditions like Stevens-Johnson syndrome or toxic epidermal necrolysis. Close monitoring and prompt intervention are vital to prevent complications and ensure patient comfort.

Gastrointestinal irAEs encompass symptoms such as diarrhea, colitis, and abdominal pain. Severe cases may progress to bowel perforation or gastrointestinal bleeding. Early recognition and management, including close monitoring of stool frequency and consistency, are essential to prevent dehydration and sepsis.

Hepatotoxicity is another important irAE, with potential manifestations ranging from mild elevation of liver enzymes to severe liver damage. Regular monitoring of liver function tests is crucial to detect hepatotoxicity early and implement appropriate interventions.

Pneumonitis is a potentially life-threatening irAE that presents with symptoms like cough, dyspnea, and chest pain. It is crucial to assess respiratory status regularly and promptly investigate any suspicious symptoms to initiate corticosteroid therapy. Collaboration with the healthcare team is essential to ensure timely intervention.

Endocrine irAEs can lead to various hormonal imbalances, including thyroid dysfunction, adrenal insufficiency, or hypophysitis. Monitoring hormone levels and promptly addressing any imbalances is crucial to prevent complications such as myxedema coma or adrenal crisis.

Musculoskeletal irAEs may manifest as arthralgias, myalgias, or autoimmune myositis. Careful evaluation and collaboration with physical and occupational therapists can optimize patient comfort and maximize functional abilities.

Management of irAEs involves a multidisciplinary approach, including close collaboration with **physician**s, pharmacists, and other healthcare providers. Treatment often involves the use of immunosuppressive medications, such as corticosteroids. However, it is important to balance the control of irAEs with the potential impact on the antitumor immune response.

Continuous education and awareness regarding irAEs among oncology nursing **professional**s are paramount. Keeping up with the latest evidence-based practices and guidelines can help ensure the delivery of high-quality care to patients undergoing immunotherapy.

5.16 Venous thromboembolism

Venous thromboembolism is a significant concern in oncology patients. It refers to the formation of blood clots, known as thrombi, in the veins, which can then break loose and travel to other parts of the body, causing potentially life-threatening complications.

One of the major risk factors for venous thromboembolism in cancer patients is the hypercoagulable state, which is attributed to various factors like tumor cells releasing procoagulant substances. Additionally, certain chemotherapeutic agents can damage the blood vessel walls, further increasing the risk. Bed rest and immobilization during treatment, as well as central venous catheters, also contribute to the increased risk.

Deep vein thrombosis (DVT) is the most common form of venous thromboembolism. It typically occurs in the lower extremities and presents with symptoms such as pain, swelling, and redness in the affected limb. Pulmonary embolism (PE) is another potentially life-threatening complication, which occurs when a blood clot from the lower extremities travels to the lungs, causing shortness of breath, chest pain, and sometimes even sudden death.

Early detection and prompt treatment are vital in managing venous thromboembolism in oncology patients. Diagnostic tools like ultrasound, venography, and computed tomography (CT) scans are used to confirm the presence of blood clots. Anticoagulant therapy, including both heparin and oral anticoagulants like warfarin or direct oral anticoagulants (DOACs), is the mainstay of treatment. These medications prevent further clotting and help dissolve existing clots.

In certain high-risk situations, like active bleeding or gastrointestinal tumors, the placement of an inferior vena cava (IVC) filter may be considered. This device helps prevent blood clots from reaching the lungs, but it does not treat the underlying cause of the clot.

Preventive measures are crucial to minimize the occurrence of venous thromboembolism in oncology patients. These include early mobilization, leg exercises, and mechanical compression devices to improve blood flow. Prophylactic anticoagulation may also be considered in high-risk patients, depending on the specific situation.

As an oncology **nurse**, it is crucial to be aware of the risk factors, signs, and symptoms of venous thromboembolism. Regular assessment and close monitoring of patients' clinical status are essential for early detection and appropriate intervention. Patient education about the signs and symptoms of blood clot formation and the importance of compliance with prescribed medications are also crucial aspects of nursing care in managing venous thromboembolism in oncology patients.

6 Psychosocial Dimensions of Care

6.1 Cultural, spiritual, and religious diversity

Cultural, spiritual, and religious diversity is a critical aspect of providing psychosocial care to oncology patients. As an oncology **nurse**, it is crucial to understand and respect the diverse cultural backgrounds, spiritual beliefs, and religious practices of each patient. This awareness helps in tailoring care to meet their individual needs and ensure a holistic approach to treatment.

Cultural diversity involves recognizing and appreciating the differences in traditions, customs, values, and beliefs among patients. This includes understanding various languages, dietary needs, and family dynamics. Taking the time to learn about different cultures can enhance communication and foster trust between the **nurse** and the patient, leading to improved patient outcomes.

Spirituality plays a significant role in the lives of many oncology patients, regardless of their religious affiliation. Some may find solace in their spiritual beliefs, finding strength and meaning in their faith. It is essential for the oncology **nurse** to be respectful and open-minded, creating a safe space for patients to express their spiritual needs and address any concerns they may have. By encouraging open dialogue, the **nurse** can provide appropriate resources and support tailored to the patient's spiritual beliefs.

Religious diversity encompasses the different religious affiliations patients may identify with. Understanding the basic practices, rituals, and beliefs of various religions can aid in providing appropriate support and accommodating their needs. This can range from dietary restrictions to scheduling treatments around prayer times or arranging for spiritual leaders to visit patients in the hospital.

Addressing cultural, spiritual, and religious diversity in oncology care also involves recognizing and overcoming potential stereotypes or biases that may impact the quality of care. Patients should feel comfortable and respected, free from discrimination based on their cultural or religious background. By promoting inclusivity and embracing diversity, **nurse**s can create an environment that fosters trust, improves patient satisfaction, and contributes to positive healthcare outcomes.

6.2 Financial concerns

Financial concerns are a significant aspect of the psychosocial dimensions of care for oncology patients. Dealing with a cancer diagnosis can be emotionally and mentally taxing for patients and their families, and financial worries only add to the stress. It is vital for oncology **nurse**s to address these concerns and provide support to help patients navigate through this challenging aspect of their cancer journey.

One of the main financial concerns for cancer patients is the cost of treatment. Cancer treatments, including chemotherapy, radiation therapy, and targeted therapies, can be extremely expensive. Many patients struggle to cover the costs of medications, doctor visits, hospital stays, and other medical expenses. As an oncology **nurse**, it is essential to be aware of the financial resources available to patients, such as insurance coverage, state and federal assistance programs, and nonprofit organizations that provide financial aid.

Additionally, an oncology **nurse** should help patients understand their insurance coverage and navigate the complex healthcare system. This involves assisting patients in understanding their insurance benefits, including copays, deductibles, and out-of-pocket expenses. Furthermore, oncology **nurse**s must be knowledgeable about available financial assistance programs and help patients explore potential options.

Transportation costs can also pose a significant financial burden for cancer patients. Many individuals require frequent trips to the hospital or clinic for treatment, which may involve long distances and transportation expenses. It is important for oncology **nurse**s to connect patients with transportation resources, such as local volunteer driver programs or discounted transportation services.

Moreover, the financial impact of cancer extends beyond treatment costs. Cancer patients often face a loss of income due to their illness. Frequent medical appointments and treatment schedules may result in reduced work hours or the inability to work altogether. Oncology **nurse**s should advise patients on available resources for financial assistance, such as disability benefits, paid leave options, or social security support.

In addition to the practical aspects of financial concerns, oncology **nurse**s should also provide emotional support to patients as they grapple with the financial stress of cancer. This can involve active listening, empathy, and guidance on coping strategies. Patients may feel overwhelmed by their financial situation, and offering emotional support can significantly alleviate their distress

6.2.1 Employment

Employment is a key aspect of financial concerns and psychosocial dimensions of care in the field of oncology nursing. It encompasses various important aspects that affect both the **nurse**s and the patients.

One important aspect of employment is job stability and security. Oncology **nurse**s often face the fear of losing their jobs due to economic fluctuations, organizational restructuring, or budget cuts. This can create a sense of insecurity and stress among the **nurse**s, affecting their overall well-being. It is essential for organizations to ensure job security for oncology **nurse**s to promote a stable and supportive work environment.

Another aspect is the compensation and benefits offered to oncology **nurse**s. These **professional**s provide critical care to cancer patients, and it is crucial that they are adequately compensated for their skills and dedication. Fair wages, health insurance coverage, retirement plans, and other benefits play a significant role in attracting and retaining skilled oncology **nurse**s. It is also essential for organizations to regularly assess and adjust compensation packages to reflect the changing demands and responsibilities in the field.

Work-life balance is another important consideration concerning employment. Oncology **nurse**s often work long hours, including night shifts and weekends, to provide round-the-clock care to their patients. This can lead to fatigue, burnout, and strained personal relationships. Therefore, organizations should promote flexible scheduling, adequate time off, and supportive policies to help oncology **nurse**s maintain a healthy work-life balance.

Professional development and growth opportunities are also crucial aspects of employment for oncology **nurse**s. Continuous education, training, and career advancement opportunities not only enhance **nurse**s' knowledge and skills but also boost their morale and job satisfaction. Organizations should provide access to conferences, workshops, certifications, and other resources to support **nurse**s' **professional** growth and keep them updated with the latest advancements in oncology care.

Additionally, workplace culture and support systems are vital for the well-being of oncology **nurse**s. A positive and collaborative work environment that encourages teamwork, open communication, and mutual respect fosters a sense of belonging and job satisfaction. Organizations should also provide emotional support programs, counseling services, and resources to help **nurse**s cope with the emotional toll of working with cancer patients.

6.2.2 Insurance

Insurance is a key consideration in the realm of financial concerns for oncology **nurse**s. It entails a system of protection wherein individuals or organizations can safeguard themselves against potential financial loss resulting from uncertain events. The concept of insurance involves transferring risk to an insurance company in exchange for a financial arrangement known as a premium.

There are various types of insurance policies available, each catering to different needs. Health insurance, for instance, covers medical expenses incurred by individuals, including consultations, hospital stays, and medications. This type of insurance is particularly pertinent to oncology **nurse**s as it directly impacts their patients' access to cancer treatments and supportive care.

Insurance coverage may also extend to life insurance, which provides a payout to policy beneficiaries upon the policyholder's death. This can offer financial relief to the family of an oncology **nurse** who may have dependents relying on their income. Disability insurance, another insurance option, provides income replacement in the event that an individual becomes temporarily or permanently unable to work due to illness or injury. This type of coverage can be crucial for oncology **nurse**s who face occupational hazards and require protection against potential income loss.

Diving deeper into the realm of health insurance, there are two primary types of coverage: private insurance and government-sponsored insurance programs. Private insurance is obtained through employers, purchased independently, or provided by **professional** organizations. Government-sponsored programs include Medicare for individuals aged **65** and older, and Medicaid for low-income individuals and families. These programs often have specific eligibility criteria and cover different aspects of healthcare services for those who qualify.

Insurance policies can have different structures and provisions. Some policies operate on a fee-for-service basis, where the insurer reimburses the healthcare provider for the cost of each service rendered. Other policies employ a managed care approach, such as health maintenance organizations (HMOs) or preferred provider organizations (PPOs), which involve contracted providers and specific networks to manage costs and ensure coordinated care.

For oncology **nurse**s, understanding the intricacies of insurance is crucial when advocating for their patients. It involves understanding coverage limitations, pre-authorization processes, and the reimbursement mechanisms associated with different insurance policies. Navigating insurance claims and ensuring that patients receive appropriate coverage and timely access to oncology treatments can greatly impact outcomes and the patient's financial well-being.

6.2.3 Resources

Resources are an essential aspect of financial concerns and the psychosocial dimensions of care in the field of oncology nursing. These resources encompass various elements that aid in providing comprehensive support to patients and their families throughout their cancer journey.

One significant aspect of resources is financial assistance. Many individuals facing cancer encounter financial challenges due to the high costs associated with treatment, medication, and supportive care. Therefore, it is crucial for oncology **nurse**s to be familiar with different financial resources available to patients. These resources may include government programs, non-profit organizations, and pharmaceutical assistance programs that can provide financial aid for medical expenses.

Another vital resource is information. Oncology **nurse**s play a pivotal role in educating patients and their families about their diagnosis, treatment options, and available support services. They provide information regarding local support groups, counseling services, and organizations that offer emotional and psychological support. By equipping patients with knowledge, **nurse**s empower them to make informed decisions and navigate their cancer journey more confidently.

Psychosocial resources are also essential in providing holistic care to cancer patients. These resources encompass emotional support, counseling services, and opportunities to engage in support groups. Oncology **nurse**s should be knowledgeable about local resources and organizations that offer these services, as they contribute significantly to the psychosocial well-being of patients and their families. These resources help patients cope with the emotional and psychological challenges that arise from their diagnosis and treatment.

In addition to financial and psychosocial resources, physical resources come into play when caring for oncology patients. These include medical equipment, medication, and facilities required for various diagnostic and therapeutic procedures. Efficient management of physical resources is essential to ensure prompt and effective treatment delivery.

Furthermore, time is a valuable resource for both oncology **nurse**s and their patients. **Nurse**s must prioritize their tasks and manage their time efficiently to provide adequate care to all patients. Proper time management ensures that patients receive timely interventions, including appointments, medication administration, and emotional support.

6.3 Altered Body Image

Altered body image is a significant psychosocial dimension of care that oncology **nurse**s need to address when caring for patients undergoing cancer treatment or experiencing the aftermath of treatment. This **topic** encompasses the changes in appearance and physical functioning that cancer patients may go through as a result of their disease or its treatment, which can greatly impact their self-perception and overall well-being.

One important aspect of altered body image is the physical changes that cancer patients may experience. For instance, patients undergoing chemotherapy may lose their hair, whereas those who have undergone surgery may have scars or loss of body parts. Additionally, radiation therapy may cause changes in skin texture and pigmentation. These physical alterations can lead to feelings of unattractiveness, shame, and embarrassment, resulting in a negative body image.

Another aspect to consider is the impact of altered body image on the patient's emotional and psychological well-being. Cancer patients may experience a range of emotions such as depression, anxiety, and anger due to the changes in their physical appearance. They may struggle with accepting their new self-image or feel socially isolated and misunderstood by others. These emotional challenges can further contribute to a poor body image and affect their overall quality of life.

Communication and support are essential in addressing altered body image concerns. Oncology **nurse**s should create a safe space for patients to express their feelings and concerns about their changed appearance. Providing empathetic listening and validating their emotions can help patients feel understood and supported. **Nurse**s can also employ therapeutic interventions like counseling, support groups, or referrals to mental health **professional**s to assist patients in managing their emotions and building resilience.

It is crucial for oncology **nurse**s to provide education and resources to patients about coping strategies and self-care techniques that can improve body image and self-esteem. Encouraging the use of prosthetics, wigs, or scarves can help patients regain a sense of normalcy and enhance their self-confidence. Promoting the involvement of supportive family members or friends during the recovery process can also facilitate emotional healing and acceptance.

6.4 Learning preferences and barriers to learning

Learning preferences and barriers to learning are crucial aspects of providing care as an oncology **nurse**. Understanding how patients prefer to learn and identifying the obstacles they face can greatly enhance the educational experiences and outcomes for both patients and healthcare providers.

When it comes to learning preferences, individuals have unique ways of acquiring and processing information. Some patients prefer visual aids, such as diagrams or videos, while others may prefer auditory methods, such as listening to explanations or participating in discussions. Additionally, some patients learn best through hands-on experiences or practical demonstrations. Recognizing these preferences can help tailor educational materials and presentations to better meet the needs of patients.

Another important consideration is the barriers that may hinder patients' ability to learn. One major obstacle is the patients' emotional state. A cancer diagnosis can be overwhelming and emotionally draining, making it difficult for patients to focus and retain information. Addressing patients' emotional needs and providing support can help alleviate this barrier to learning.

Furthermore, language and cultural barriers can impede learning. Patients who speak a different language or come from diverse cultural backgrounds may struggle to fully comprehend medical information presented in a different language or context. To overcome this barrier, healthcare providers can utilize language interpreters, translate educational materials, or enlist the help of cultural liaisons to bridge the communication gap.

Health literacy is another critical factor that can influence the learning process. Many patients have limited health literacy skills, which means they may struggle to understand medical jargon, navigate complex healthcare systems, or adhere to treatment plans. **Nurse**s can address this barrier by using clear and simple language, providing written materials in plain English or other accessible formats, and offering repeated explanations or demonstrations to reinforce understanding.

Time constraints and competing priorities may also hinder patients' ability to learn. Many patients undergoing cancer treatment may have demanding schedules due to medical appointments, treatments, and other responsibilities. As an oncology **nurse**, it is important to recognize these competing priorities and find flexible ways to deliver educational information, such as offering online resources or providing materials for patients to review at their own pace.

6.5 Social relationships and family dynamics

Social relationships and family dynamics play a crucial role in the psychosocial dimensions of care for oncology patients. These aspects encompass the interactions and support systems within a patient's social circle, including family, friends, and the broader community.

One important aspect of social relationships is the emotional support provided by loved ones. Having a strong support system can significantly impact a patient's psychological well-being throughout their cancer journey. The encouragement, empathy, and understanding from family and close friends can help alleviate anxiety, depression, and feelings of isolation.

Family dynamics also influence the caregiving process. In many cases, family members assume the role of primary caregivers, offering physical and emotional care to the patient. It is vital for oncology **nurse**s to assess the family's dynamics and provide appropriate guidance and support, especially when conflicts or communication breakdowns occur.

Supporting the patient's social relationships and family dynamics involves fostering open lines of communication among all parties involved. This can help address conflicts, manage expectations, and ensure everyone understands the patient's needs and wishes. Effective communication is also crucial for ensuring accurate information is shared, enhancing the shared decision-making process.

Maintaining healthy relationships and family dynamics can reduce stress levels for both the patient and their caregivers. Encouraging mutual respect, empathy, and understanding among all members helps create a positive and supportive environment for the patient. This positivity can improve the patient's overall well-being and potentially enhance treatment outcomes.

Understanding cultural and social factors that influence social relationships and family dynamics is also important for oncology **nurse**s. Different cultures may have varying perspectives on illness, caregiving, and family roles. Being sensitive to these differences can help **nurse**s provide appropriate support tailored to each patient's cultural background.

In some cases, cancer may strain social relationships and family dynamics due to the challenges it presents. Role changes, financial burdens, and increased dependency on caregivers can be sources of stress. Oncology **nurse**s must be prepared to address these challenges by offering counseling services, connecting patients and their families with support groups, and providing resources for financial assistance.

By recognizing the significance of social relationships and family dynamics, oncology **nurse**s can better meet the holistic needs of their patients. By fostering and supporting healthy relationships, they contribute to the patient's overall well-being and enhance the patient's experience throughout their cancer journey.

6.6 Coping mechanisms and skills

Coping mechanisms and skills are extremely important for those working in the field of oncology nursing. As oncology **nurse**s provide care and support to patients with cancer, they often witness and experience emotional, psychological, and social challenges. It is vital for these **nurse**s to possess coping mechanisms and skills to deal with the stress and demands of their profession effectively.

One coping mechanism that is crucial for oncology **nurse**s is self-care. Taking care of oneself is essential in maintaining physical and emotional well-being. Engaging in activities that promote relaxation, such as exercise, meditation, or hobbies, can help **nurse**s manage stress and prevent burnout. Additionally, seeking support from friends, family, or **professional** counselors can provide a valuable outlet for **nurse**s to express their emotions and concerns.

Another important coping skill for oncology **nurse**s is effective communication. Being able to communicate with patients, their families, and the healthcare team is vital in providing quality care. Oncology **nurse**s must develop strong listening and empathetic skills to understand patients' needs and concerns. They should also be able to effectively convey medical information to patients in a compassionate and understandable manner.

Resilience is another essential coping mechanism for oncology **nurse**s. It refers to the ability to adapt and bounce back from challenging situations. Resilient **nurse**s are better equipped to handle the emotional ups and downs of providing care to cancer patients. They can maintain a positive attitude, remain focused on their goals, and find meaning in their work, even in the face of adversity.

Furthermore, problem-solving skills are vital for oncology **nurse**s. They often encounter complex situations that require critical thinking and decision-making. Developing effective problem-solving skills allows **nurse**s to assess different situations, identify potential challenges, and find appropriate solutions. This skill helps them navigate difficult situations and provide the best possible care for their patients.

In addition to these coping mechanisms and skills, self-reflection is essential for oncology **nurse**s. Taking time to reflect on their experiences, emotions, and **professional** growth can enhance self-awareness and promote personal development. It allows **nurse**s to recognize their strengths and weaknesses, make necessary adjustments, and continually improve their practice.

6.7 Support

As an oncology **nurse**, providing support is an essential part of caring for patients. Support can come in various forms and is pivotal in addressing the psychosocial dimensions of care.

One important aspect of support is emotional support. This involves being empathetic, compassionate, and understanding towards patients and their families. By being a source of emotional support, oncology **nurse**s can provide comfort and alleviate anxiety and fear that patients may experience.

Another crucial form of support is informational support. Oncology **nurse**s play a vital role in educating patients and their families about the nature of their illness, treatment options, potential side effects, and available resources. By providing clear and accurate information, **nurse**s help patients make informed decisions and empower them to actively participate in their care.

Practical support is also essential. This includes assisting patients with activities of daily living, providing resources for transportation and accommodation, and facilitating communication with the healthcare team. By addressing practical needs, **nurse**s can lighten the burden on patients and their families, allowing them to focus on their well-being.

Support groups are another valuable resource for patients and their families. These groups provide a platform for individuals with similar experiences to come together, share their challenges, seek advice, and offer support to one another. Oncology **nurse**s can encourage patients to join support groups, as they provide a sense of belonging and can help alleviate feelings of isolation.

Collaboration with other healthcare **professional**s is crucial in providing comprehensive support. By working closely with social workers, psychologists, palliative care teams, and other specialists, oncology **nurse**s can ensure that patients receive holistic care that addresses their psychosocial needs.

Lastly, self-care for oncology **nurse**s is vital in effectively supporting patients. Taking care of one's physical and emotional well-being allows **nurse**s to stay resilient and provide the best possible care. By seeking support from colleagues, practicing self-reflection, and setting boundaries, **nurse**s can maintain their own mental health while supporting others.

6.7.1 Patient (i.e., individual and group)

The **topic** of "Patient (i.e., individual and group)" within the broad **topic** of "Support, Psychosocial Dimensions of Care" is crucial for oncology **nurse**s to understand. This **topic** encompasses various aspects of patient care and highlights the unique needs of individual patients and groups in the oncology setting.

Patients in oncology care can be viewed as individuals who require tailored support and assistance throughout their cancer journey. Each patient has unique physical, emotional, and psychological needs, which must be addressed by the oncology **nurse**. These needs can include pain management, symptom control, and addressing concerns about treatment side effects.

Furthermore, patients are not isolated individuals, but they also belong to various groups that influence their experiences and support systems. These groups can include family members, friends, and other patients facing similar diagnoses. The oncology **nurse** plays a pivotal role in understanding and addressing the needs of both the individual patient and their support networks.

In caring for individual patients, oncology **nurse**s need to provide empathetic and compassionate care. This involves acknowledging and validating the patient's emotions, fears, and concerns related to their diagnosis and treatment. The **nurse** should actively listen to the patient, encourage open communication, and foster a trusting relationship.

Additionally, the **nurse** should assess and address the psychosocial well-being of the patient. This includes evaluating the patient's coping strategies, assessing their social support systems, and identifying any mental health concerns that may arise during the course of treatment. The **nurse** should be knowledgeable about available resources, such as support groups, counseling services, and financial assistance programs, to help meet the patient's psychosocial needs.

In recognizing the importance of group dynamics, the oncology **nurse** should facilitate opportunities for patients to connect and share their experiences. Group interventions, such as support groups or educational sessions, can help patients feel less isolated, provide a platform for mutual support, and foster a sense of belonging.

Addressing the needs of both the individual and group also involves advocating for the patient's rights and facilitating communication between the patient and their healthcare team. The oncology **nurse** should empower patients to actively participate in their own care, ensuring their voices are heard and their preferences are respected.

6.7.2 Caregiver (including family)

The **topic** of caregiving in oncology focuses on the important role that caregivers, including family members, play in supporting patients throughout their cancer journey. Caregivers provide physical, emotional, and practical support to those affected by cancer, and their contribution is vital to the overall well-being of the patient.

One aspect of caregiving is the physical support provided by caregivers. This can include assisting with activities of daily living such as bathing, dressing, and feeding the patient. Caregivers often accompany patients to medical appointments and help manage medications and treatment regimens. They may also be responsible for monitoring and reporting any changes in the patient's condition to the healthcare team.

Another important dimension of caregiving is the emotional support caregivers offer to patients. Cancer diagnosis and treatment can be emotionally overwhelming, and caregivers play a key role in providing a listening ear, empathy, and reassurance. They offer comfort through words and gestures, helping patients navigate the emotional challenges that come with cancer.

Caregivers also provide practical support, such as coordinating logistics and appointments. They may handle financial matters, transportation, and meal preparation to alleviate stress for the patient. Caregivers act as advocates, ensuring that the patient's needs and concerns are addressed by the healthcare team.

Furthermore, caregivers also face their own unique challenges and psychosocial needs. They may experience emotional distress, fatigue, and burnout due to the demands of caregiving. Providing support to caregivers is essential to help them maintain their own mental and physical well-being. Support groups, counseling services, and respite care are valuable resources that can assist caregivers in coping with their caregiving responsibilities.

It is crucial for oncology **nurse**s to recognize the pivotal role that caregivers, including family members, play in the care of patients. By acknowledging and involving caregivers in the treatment process, **nurse**s can enhance the quality of care and improve patient outcomes. Providing education and resources to caregivers can empower them to effectively fulfill their caregiving roles.

6.8 Psychosocial distress

Psychosocial distress is a critical aspect of the psychosocial dimensions of care that oncology **nurse**s need to address. It refers to the emotional, psychological, and social challenges experienced by individuals facing a cancer diagnosis and treatment. This distress can arise due to various factors such as fear of the unknown, uncertainty about prognosis, concerns about treatment outcomes, body image issues, financial burden, changes in roles and relationships, and social isolation.

One important aspect of psychosocial distress is the emotional impact of cancer. Patients often experience a range of emotions including fear, anxiety, sadness, anger, and grief. They may worry about the future and the impact of cancer on their lives. Oncology **nurse**s play a crucial role in providing emotional support, listening to patients' concerns, normalizing their feelings, and helping them cope with their emotions.

Another aspect of psychosocial distress is the psychological impact. Cancer can significantly affect an individual's self-esteem and body image. Physical changes resulting from treatment, such as hair loss, weight gain or loss, and scars, can have a profound impact on patients' self-image. Oncology **nurse**s can offer reassurance, provide resources for wig and prosthetic options, and refer patients to support groups or counseling services to help them navigate these challenges.

Social distress is yet another important aspect to consider. Many cancer patients experience social isolation due to the disruption of their daily routines, work, and social activities. They may face stigma or discrimination from their community or experience difficulties in maintaining relationships. Oncology **nurse**s can identify patients' social needs, provide education on support resources, and facilitate connections with support groups or counseling services to help patients rebuild their social networks.

In addition to these primary aspects of psychosocial distress, several sub**topic**s contribute to the overall well-being of cancer patients. These include family dynamics, caregiver stress, financial concerns, spiritual and existential distress, and the impact of cancer on sexuality. Each of these areas requires careful assessment, support, and intervention from oncology **nurse**s to address the holistic needs of patients.

6.8.1 Anxiety

Anxiety is a common psychosocial distress experienced by individuals, particularly those undergoing cancer treatment. It is characterized by feelings of fear, unease, worry, and nervousness. Oncology **nurse**s play a crucial role in identifying and addressing anxiety in their patients. Understanding the various aspects of anxiety can help **nurse**s provide effective care and support.

One important aspect of anxiety is its prevalence among cancer patients. Studies have shown that up to **40**% of cancer patients experience significant levels of anxiety. This highlights the need for **nurse**s to be vigilant in assessing and addressing anxiety in their patients. By recognizing the signs and symptoms of anxiety, **nurse**s can intervene early and provide appropriate interventions.

Anxiety can manifest in various ways, including physical symptoms. Patients may experience rapid heartbeat, shortness of breath, trembling, sweating, and gastrointestinal distress. **Nurse**s should be aware of these physical manifestations and inquire about them during patient assessments. By addressing these physical symptoms, **nurse**s can help alleviate the distress experienced by patients.

Another important aspect of anxiety is its impact on the psychological well-being of patients. Anxiety can lead to increased feelings of sadness, irritability, and difficulty concentrating. It can also exacerbate existing mental health conditions, such as depression. Oncology **nurse**s should have a comprehensive understanding of the psychological impact of anxiety in order to provide appropriate emotional support and referrals to mental health **professional**s if needed.

The causes of anxiety in cancer patients are multifactorial. The uncertainty surrounding cancer diagnosis and treatment, fear of pain, worries about prognosis and the future, and the disruption of daily life can all contribute to anxiety. **Nurse**s should be empathetic listeners, providing a safe space for patients to express their concerns and fears. By validating these feelings, **nurse**s can help patients cope with anxiety more effectively.

Treatment for anxiety may include pharmacological interventions, such as anxiolytic medications, as prescribed by the healthcare provider. Non-pharmacological interventions, such as cognitive-behavioral therapy, relaxation techniques, and support groups, can also be beneficial. **Nurse**s should educate patients about these treatment options and provide appropriate referrals.

6.8.2 Loss and grief

Loss and grief are common experiences in the field of oncology. As an oncology **nurse**, understanding and addressing these psychosocial dimensions of care is crucial.

Loss refers to the experience of being deprived of someone or something of value. In the context of cancer, patients may experience loss in various ways. This can include loss of physical abilities, loss of independence, loss of self-image, and even loss of life.

Grief, on the other hand, is the emotional response to loss. It is a complex and individual process that can manifest in different ways. Some patients may feel overwhelming sadness, while others may experience anger, guilt, or even numbness.

Recognizing and acknowledging the experience of loss and grief is essential for providing holistic care to oncology patients. It is important to create a safe and supportive environment where patients feel comfortable expressing their emotions.

One sub**topic** within loss and grief is anticipatory grief. This type of grief occurs before an actual loss takes place, often when patients are aware that their condition is terminal. Anticipatory grief can have a significant impact on patients and their families, as they grapple with the impending loss and the accompanying emotions.

Another sub**topic** is complicated grief. This occurs when the grief process becomes prolonged or debilitating. It may manifest as intense and persistent feelings of sorrow, difficulty accepting the loss, or an inability to engage in daily activities. Recognizing signs of complicated grief is important to provide appropriate support and intervention.

Additionally, cultural and spiritual beliefs play a significant role in how individuals experience and express grief. It is crucial for oncology **nurse**s to be culturally sensitive and respectful of these beliefs, as they can greatly influence the grieving process.

Support groups and counseling services are valuable resources for patients and their families dealing with loss and grief. These provide a space for individuals to share their experiences, learn coping strategies, and receive emotional support from others who have gone through similar challenges.

As an oncology **nurse**, it is important to assess and address the psychosocial distress of patients experiencing loss and grief. This involves active listening, empathy, and providing appropriate interventions and referrals. Collaborating with the interdisciplinary team, including social workers and psychologists, can also enhance the support provided to patients and their families during this challenging time.

6.8.3 Depression

Depression is a common psychological condition that often accompanies a diagnosis of cancer. It is considered as a psychosocial distress and falls under the psychosocial dimensions of care for an Oncology **Nurse**. Depression can greatly impact the overall well-being and quality of life of cancer patients. It is crucial for oncology **nurse**s to have a comprehensive understanding of depression in order to effectively support their patients.

Depression, in the context of cancer, is characterized by persistent feelings of sadness, hopelessness, fatigue, and loss of interest in activities. It can affect patients at any stage of the cancer journey, from diagnosis to treatment and survivorship. The causes of depression in cancer patients are multifactorial, including biological, psychological, and social factors.

One important aspect of depression to consider is the screening and assessment process. Oncology **nurse**s play a crucial role in identifying patients who may be experiencing depression. This involves using validated screening tools and conducting thorough assessments to determine the severity and impact of depression on the patient's daily life.

Once depression is identified, appropriate interventions can be implemented. Psychosocial support is a key component of managing depression in cancer patients. This may include counseling, psychotherapy, and support groups. Collaborating with other healthcare **professional**s, such as psychologists and psychiatrists, can further enhance the effectiveness of these interventions.

Additionally, education and self-management strategies are vital in empowering patients to cope with depression. Oncology **nurse**s can provide information and resources about depression, its symptoms, and available treatment options. Encouraging patients to engage in self-care activities, such as exercise, relaxation techniques, and maintaining a support network, can also be beneficial.

Furthermore, it is essential for oncology **nurse**s to address the stigma and misconceptions surrounding depression. Patients may feel reluctant to seek help due to societal attitudes or fear of being labeled as weak. Educating patients, families, and the wider community about the psychological impact of cancer and the importance of seeking support can help reduce stigma.

Lastly, ongoing follow-up and monitoring of depression symptoms is crucial. Regular assessments can determine if interventions are effective and if any adjustments need to be made. Oncology **nurse**s should also be vigilant for signs of suicidal ideation or worsening depression, as immediate intervention may be necessary.

6.8.4   Loss of personal control

Loss of personal control is a significant psychosocial distress experienced by oncology patients. This **topic** encompasses various aspects that can greatly affect the well-being of individuals undergoing cancer treatment. It involves a loss of autonomy, independence, and self-determination, which can have a profound emotional and psychological impact.

One of the primary factors contributing to the loss of personal control is the invasive nature of cancer treatments. Patients often have to undergo surgeries, chemotherapy, radiation therapy, and other invasive procedures, which can leave them feeling helpless and powerless. These interventions disrupt their daily routines, independence, and ability to make decisions about their own bodies.

The loss of personal control also manifests in the form of treatment-related side effects. Patients may experience symptoms such as pain, fatigue, nausea, and hair loss, which further diminish their sense of control over their bodies and their lives. These physical changes can negatively impact their self-image and self-esteem, leading to emotional distress and a loss of confidence.

Furthermore, the diagnosis of cancer itself can impose a sense of powerlessness. Patients may feel overwhelmed by the uncertainty of their prognosis, the fear of recurrence, and the potential loss of life. They may also face the need to rely on others for emotional and practical support, which can challenge their independence and self-sufficiency.

In addition to these broader factors, specific sub**topic**s contribute to the loss of personal control in the context of oncology care. These include the loss of control over treatment decisions, financial burdens associated with medical expenses, the impact on personal relationships and social support, and the loss of control over future plans and aspirations.

As an oncology **nurse**, understanding the psychosocial distress caused by the loss of personal control is crucial for providing holistic care. By acknowledging and addressing these concerns, **nurse**s can empower patients to regain a sense of control and autonomy in their cancer journey. This can be achieved through effective communication, providing education about treatment options, involving patients in shared decision-making, providing emotional support, and connecting patients with resources to help them cope with the financial and social challenges they may face

6.8.5   Spiritual distress

Spiritual distress is a significant aspect of psychosocial distress that oncology **nurse**s need to address when providing care to patients. It refers to the inner turmoil or conflict experienced by individuals when their spiritual beliefs or values are challenged or compromised due to their illness or the treatments they undergo.

One important aspect of spiritual distress is the loss of meaning or purpose in life. Patients facing a cancer diagnosis may question the meaning of their illness and struggle to find a sense of purpose in their current circumstances. This can lead to feelings of hopelessness and despair.

Another aspect of spiritual distress is a loss of faith or trust in their religious or spiritual beliefs. Patients may question why they are suffering from cancer despite their strong faith or may feel abandoned by their higher power. Such doubts can create feelings of guilt, anger, or resentment

Furthermore, spiritual distress may manifest as a loss of connection to oneself, others, or the world. Patients may feel disconnected from their own bodies, experiencing a loss of control or a sense of betrayal by their own bodies. They may also feel isolated or alone, struggling to find support or understanding from those around them.

Coping with spiritual distress requires a holistic approach that acknowledges and addresses patients' spiritual needs. Oncology **nurse**s can provide support by actively listening to patients' concerns, encouraging open conversations about spirituality, and involving chaplains or spiritual leaders when appropriate.

Assessment is a crucial step in identifying spiritual distress. **Nurse**s can use various assessment tools to evaluate patients' spiritual well-being and identify specific areas of concern. These tools may include questions about religious beliefs, meaning and purpose in life, sources of strength, and the impact of illness on spirituality.

Interventions to address spiritual distress may involve providing emotional support, facilitating discussions on spirituality, assisting patients in finding meaning and purpose, and connecting patients with appropriate spiritual resources. This can include referrals to chaplains, pastoral care services, support groups, or counseling services.

Finally, ongoing evaluation and reassessment are important in ensuring that patients' spiritual needs are continuously met. By regularly checking in with patients and offering ongoing support, **nurse**s can help patients navigate their spiritual distress and find a sense of peace and comfort amidst their cancer journey.

6.8.6 Caregiver fatigue

Caregiver fatigue refers to the physical, emotional, and mental exhaustion experienced by individuals who provide care for cancer patients. Being an oncology **nurse**, it is crucial to understand this **topic** as it directly impacts the well-being of caregivers and their ability to provide effective care.

One of the contributing factors to caregiver fatigue is the demanding nature of caregiving itself. Oncology **nurse**s who care for cancer patients often face long working hours and high job demands. This can lead to chronic fatigue, sleep disturbances, and reduced energy levels.

Emotional stress is another significant aspect of caregiver fatigue. Witnessing the suffering of cancer patients on a daily basis can take a toll on the mental health of caregivers. They may experience feelings of sadness, anxiety, and helplessness. This emotional burden can manifest as burnout and lead to decreased motivation and engagement in caregiving tasks.

Additionally, caregivers often neglect their own self-care needs in the process of caring for others. They may sacrifice their personal lives, relationships, and hobbies, which further contributes to their exhaustion. The lack of time for relaxation and self-care activities can lead to chronic stress and feelings of overwhelm.

Furthermore, the role of caregivers can be emotionally and physically demanding. They may be responsible for managing medications, coordinating medical appointments, and providing physical assistance to patients. This constant responsibility and pressure can result in physical strain, such as musculoskeletal injuries or chronic pain.

To address caregiver fatigue, it is vital for oncology **nurse**s to prioritize caregiver well-being. This can be done through providing education, support, and resources. **Nurse**s can educate caregivers on the importance of self-care and stress management techniques. They can also facilitate support groups or counseling services to help caregivers cope with their emotional challenges. Moreover, **nurse**s can encourage caregivers to seek respite and take breaks from their caregiving responsibilities to rest and recharge.

Collaboration with a multidisciplinary team is essential to address caregiver fatigue comprehensively. This may involve coordinating with social workers, psychologists, and other healthcare **professional**s who can provide additional support and resources to caregivers

6.8.7 Crisis management (e.g., domestic violence, suicidal ideation)

Crisis management is a crucial aspect of providing psychosocial care to oncology patients. It involves addressing various psychosocial distress situations, such as domestic violence and suicidal ideation, which can significantly impact the overall well-being of individuals facing cancer.

Domestic violence, an intensely distressing issue, refers to any form of abusive behavior within a family or intimate relationship. It can manifest as physical, emotional, sexual, or financial abuse. In the context of oncology, patients may experience heightened vulnerability and stress, potentially increasing the risk of domestic violence. As an oncology **nurse**, it is important to identify signs of domestic violence, such as unexplained injuries, frequent absences from appointments, changes in behavior, or reluctance to involve family members in their care. By recognizing these signs, the **nurse** can provide the necessary support and resources, including referrals to social workers, counselor, or helplines specializing in domestic violence.

Suicidal ideation, another critical psychosocial distress issue, involves thoughts and contemplation of self-harm or ending one's life. Oncology patients may experience heightened feelings of hopelessness, despair, or a loss of control, leading to suicidal thoughts. As an oncology **nurse**, it is vital to be vigilant for signs of suicidal ideation, like expressions of hopelessness, withdrawal, giving away personal belongings, or mentioning suicide directly or indirectly. If such signs arise, it is crucial to maintain a non-judgmental approach and actively listen to the patient. Promptly involving mental health **professional**s, such as psychologists or psychiatrists, can help in assessing the risk and developing an appropriate crisis management plan.

To address crisis situations like domestic violence and suicidal ideation effectively, oncology **nurse**s must possess strong communication and interpersonal skills. Developing a trusting relationship with patients is vital, as this creates an environment where individuals feel safe to share their concerns and seek help. Active listening, empathy, and validation of emotions can significantly assist in crisis management situations.

In addition to creating a supportive environment, oncology **nurse**s should also be knowledgeable about local resources and support services available in their healthcare facility or community. Collaborating with social workers, mental health **professional**s, and community organizations can provide a comprehensive network of support and assistance for patients experiencing psychosocial distress.

6.9 Sexuality

Sexuality is an important aspect of psychosocial care for oncology **nurse**s to address. It encompasses an individual's sexual identity, orientation, desires, and behaviors. Supporting patients in their sexual well-being can positively impact their overall quality of life and emotional well-being during their oncology journey.

One key aspect of sexuality is understanding and respecting each patient's sexual identity. Oncology **nurse**s should recognize that individuals may identify as heterosexual, homosexual, bisexual, or different genders. It is vital to provide a non-judgmental and inclusive environment where patients feel comfortable expressing their sexual orientation.

Another important consideration is the impact of cancer and its treatments on sexual functioning. Many cancer treatments can lead to physical changes in the body, such as surgical scars, changes in body image, or side effects like fatigue and pain, which can affect sexual desire and function. Oncology **nurse**s should be knowledgeable about these potential effects and provide information and support to patients.

Communication plays a crucial role in addressing patients' sexual concerns. Oncology **nurse**s should create an open dialogue with patients, allowing them to express their worries and ask questions regarding sexual health. This communication should include discussions about sexual activities, contraception, fertility preservation, and potential concerns related to intimacy and relationships during and after treatment.

Education forms another essential component of addressing sexuality in oncology care. **Nurse**s can provide patients with resources, such as pamphlets or websites that discuss sexual health during and after cancer treatment. These resources should cover **topic**s like managing sexual side effects, counseling services, and support groups available to help patients navigate their sexual concerns.

Counseling and psychological support are crucial for addressing the psychosocial dimensions of sexuality in oncology care. Oncology **nurse**s should identify patients who may benefit from **professional** counseling to cope with emotional and psychological issues related to their sexual health. This support can help patients improve their self-esteem, body image, and overall well-being.

It's important for oncology **nurse**s to work collaboratively with other healthcare **professional**s, including oncologists and psychologists, to ensure comprehensive care for patients' sexual concerns. By taking the lead in addressing sexuality, oncology **nurse**s can play a crucial role in enhancing patients' overall well-being and quality of life during their cancer journey.

6.9.1 Reproductive issues (e.g., contraception, fertility)

Reproductive issues are a significant concern for individuals undergoing cancer treatment, and as an oncology **nurse**, it is crucial to provide comprehensive support and guidance in this area. Reproductive issues encompass a range of **topic**s, including contraception and fertility preservation.

Contraception is essential for patients of reproductive age who wish to prevent pregnancy during their cancer treatment. It is important to discuss various contraceptive options with patients and their partners, taking into account the potential interactions between contraception and cancer therapy. Barrier methods, such as condoms or diaphragms, are generally safe to use, while hormonal methods like birth control pills or patches may have contraindications or require adjustments in dosage due to potential drug interactions.

For patients interested in preserving their fertility, it is crucial to explore fertility preservation options before starting cancer treatment. This is especially important for patients who may experience fertility-related side effects, such as damage to the ovaries or testes, as a result of certain treatment modalities. Fertility preservation methods include sperm or egg cryopreservation, embryo freezing, or ovarian tissue preservation. These options should be discussed with patients, taking into account their specific diagnosis, treatment plan, and personal preferences.

It is important for oncology **nurse**s to address the emotional and psychosocial aspects associated with reproductive issues. Patients may experience anxiety, fear, or sadness when considering contraception or fertility preservation. Providing empathetic and supportive care is crucial during these conversations, helping patients understand their options and cope with their desires and concerns about future parenthood.

Moreover, education on alternative reproductive options, such as adoption or surrogacy, should be provided to patients who may face permanent infertility due to cancer treatment. These discussions should be approached with sensitivity and respect, allowing patients to explore these options while acknowledging their unique circumstances and desires.

Continued follow-up and support are essential throughout the patient's cancer journey. Information on resources and support groups for patients dealing with reproductive issues can be provided to ensure ongoing assistance and guidance. Collaborating with other members of the healthcare team, such as oncologists, fertility specialists, or reproductive endocrinologists, can also enhance patient care in this domain

6.9.2 Sexual dysfunction (e.g., physical and psychological effects)

Sexual dysfunction refers to difficulties or problems that a person may experience in their sexual life. In the context of oncology, sexual dysfunction can occur as a result of both physical and psychological effects.

Physical effects of cancer and its treatment can contribute to sexual dysfunction. For example, certain cancer treatments such as surgery, radiation therapy, and chemotherapy may lead to changes in hormone levels, physical discomfort, or damage to sexual organs. These physical changes can result in pain during intercourse, loss of libido, difficulty achieving or maintaining an erection (erectile dysfunction), or difficulty reaching orgasm.

Psychological effects can also play a significant role in sexual dysfunction among oncology patients. A cancer diagnosis can cause anxiety, depression, body image issues, and stress, which can negatively impact sexual desire and function. Fear of recurrence, relationship changes, and concerns about fertility or sexual attractiveness can further contribute to sexual problems.

It is important for oncology **nurse**s to address sexual dysfunction in their patients because it can have a profound impact on their overall quality of life. Open communication and education about sexual health are crucial. **Nurse**s should create a safe and non-judgmental environment where patients feel comfortable discussing their concerns and seeking help.

Treatment options for sexual dysfunction may vary depending on the underlying cause. For example, if the dysfunction is primarily due to physical factors, medical interventions such as hormone replacement therapy or medications for erectile dysfunction may be considered. Non-pharmacological interventions, such as pelvic floor exercises, lubricants, or sex therapy, can also be beneficial.

Psychological support and counseling are essential components of managing sexual dysfunction caused by psychological factors. Oncology **nurse**s can provide emotional support, refer patients to psychologists or counselors who specialize in sexual health, and help patients explore strategies to improve body image and reduce anxiety or depression.

6.9.3 Intimacy

Intimacy is a crucial aspect of sexuality that plays a significant role in the psychosocial dimensions of care for Oncology **Nurse**s. It encompasses various components, including emotional, physical, and sexual connections between individuals. As an Oncology **Nurse**, understanding and addressing issues related to intimacy can greatly impact the overall well-being of patients.

Emotional intimacy involves establishing a deep connection and trust with the patient. It is vital for Oncology **Nurse**s to create a safe and supportive environment where patients feel comfortable expressing their emotions and fears. Engaging in active listening, empathy, and providing emotional support can foster a sense of intimacy and build a strong therapeutic relationship.

Physical intimacy refers to non-sexual touch that can be comforting, such as holding a patient's hand or providing a gentle massage. These gestures can promote a sense of closeness and provide comfort during difficult times. Oncology **Nurse**s should be mindful of patients' comfort levels and cultural differences when engaging in physical intimacy.

Sexual intimacy is often impacted by cancer and its treatments. Cancer and its treatments can lead to physical changes that affect one's sexual health and function. As an Oncology **Nurse**, it is important to address these concerns sensitively and provide information about possible solutions, such as medication or therapy. **Nurses** can collaborate with other healthcare **professionals**, such as psychologists or sexual health specialists, to ensure patients receive comprehensive care.

Communication is key in addressing intimacy-related concerns. Oncology **Nurse**s should encourage open dialogue with patients, allowing them to express their questions, concerns, or fears regarding intimacy. By providing accurate and appropriate information, **nurses** can help patients navigate through the challenges they may face and offer guidance to maintain intimacy during treatment and recovery.

Couples counseling can be beneficial for patients and their partners, as cancer can impact both individuals and their relationship. It offers a supportive space to address intimacy-related concerns, relationship challenges, and explore methods to enhance intimacy. Providing resources or referrals to couples counseling services can be beneficial for patients and their partners.

6.9.4   Considerations for sexual and gender minorities

Considerations for sexual and gender minorities are crucial in providing comprehensive and inclusive care for oncology patients. These individuals may face unique psychosocial challenges related to their sexual orientation or gender identity, which can significantly impact their quality of life and healthcare experiences.

One of the key considerations for oncology **nurse**s is to create a safe and nonjudgmental environment that respects diversity and promotes inclusivity. This involves being sensitive to the personal preferences, pronouns, and identities of sexual and gender minorities. It is important for **nurse**s to use appropriate language and terminology when communicating with these individuals, ensuring that their experiences and identities are validate

Addressing the specific healthcare needs of sexual and gender minorities is another important consideration. These individuals may have higher rates of certain cancers, such as breast, cervical, and anal cancer, due to unique risk factors or barriers to screening and prevention services. Oncology **nurse**s should be knowledgeable about these disparities and provide tailored education and support regarding cancer prevention, screening, and treatment options.

In addition, sexual and gender minorities may face additional psychosocial challenges related to their cancer diagnosis. They may experience discrimination, stigma, and social isolation, which can lead to heightened anxiety, depression, and distress. Oncology **nurse**s should be proactive in identifying and addressing these psychosocial concerns, providing appropriate emotional support and referral to mental health services when necessary.

Cultural competence is another crucial consideration when caring for sexual and gender minorities. **Nurse**s should strive to understand the specific cultural contexts and needs of these individuals, as they may come from different racial or ethnic backgrounds or have intersecting identities. This includes recognizing the impact of cultural and religious beliefs on their healthcare decision-making and incorporating culturally sensitive practices into their care.

Finally, oncology **nurse**s should be aware of the unique legal and policy considerations that may affect sexual and gender minorities. This includes understanding the rights and protections afforded to these individuals, such as anti-discrimination laws and access to gender-affirming healthcare. **Nurse**s should advocate for equitable and accessible healthcare services for sexual and gender minorities, including appropriate insurance coverage and inclusive healthcare policies.

OCN Practice Questions [SET 1]

Question 1: Scenario: Michael, a 70-year-old male with prostate cancer, presents with lower abdominal pain, bloating, and difficulty passing urine. On examination, there is suprapubic tenderness and a palpable bladder. What is the likely complication?
A) Bowel obstruction
B) Urinary retention
C) Gastric ulcer
D) Appendicitis

Question 2: Mr. Johnson, a 65-year-old patient with advanced cancer, is experiencing severe breakthrough pain despite being on around-the-clock opioid therapy. Which pharmacologic intervention would be most appropriate for managing his breakthrough pain?
A) Adding a short-acting opioid analgesic
B) Increasing the dose of the long-acting opioid
C) Administering a nonsteroidal anti-inflammatory drug (NSAID)
D) Initiating a tricyclic antidepressant

Question 3: Mr. Brown, a 50-year-old patient, has a family history of colorectal cancer. Which preventive health practice should the nurse recommend for Mr. Brown?
A) Annual prostate exam
B) Low-dose aspirin regimen
C) Colonoscopy every 5 years
D) Lung cancer screening

Question 4: Scenario: Emily, a 45-year-old female with cervical cancer, develops abdominal distension, nausea, and vomiting. On examination, there is a palpable mass in the lower abdomen. What is the most likely cause of her symptoms?
A) Urinary incontinence
B) Bowel obstruction
C) Peptic ulcer disease
D) Pelvic inflammatory disease

Question 5: Which immune-related adverse event is associated with inflammation of the lungs and can present with symptoms like cough, shortness of breath, and chest pain in patients on immunotherapy?
A) Nephritis
B) Pneumonitis
C) Thyroiditis
D) Arthritis

Question 6: Mr. Lee, a 60-year-old male with a history of prostate cancer, presents with abdominal discomfort. Imaging reveals metastasis to the bones. Which site is a common location for prostate cancer metastasis?
A) Brain
B) Bones
C) Liver
D) Colon

Question 7: Mr. Patel, a 60-year-old patient with terminal lung cancer, is experiencing anticipatory grief as he prepares for the end-of-life stage. Which nursing intervention would be most beneficial in supporting Mr. Patel through his anticipatory grief?
A) Avoiding discussions about death and dying
B) Providing opportunities for Mr. Patel to reminisce about his life
C) Discouraging Mr. Patel from expressing his emotions
D) Minimizing the impact of his impending loss

Question 8: Which healthcare professional is typically responsible for coordinating follow-up care for oncology patients?
A) Oncology nurse
B) Radiology technician
C) Physical therapist
D) Nutritionist

Question 9: Scenario: Mark, a 55-year-old patient with lung cancer, is considering palliative care options. How can the Oncology Certified Nurse facilitate effective communication with Mark and his family during this decision-making process?
A) Avoiding discussions about end-of-life care
B) Including only medical jargon in conversations
C) Encouraging shared decision-making and addressing concerns
D) Providing limited information to avoid overwhelming the family

Question 10: Which of the following is a primary function of the immune system in cancer patients?
A) Promoting tumor growth
B) Suppressing immune response
C) Recognizing and destroying cancer cells
D) Enhancing cancer cell proliferation

Question 11: What distinguishes late symptoms from acute and chronic symptoms in oncology patients?
A) Resolves spontaneously
B) Occurs during active treatment
C) Develops months to years after treatment
D) Requires immediate intervention

Question 12: Sarah, a 30-year-old leukemia patient, is experiencing distress due to her treatment regimen. How can the nurse help Sarah regain a sense of personal control?
A) Dictating her daily schedule
B) Allowing her to participate in treatment decisions
C) Withholding information about her condition
D) Excluding her from discussions about her care

Question 13: Scenario: Mark, a 55-year-old cancer patient, is struggling with anger and frustration following a recent treatment setback. Which coping strategy should the nurse recommend to help Mark manage his emotions effectively?
A) Expressing emotions through journaling
B) Suppressing emotions
C) Engaging in risky behaviors
D) Blaming others for the setback

Question 14: What is the primary mechanism of action of biotherapy in cancer treatment?
A) Inhibiting cell division
B) Enhancing the immune response
C) Blocking blood vessel formation
D) Inducing DNA damage

Question 15: Which medication is commonly used for prophylaxis against tumor lysis syndrome in high-risk patients?
A) Allopurinol
B) Spironolactone
C) Metoprolol
D) Ondansetron

Question 16: How can oncology nurses promote spiritual well-being in patients experiencing distress?
A) Disregarding patients' spiritual beliefs to focus on medical care
B) Encouraging patients to suppress their emotions to stay strong
C) Facilitating access to spiritual support services and resources
D) Minimizing the importance of addressing spiritual concerns

Question 17: Which of the following is a recommended approach to promoting healthy survivorship outcomes in cancer patients?
A) Isolating oneself from social support
B) Ignoring any physical symptoms

C) Engaging in regular physical activity
D) Avoiding follow-up appointments

Question 18: Mr. Patel, a 70-year-old patient with metastatic lung cancer, is experiencing dyspnea at rest. Which of the following interventions is most appropriate for managing his symptom in palliative care?
A) Initiate supplemental oxygen therapy
B) Administer a diuretic
C) Start high-dose chemotherapy
D) Increase the dose of opioid analgesics

Question 19: Scenario: Sarah, a 55-year-old caregiver, is taking care of her husband who is in the advanced stages of cancer. She is feeling overwhelmed and exhausted. Which of the following interventions would be most appropriate to support Sarah in this situation?
A) Encouraging Sarah to solely focus on her husband's needs
B) Providing Sarah with information on local caregiver support groups
C) Advising Sarah to avoid seeking help and manage everything on her own
D) Suggesting Sarah to prioritize her husband's medical needs over her own well-being

Question 20: Mr. Lee, a 70-year-old male with lung cancer, develops sudden onset paralysis of both legs and loss of bowel and bladder control. What is the priority nursing action in this situation?
A) Initiating range of motion exercises
B) Applying heat packs to the legs
C) Elevating the legs
D) Ensuring airway patency and calling for immediate medical assistance

Question 21: Scenario: Michael, a 60-year-old patient undergoing chemotherapy, is experiencing chemotherapy-induced peripheral neuropathy. Which non-pharmacologic comfort measure would be most appropriate for Michael?
A) Topical capsaicin cream
B) Administering pain medication
C) Acupuncture therapy
D) Hot and cold therapy

Question 22: Ms. Johnson, a 50-year-old female with breast cancer, is found to have hypercalcemia with a calcium level of 13.2 mg/dL. Which of the following medications should be avoided in the management of her hypercalcemia?
A) Prednisone
B) Thiazide diuretics
C) Lithium
D) Vitamin D supplements

Question 23: A patient with melanoma is being treated with a checkpoint inhibitor. Which of the following is a common side effect associated with checkpoint inhibitors?
A) Hypertension
B) Hypothyroidism
C) Osteoporosis
D) Anemia

Question 24: Scenario: John, a 55-year-old prostate cancer patient, is experiencing anxiety and depression due to his diagnosis. Which resource can provide support for John's psychosocial needs?
A) Oncology nurse
B) Palliative care team
C) Oncology pharmacist
D) Psychologist

Question 25: In the context of end-of-life care within the oncology setting, which member of the interdisciplinary team plays a crucial role in providing spiritual support to patients and their families?
A) Social Worker
B) Physical Therapist
C) Dietitian
D) Chaplain

Question 26: What is a significant treatment-related consideration for oncology patients receiving radiation therapy?
A) Skin care
B) Dental hygiene
C) Hearing tests
D) Eye examinations

Question 27: Ms. Johnson, a 58-year-old patient with advanced breast cancer, presents with a painful, open wound on her chest due to tumor infiltration. Which intervention is most appropriate for managing this wound?
A) Applying a hydrocolloid dressing
B) Using a transparent film dressing
C) Packing the wound with alginate dressing
D) Administering topical antibiotics

Question 28: Scenario: John, a 60-year-old male, is undergoing treatment for lung cancer. The nurse explains to him the role of carcinogens in the development of cancer. Which of the following is a known carcinogen associated with lung cancer?
A) Asbestos
B) Vitamin C
C) Calcium
D) Iron

Question 29: How can cancer survivors improve intimacy post-treatment?
A) Avoiding open communication
B) Ignoring emotional needs
C) Seeking counseling or therapy
D) Isolating themselves from loved ones

Question 30: Which psychological aspect is commonly associated with intimacy challenges in cancer patients?
A) Increased self-esteem
B) Fear of rejection
C) Enhanced body image
D) Strong social support

Question 31: Mr. Garcia, a 55-year-old patient with Hodgkin lymphoma, is undergoing chemotherapy. He develops febrile neutropenia. Which of the following interventions is essential in the management of febrile neutropenia?
A) Initiating prophylactic antibiotics
B) Administering erythropoietin
C) Encouraging raw food consumption
D) Avoiding hand hygiene

Question 32: Which of the following is a non-modifiable risk factor for cancer?
A) Smoking
B) Obesity
C) Age
D) Physical inactivity

Question 33: Which of the following is a common site for venous thromboembolism (VTE) in cancer patients?
A) Femoral artery
B) Radial vein
C) Popliteal vein
D) Brachial artery

Question 34: What is an essential component of survivorship care plans in oncology follow-up care?
A) Psychological support resources

B) Performing surgical procedures
C) Administering radiation therapy
D) Conducting laboratory tests

Question 35: Mr. Johnson, a 65-year-old patient with acute myeloid leukemia (AML), presents with severe anemia. Which of the following symptoms is most commonly associated with anemia in patients with AML?
A) Easy bruising and bleeding
B) Fatigue and weakness
C) Bone pain
D) Headaches and dizziness

Question 36: Which of the following is a common side effect of radiation therapy in cancer patients undergoing treatment?
A) Hypertension
B) Hair loss
C) Weight gain
D) Anemia

Question 37: Which modifiable risk factor is linked to a higher risk of cancer recurrence and poorer treatment outcomes in cancer patients?
A) Exercise
B) Occupation
C) Smoking
D) Diet

Question 38: Mr. Smith, a 58-year-old patient with lung cancer, develops a severe rash, itching, and shortness of breath shortly after receiving his first dose of chemotherapy. Which type of hypersensitivity reaction is he most likely experiencing?
A) Type I
B) Type II
C) Type III
D) Type IV

Question 39: Which genitourinary alteration is a side effect of cisplatin chemotherapy?
A) Urinary retention
B) Polyuria
C) Hematuria
D) Renal failure

Question 40: Scenario: Emily, an Oncology Nurse, works at a hospital aiming to achieve Magnet Recognition for nursing excellence. What is a significant characteristic of Magnet Recognition in oncology nursing practice?
A) High Patient Mortality Rates
B) Empirical Nursing Practice
C) Interdisciplinary Collaboration
D) Limited Staff Training

Question 41: Which hematologic disorder is characterized by the overproduction of abnormal white blood cells in the bone marrow?
A) Thrombocytopenia
B) Leukemia
C) Anemia
D) Lymphoma

Question 42: Mrs. Lee, a 70-year-old patient with colorectal cancer, is undergoing surgery. Which of the following preoperative considerations should the nurse prioritize to ensure safe perioperative care?
A) Administering high-dose vitamin supplements
B) Ensuring the patient is well-hydrated
C) Allowing the patient to eat a heavy meal before surgery
D) Encouraging smoking before surgery

Question 43: Which of the following is a potential challenge faced by cancer survivors in terms of family and social support concerns?
A) Increased emotional support from family
B) Financial burden due to treatment costs
C) Enhanced communication within the family
D) Strong social network post-treatment

Question 44: Which molecular test is used to identify HER2-positive breast cancer patients who may benefit from targeted therapy?
A) FISH
B) PCR
C) ELISA
D) Western blot

Question 45: When should advance care planning discussions take place?
A) Only when an individual is diagnosed with a terminal illness
B) Only when an individual is admitted to the hospital
C) At any stage of life, especially during significant life events or changes in health status
D) Only when an individual is over the age of 80

Question 46: Mr. Johnson, a 58-year-old patient with advanced colorectal cancer, is experiencing severe diarrhea as a side effect of chemotherapy. Which of the following interventions is most appropriate for managing his symptoms?
A) Administering loperamide for symptomatic relief
B) Increasing the dose of chemotherapy to combat the cancer
C) Encouraging the patient to consume high-fiber foods
D) Withholding fluids to reduce the frequency of bowel movements

Question 47: Which symptom is commonly associated with gastrointestinal alterations in cancer patients?
A) Constipation
B) Hypertension
C) Insomnia
D) Allergic reaction

Question 48: Which of the following is a common type of biotherapy used in cancer treatment?
A) Chemotherapy
B) Radiation therapy
C) Immunotherapy
D) Surgery

Question 49: What is a characteristic of complicated grief?
A) Resuming daily activities promptly
B) Intense feelings of sadness gradually subsiding
C) Prolonged and persistent yearning for the deceased
D) Seeking social support and expressing emotions openly

Question 50: Scenario: David, a 60-year-old Caucasian patient, is diagnosed with lung cancer and expresses interest in exploring alternative healing practices such as acupuncture. How should the oncology nurse best respond to David's interest in alternative healing?
A) Discourage David from exploring alternative healing practices.
B) Support David's interest in alternative healing and provide information on reputable practitioners.
C) Ignore David's interest in alternative healing as it is not evidence-based.
D) Inform David that alternative healing practices have no benefit in cancer treatment.

Question 51: Scenario: John, a 50-year-old male patient undergoing cancer treatment, expresses thoughts of hopelessness and mentions feeling like a burden to his family. What is the most appropriate response by the nurse?
A) Dismiss John's feelings as common during cancer treatment.
B) Refer John to a mental health professional for evaluation.

C) Tell John to focus on his treatment and not dwell on negative thoughts.
D) Advise John to keep his feelings to himself to avoid worrying his family.

Question 52: How can caregivers alleviate caregiver fatigue?
A) Avoid seeking help from others
B) Neglect self-care practices
C) Engage in regular physical activity
D) Isolate themselves from social support

Question 53: Scenario: John, a 60-year-old patient undergoing chemotherapy, is experiencing severe side effects and is hesitant to continue treatment. What communication approach should the Oncology Certified Nurse adopt to address John's concerns effectively?
A) Dismissing John's fears
B) Providing factual information only
C) Encouraging open dialogue
D) Rushing through the conversation

Question 54: Mr. Patel, a lymphoma survivor, reports feeling discriminated against by his healthcare provider due to his cultural background. What should the Oncology Certified Nurse prioritize in this situation?
A) Acknowledge Mr. Patel's feelings and concerns
B) Dismiss Mr. Patel's claims as misunderstandings
C) Avoid discussing cultural issues with Mr. Patel
D) Refer Mr. Patel to a different healthcare provider

Question 55: Which dietary recommendation is appropriate for a patient experiencing taste changes due to chemotherapy?
A) Increase intake of spicy foods
B) Avoid using plastic utensils
C) Consume foods at extreme temperatures
D) Opt for citrus fruits and marinades

Question 56: Which of the following is a common financial concern for cancer patients undergoing treatment?
A) Transportation costs to and from medical appointments
B) Free access to all medications
C) No impact on employment status
D) No need for additional support services

Question 57: Scenario: Emily, a cancer survivor, is struggling with survivorship issues and seeks guidance on lifestyle modifications and follow-up care. Which team member is most qualified to assist Emily in navigating survivorship challenges?
A) Radiology Technologist
B) Genetic Counselor
C) Survivorship Nurse
D) Occupational Therapist

Question 58: Ms. Johnson, a 32-year-old female with breast cancer, is concerned about her fertility preservation options before starting chemotherapy. Which of the following methods is NOT recommended for fertility preservation in female cancer patients?
A) Ovarian transposition
B) Oocyte cryopreservation
C) In vitro fertilization (IVF) with embryo cryopreservation
D) Hormonal contraception

Question 59: Which of the following is a preventive health practice to reduce the risk of cervical cancer?
A) Getting regular Pap smears
B) Avoiding HPV vaccination
C) Engaging in unprotected sexual activity
D) Smoking cigarettes

Question 60: Mr. Brown, a 55-year-old male, has a family history of skin cancer. Which screening method is recommended for Mr. Brown to detect early signs of skin cancer?
A) Colonoscopy
B) Skin self-examination
C) Mammography
D) Prostate-specific antigen (PSA) test

Question 61: Which of the following is a common symptom of anxiety in oncology patients?
A) Increased appetite
B) Decreased heart rate
C) Difficulty concentrating
D) Excessive sleepiness

Question 62: Which of the following factors can contribute to fatigue in cancer patients?
A) Increased physical activity
B) Adequate rest and sleep
C) Emotional distress
D) Balanced diet

Question 63: Mr. Patel, a 60-year-old prostate cancer survivor, is due for his follow-up appointment. Which of the following tests is most appropriate for monitoring his prostate cancer recurrence?
A) CA-125 blood test
B) PSA blood test
C) Thyroglobulin blood test
D) CEA blood test

Question 64: Scenario: David, a 50-year-old colorectal cancer patient, is struggling to afford his medications post-surgery. Which resource can help David explore financial assistance programs for his medications?
A) Oncology social worker
B) Oncology dietician
C) Oncology navigator
D) Oncology genetic counselor

Question 65: Scenario: Mr. Brown, a patient with prostate cancer, is discussing with his oncology nurse about the role of radiation therapy in his treatment plan. The nurse explains that the goal of radiation therapy is to:
A) Remove the tumor completely
B) Prevent cancer spread to other organs
C) Relieve pain and discomfort
D) Destroy cancer cells while minimizing damage to healthy tissue

Question 66: Scenario: John, a 60-year-old prostate cancer patient, requires regular blood tests to monitor his treatment response. The nurse observes that multiple blood samples are being collected unnecessarily, leading to increased resource utilization. What should the nurse do to address this issue?
A) Continue with the current blood collection protocol
B) Educate the healthcare team on appropriate blood test frequency
C) Disregard the excess blood samples as part of standard practice
D) Implement a new blood collection procedure

Question 67: Mr. Garcia, a 60-year-old patient with metastatic breast cancer, has been receiving hospice care for palliative symptom management. He has expressed a desire to spend his remaining days at home surrounded by his family. As the hospice nurse, what is a key aspect to consider when supporting Mr. Garcia's wish for home-based care?
A) Arrange for frequent hospital visits to monitor his condition
B) Ensure access to 24/7 hospice support and guidance

C) Encourage him to consider transferring to an inpatient hospice facility
D) Limit family involvement to prevent caregiver burnout

Question 68: What is an effective strategy for healthcare professionals to help individuals cope with bereavement in the care continuum?
A) Rushing the grieving process
B) Encouraging avoidance of emotions
C) Providing grief counseling and support groups
D) Minimizing acknowledgment of the loss

Question 69: Scenario: John, an Oncology Nurse, is preparing to administer a new chemotherapy drug to a patient. The drug requires a specific certification for administration. What should John do?
A) Proceed with the administration based on his experience.
B) Ask a colleague to administer the drug instead.
C) Obtain the necessary certification before administering the drug.
D) Document the administration without mentioning the certification.

Question 70: When collaborating with the interdisciplinary team in oncology care, the oncology nurse serves as the:
A) Sole decision-maker
B) Information gatekeeper
C) Treatment prescriber
D) Team coordinator

Question 71: Scenario: David, a 50-year-old male with advanced melanoma, is exploring targeted therapy options with his healthcare team. Which of the following is a challenge associated with targeted therapies in cancer treatment?
A) Resistance development by cancer cells
B) Broad effectiveness across different cancer types
C) Minimal impact on tumor growth
D) Limited specificity for cancer cells

Question 72: Which neurological symptom is commonly associated with brain metastases in cancer patients?
A) Muscle weakness
B) Visual disturbances
C) Hearing loss
D) Skin rash

Question 73: How can healthcare providers assess the severity of fatigue in cancer patients?
A) Blood pressure measurement
B) Physical fitness test
C) Fatigue severity scale
D) X-ray imaging

Question 74: Ms. Johnson, a 60-year-old patient with leukemia, is scheduled for a bone marrow transplant. Which type of immunity will be primarily restored through this procedure?
A) Innate immunity
B) Passive immunity
C) Acquired immunity
D) Humoral immunity

Question 75: Scenario: Sarah, a 55-year-old female patient with metastatic lung cancer, is scheduled to start immunotherapy. Which of the following mechanisms is the primary mode of action of immunotherapy in cancer treatment?
A) Activation of the immune system to target cancer cells
B) Inhibition of cancer cell division
C) Promotion of angiogenesis
D) Induction of cancer cell apoptosis

Question 76: Scenario: John, a 60-year-old male patient with melanoma, is receiving checkpoint inhibitor immunotherapy. Which of the following is a common side effect associated with checkpoint inhibitors?
A) Fatigue
B) Hair loss
C) Nausea
D) Muscle pain

Question 77: Scenario: Sarah, an oncology nurse, is preparing to administer chemotherapy to a patient. She notices that the medication dosage seems higher than the prescribed amount. What should Sarah do first?
A) Administer the medication as prescribed
B) Double-check the medication order with another nurse
C) Consult the physician for clarification
D) Inform the patient about the potential error

Question 78: Ms. Garcia, a 60-year-old patient with pancreatic cancer, is experiencing difficulty with decision-making and problem-solving. Which nursing intervention can support her cognitive function?
A) Providing excessive choices
B) Encouraging independence in decision-making
C) Limiting social interactions
D) Minimizing cognitive stimulation

Question 79: Which insurance plan requires patients to choose a primary care physician and obtain referrals to see specialists?
A) Health Maintenance Organization (HMO)
B) Preferred Provider Organization (PPO)
C) Exclusive Provider Organization (EPO)
D) High Deductible Health Plan (HDHP)

Question 80: James, a 55-year-old prostate cancer survivor, struggles with intimacy issues with his partner following treatment. How can the nurse best address James' concerns regarding his altered body image?
A) Advise James to avoid discussing intimacy concerns with his partner
B) Encourage open communication and exploration of alternative forms of intimacy
C) Suggest that James should prioritize physical recovery over emotional concerns
D) Discourage James from seeking professional support for intimacy issues

Question 81: What psychological effect is commonly associated with sexual dysfunction in cancer survivors?
A) Decreased anxiety
B) Enhanced self-esteem
C) Depression
D) Improved body image

Question 82: How can the psychosocial dimensions of care impact an oncology patient's ability to work?
A) Providing emotional support can improve work performance
B) Social isolation has no effect on work productivity
C) Lack of communication skills is beneficial in the workplace
D) Avoiding stress has no impact on work-life balance

Question 83: Which electrolyte imbalance is typically seen in patients with Syndrome of Inappropriate Antidiuretic Hormone Secretion (SIADH)?
A) Hypernatremia
B) Hypokalemia
C) Hyperkalemia
D) Hyponatremia

Question 84: Which non-pharmacologic comfort measure focuses on creating a soothing environment through the use of soft music, dim lighting, and aromatherapy?

A) Acupuncture
B) Massage Therapy
C) Environmental Manipulation
D) Radiation Therapy

Question 85: Mr. Patel, a 72-year-old patient with end-stage lung cancer, has been receiving hospice care for the past three months. His family expresses concerns about his increasing restlessness and agitation, especially during the evenings. As the hospice nurse, what is the most appropriate action to address this issue?
A) Administer a higher dose of the current sedative medication
B) Implement music therapy during the evening hours
C) Evaluate for any underlying causes of restlessness
D) Recommend a change in the patient's diet

Question 86: Scenario: John, a 60-year-old prostate cancer survivor, is experiencing anxiety related to the fear of cancer recurrence. He expresses concerns about his future health and well-being. Which approach would be most beneficial for the nurse to use when addressing John's anxiety?
A) Dismissing John's fears as irrational and unfounded
B) Providing education about the statistics of cancer recurrence to alleviate his anxiety
C) Offering empathetic listening and emotional support to validate John's feelings
D) Ignoring John's anxiety and focusing solely on his physical health status

Question 87: Ms. Johnson, a 55-year-old female, was recently diagnosed with breast cancer. Which of the following factors is considered a primary prevention strategy in reducing the incidence of breast cancer?
A) Mammography screening every 2 years for women aged 50-74
B) Genetic testing for BRCA1 and BRCA2 mutations in high-risk individuals
C) Smoking cessation programs for women with breast cancer
D) Regular physical activity and maintaining a healthy weight

Question 88: Ms. Smith, a 45-year-old patient with lung cancer, develops hypothyroidism following treatment with immune checkpoint inhibitors. Which immune-related adverse event is she experiencing?
A) Hypophysitis
B) Thyroiditis
C) Adrenal insufficiency
D) Nephritis

Question 89: Ms. Johnson, a 55-year-old breast cancer survivor, completed her adjuvant chemotherapy six months ago. She is scheduled for her first follow-up visit. Which of the following is an essential component of her follow-up care?
A) Mammogram every 5 years
B) Bone density scan every 2 years
C) Routine blood tests every month
D) Clinical breast exam every 6-12 months

Question 90: James, a 55-year-old patient, is experiencing disenfranchised grief due to societal stigma surrounding his cancer diagnosis. How can the nurse best address James' disenfranchised grief?
A) Ignoring James' feelings to prevent further distress
B) Validating James' emotions and acknowledging his unique experience
C) Encouraging James to conform to societal expectations
D) Minimizing the impact of societal stigma on James' grief

Question 91: Scenario: Sarah, a 55-year-old patient with advanced cancer, is experiencing severe breakthrough pain despite being on around-the-clock opioid therapy. She reports the pain as sharp and stabbing, localized in her lower back, with a pain score of 8/10. Which intervention would be most appropriate for managing Sarah's breakthrough pain?
A) Increasing the dose of her current around-the-clock opioid medication
B) Adding a short-acting opioid for breakthrough pain
C) Switching to a different class of analgesic medication
D) Implementing non-pharmacological pain management techniques

Question 92: Ms. Brown, a 55-year-old patient with bladder cancer, develops shortness of breath, cough, and fever after receiving immune checkpoint inhibitors. Which immune-related adverse event is she experiencing?
A) Pneumonitis
B) Myocarditis
C) Arthritis
D) Encephalitis

Question 93: Which of the following is a potential complication of a blood and marrow transplant?
A) Increased appetite
B) Hair growth
C) Graft-versus-host disease
D) Improved energy levels

Question 94: Which of the following is NOT a common symptom of pneumonitis in oncology patients?
A) Cough
B) Shortness of breath
C) Chest pain
D) Hematuria

Question 95: Mr. Patel, a 65-year-old patient with prostate cancer, underwent radiation therapy two years ago. He now complains of persistent diarrhea and abdominal cramping. Which chronic side effect is most likely responsible for his symptoms?
A) Fatigue
B) Nausea
C) Diarrhea
D) Anemia

Question 96: Scenario: Lisa, a 45-year-old female with metastatic colorectal cancer, is considering targeted therapy as part of her treatment plan. Which of the following is a potential mechanism of action for targeted therapies in cancer treatment?
A) Inhibiting angiogenesis
B) Stimulating cell division
C) Promoting DNA repair
D) Enhancing inflammation

Question 97: Which of the following is a recommended approach to addressing the unique challenges faced by sexual and gender minorities in cancer care?
A) Providing standardized care without customization
B) Offering support groups exclusively for heterosexual patients
C) Acknowledging and validating diverse identities and experiences
D) Avoiding discussions about sexual health

Question 98: Which action demonstrates effective resource utilization by an OCN in oncology nursing practice?
A) Ignoring patient preferences in treatment decisions
B) Engaging in continuous education to stay updated on best practices
C) Stockpiling supplies for personal use
D) Disregarding institutional policies on resource allocation

Question 99: Mrs. Lee, an 80-year-old patient with metastatic cancer, is nearing the end of life and is experiencing

dyspnea. Which nursing intervention is appropriate to help Mrs. Lee breathe more comfortably?
A) Elevating the head of the bed
B) Limiting fluid intake
C) Administering oxygen at a high flow rate
D) Encouraging deep breathing exercises

Question 100: Mrs. Thompson, a 70-year-old patient with lung cancer, completed her immunotherapy treatment a year ago. She now presents with shortness of breath and a persistent cough. Which chronic side effect is she likely experiencing?
A) Fatigue
B) Pneumonitis
C) Mucositis
D) Cardiomyopathy

Question 101: Which of the following is a key factor contributing to the development of site-specific cancers?
A) Genetic predisposition
B) Regular physical exercise
C) High intake of antioxidants
D) Low exposure to environmental toxins

Question 102: James, a 55-year-old lung cancer patient, is facing resistance from his family in accepting his treatment decisions. How can the oncology nurse best assist James in navigating this situation?
A) Advise James to prioritize his family's wishes over his own treatment preferences.
B) Encourage James to ignore his family's concerns and proceed with his treatment plan.
C) Facilitate a family meeting to address concerns and promote understanding of James' treatment choices.
D) Suggest that James cut off communication with his family to avoid conflict.

Question 103: Which of the following is an example of a targeted therapy used in oncology?
A) Methotrexate
B) Trastuzumab
C) Vincristine
D) Doxorubicin

Question 104: Scenario: John, a 70-year-old colon cancer patient, is curious about the role of precision medicine in oncology. The nurse explains the concept of personalized treatment based on genetic factors. Which statement best describes the application of evidence-based practice in precision medicine?
A) "Precision medicine does not consider individual genetic variations in treatment decisions."
B) "Evidence-based practice in precision medicine relies solely on trial and error."
C) "Personalized treatment in precision medicine is guided by genetic testing and research evidence."
D) "There is no need for research evidence in implementing precision medicine approaches."

Question 105: Scenario: Sarah, an Oncology Certified Nurse, is conducting a professional practice evaluation. Which of the following best describes the purpose of professional practice evaluation in oncology nursing?
A) To increase workload for nurses
B) To identify areas for improvement in patient care
C) To discourage professional growth
D) To limit scope of practice

Question 106: Scenario: Mark, an OCN, is mentoring a new oncology nurse on the Standards of Practice for Oncology Nursing. Which of the following best exemplifies a Standard of Practice for an OCN?
A) Providing legal representation for oncology patients
B) Ensuring patient confidentiality in oncology care
C) Managing hospital finances for oncology services
D) Conducting psychological evaluations for oncology patients

Question 107: Scenario: During a professional practice evaluation, the oncology nurse notices a deviation from the established standards of care. What should be the nurse's immediate action?
A) Ignore the deviation
B) Document the deviation and report it to the appropriate personnel
C) Confront the colleague responsible for the deviation
D) Cover up the deviation

Question 108: Which of the following is a key goal of rehabilitation in cancer survivorship?
A) Promoting physical activity and exercise
B) Encouraging smoking cessation
C) Limiting access to support groups
D) Discouraging emotional expression

Question 109: Mr. Patel, a 60-year-old prostate cancer patient, is experiencing distress due to his recent diagnosis. Which nursing action would be most effective in supporting Mr. Patel's psychosocial well-being?
A) Scheduling additional medical tests to confirm the diagnosis.
B) Encouraging him to engage in physical activities to distract his mind.
C) Providing him with a quiet environment to process his emotions.
D) Ignoring his emotional cues to avoid making him uncomfortable.

Question 110: Which dietary instruction is suitable for a patient experiencing diarrhea as a side effect of cancer treatment?
A) Limit fluid intake
B) Increase fiber consumption
C) Avoid dairy products
D) Consume high-fat foods

Question 111: Which of the following is a common side effect of radiation therapy?
A) Fatigue
B) Hair growth stimulation
C) Weight gain
D) Increased appetite

Question 112: Which intervention is most appropriate when managing a patient experiencing suicidal ideation?
A) Providing a safe environment
B) Ignoring the patient's statements
C) Leaving the patient alone
D) Encouraging the patient to isolate

Question 113: Scenario: Emily, a 45-year-old lung cancer patient, is experiencing challenges in accessing supportive care services due to transportation issues. As an Oncology Certified Nurse, what is the most appropriate intervention to enhance navigation and coordination of care for Emily?
A) Provide Emily with a list of local supportive care services.
B) Arrange for telehealth consultations for Emily with supportive care providers.
C) Collaborate with community resources to arrange transportation assistance for Emily.
D) Advise Emily to rely on family members for transportation to appointments.

Question 114: How does immunotherapy differ from traditional cancer treatments?
A) Immunotherapy only targets cancer cells
B) Immunotherapy does not involve the use of drugs
C) Immunotherapy boosts the body's immune system to fight

cancer
D) Immunotherapy is not effective in treating advanced cancers

Question 115: Scenario: Mark, a 55-year-old male, is diagnosed with colorectal cancer. His oncologist recommends testing for microsatellite instability (MSI) to determine his response to immunotherapy. What is the significance of MSI testing in colorectal cancer?
A) MSI-high tumors are associated with a better response to immunotherapy.
B) MSI testing is primarily used to detect hormone receptor status.
C) MSI status does not impact treatment decisions in colorectal cancer.
D) MSI-low tumors have a higher mutation burden.

Question 116: Mr. Smith, a 60-year-old male, has been diagnosed with lung cancer. Which of the following statements best describes the concept of incidence rate in epidemiology?
A) The proportion of individuals with lung cancer who die within a year of diagnosis
B) The number of new cases of lung cancer diagnosed in a specific population over a defined period
C) The percentage of individuals with lung cancer who have a family history of the disease
D) The average age at which individuals are diagnosed with lung cancer

Question 117: Which of the following is a crucial aspect of providing caregiver support in end-of-life care?
A) Encouraging caregivers to prioritize their own needs
B) Discouraging open communication between caregivers and healthcare team
C) Minimizing respite care opportunities for caregivers
D) Providing limited information about the patient's condition to caregivers

Question 118: Mr. Lee, a 60-year-old male with advanced pancreatic cancer, develops hypotension, jugular venous distention, and pulsus paradoxus. He reports recent chemotherapy. What is the most likely cause of his hemodynamic instability?
A) Sepsis
B) Cardiac tamponade
C) Anaphylaxis
D) Hypovolemic shock

Question 119: Ms. Johnson, a 45-year-old breast cancer patient, expresses concerns about the impact of her diagnosis on her family relationships. Which intervention by the oncology nurse would be most appropriate to address Ms. Johnson's needs?
A) Encourage Ms. Johnson to avoid discussing her diagnosis with her family to protect them from worry.
B) Provide resources for family counseling to facilitate open communication and support.
C) Advise Ms. Johnson to isolate herself from her family to prevent emotional distress.
D) Suggest that Ms. Johnson ignore her family's concerns and focus solely on her treatment.

Question 120: Ms. Johnson, a breast cancer survivor, expresses concerns about facing discrimination at her workplace due to her medical history. As an Oncology Certified Nurse, what is the most appropriate action to take?
A) Provide Ms. Johnson with resources on legal rights for cancer survivors
B) Advise Ms. Johnson to keep her medical history confidential at work
C) Suggest Ms. Johnson to quit her job to avoid discrimination
D) Ignore Ms. Johnson's concerns as they are unfounded

Question 121: Mr. Patel, a 60-year-old prostate cancer survivor, is experiencing erectile dysfunction following treatment. Which of the following medications is commonly used to manage erectile dysfunction in cancer survivors like Mr. Patel?
A) Finasteride
B) Tadalafil (Cialis)
C) Sertraline
D) Gabapentin

Question 122: Which of the following is a classification system that categorizes tumors based on their cell differentiation and growth rate?
A) Gleason Score
B) Ann Arbor Staging System
C) Clark's Level of Invasion
D) Scarff-Bloom-Richardson Grading System

Question 123: Which of the following is NOT a recommended self-care practice for managing compassion fatigue in oncology nursing?
A) Engaging in regular physical exercise
B) Seeking professional counseling or therapy
C) Isolating oneself from colleagues and friends
D) Practicing mindfulness and meditation

Question 124: How can healthcare providers support intimacy in cancer patients?
A) Encouraging isolation
B) Avoiding discussions about intimacy
C) Providing resources for sexual health
D) Disregarding emotional needs

Question 125: Which of the following is a common sign of extravasation?
A) Numbness or tingling at the site
B) Redness and warmth
C) Swelling and pain
D) Normal blood return upon aspiration

Question 126: Which of the following is the initial step in managing an extravasation injury?
A) Apply ice pack
B) Stop the infusion immediately
C) Administer an antidote
D) Continue the infusion

Question 127: Scenario: David, a 50-year-old male patient with colon cancer, is receiving chemotherapy that can cause myelosuppression. Which of the following nursing interventions is essential to prevent infection in David?
A) Encouraging raw vegetable consumption
B) Avoiding hand hygiene
C) Placing a potted plant in the room
D) Monitoring for fever and signs of infection

Question 128: Which of the following best defines spiritual distress in the context of oncology care?
A) Feeling sad or anxious about the cancer diagnosis
B) Experiencing a crisis of faith or loss of meaning and purpose
C) Difficulty in managing treatment side effects
D) Fear of recurrence or progression of the disease

Question 129: Scenario: John, a 60-year-old male, is receiving radiation therapy for prostate cancer. He complains of fatigue and weakness. Which nursing intervention is essential in managing radiation-induced fatigue?
A) Encouraging high-intensity exercise
B) Limiting fluid intake
C) Scheduling rest periods throughout the day
D) Providing caffeine-rich beverages

Question 130: Which medication is commonly used to manage breakthrough cancer pain in patients with advanced cancer?
A) NSAIDs
B) Muscle relaxants
C) Anticonvulsants
D) Short-acting opioids

Question 131: How can oncology nurses help patients regain a sense of control in the face of their cancer diagnosis?
A) Making decisions on behalf of the patient
B) Limiting information shared with the patient
C) Encouraging patient participation in care planning
D) Avoiding discussions about treatment options

Question 132: Which phase of the nursing process involves reassessment and modification of the care plan?
A) Assessment
B) Planning
C) Implementation
D) Evaluation

Question 133: Which factor can contribute to sexual dysfunction in cancer survivors?
A) Regular exercise routine
B) Healthy diet
C) Chemotherapy side effects
D) Supportive social network

Question 134: What is the primary goal of care coordination in oncology?
A) Minimizing patient involvement in decision-making
B) Ensuring seamless communication among healthcare providers
C) Delaying treatment initiation
D) Limiting access to supportive care services

Question 135: Mrs. Lee, a 45-year-old lung cancer patient, is undergoing chemotherapy and reports feeling overwhelmed, anxious, and socially isolated. Which psychosocial intervention would be most beneficial in addressing her emotional distress and enhancing her coping skills?
A) Relaxation Techniques
B) Cognitive-Behavioral Therapy (CBT)
C) Massage Therapy
D) Acupuncture

Question 136: How can psychosocial distress impact cancer treatment outcomes?
A) It has no effect on treatment outcomes
B) It can lead to better adherence to treatment
C) It may result in treatment delays or discontinuation
D) It improves overall quality of life

Question 137: Scenario: Michael, a 55-year-old lung cancer survivor, undergoes routine follow-up imaging, which reveals a new tumor in his liver. What term best describes this new tumor?
A) Metastatic lesion
B) Benign growth
C) Recurrent cancer
D) Secondary malignancy

Question 138: Which communication skill is essential for an Oncology Certified Nurse (OCN) when interacting with patients and their families?
A) Using medical jargon
B) Active listening
C) Interrupting the patient to save time
D) Avoiding eye contact

Question 139: Which financial resource is specifically designed to help cancer patients cover medical expenses that are not typically paid by insurance?
A) Medicaid
B) Medicare
C) Social Security Disability Insurance
D) Cancer Financial Assistance

Question 140: Ms. Rodriguez, a 45-year-old patient with breast cancer, is receiving her third cycle of chemotherapy with doxorubicin. She develops facial flushing, itching, and angioedema. What is the priority nursing action for managing a suspected anaphylactic reaction in this patient?
A) Administer oxygen therapy
B) Notify the healthcare provider immediately
C) Administer intravenous fluids
D) Stop the infusion and assess vital signs

Question 141: Which vascular access device (VAD) is suitable for long-term chemotherapy administration in cancer patients?
A) Peripherally Inserted Central Catheter (PICC)
B) Midline Catheter
C) Intraosseous Catheter
D) Peripheral Intravenous Catheter

Question 142: Ms. Johnson, a 45-year-old female diagnosed with breast cancer, reports persistent back pain. Further evaluation reveals metastasis to the spine. Which site is a common location for breast cancer metastasis?
A) Lungs
B) Pancreas
C) Spine
D) Kidneys

Question 143: Scenario: Ms. Garcia, a 55-year-old patient with terminal pancreatic cancer, wants to ensure her family understands her wishes for end-of-life care. She desires a document that focuses on her values and goals rather than specific medical treatments. What would be the most suitable choice for Ms. Garcia?
A) Provider Orders for Life-Sustaining Treatment (POLST)
B) Medical Power of Attorney
C) Advance Directive
D) Do Not Intubate (DNI) Order

Question 144: Which of the following is NOT a common symptom that may require palliative care in cancer patients?
A) Fatigue
B) Nausea and Vomiting
C) Hair Loss
D) Pain

Question 145: Scenario: John, a 60-year-old prostate cancer patient, is transitioning from active treatment to survivorship care. He is unsure about the follow-up appointments and monitoring required post-treatment. What is the most appropriate action for the Oncology Certified Nurse to facilitate navigation and coordination of care for John?
A) Provide John with general information about survivorship care.
B) Schedule all follow-up appointments for John without his input.
C) Educate John about the importance of survivorship care and involve him in developing a follow-up plan.
D) Recommend John to seek alternative therapies for post-treatment care.

Question 146: What imaging modality is most commonly used to diagnose spinal cord compression in oncology patients?
A) MRI

B) X-ray
C) CT scan
D) Ultrasound

Question 147: Which of the following is a common symptom of increased intracranial pressure in oncologic emergencies?
A) Hypotension
B) Bradycardia
C) Headache
D) Low-grade fever

Question 148: Sarah, a 40-year-old patient with lung cancer, prefers hands-on activities to enhance her learning experience. Which method would best accommodate her learning preference?
A) Watching educational videos
B) Participating in group discussions
C) Engaging in role-playing scenarios
D) Listening to audio recordings

Question 149: Scenario: Emily, an oncology nurse, is caring for a patient who is participating in a clinical trial for a new cancer treatment. The patient expresses concerns about the potential side effects of the experimental drug. How should Emily respond?
A) Reassure the patient that the benefits of the trial outweigh the risks.
B) Encourage the patient to withdraw from the trial if they are uncomfortable.
C) Provide the patient with detailed information about the drug's side effects and the trial process.
D) Minimize the potential side effects to alleviate the patient's fears.

Question 150: What impact can inadequate family and social support have on cancer survivors?
A) Improved emotional well-being
B) Enhanced coping mechanisms
C) Increased risk of depression and anxiety
D) Strengthened sense of independence

ANSWER WITH DETAILED EXPLANATION SET [1]

Question 1: Correct Answer: B) Urinary retention
Rationale: Michael's symptoms of lower abdominal pain, bloating, difficulty passing urine, suprapubic tenderness, and a palpable bladder indicate urinary retention, a common issue in prostate cancer patients. Bowel obstruction (Option A) presents with different symptoms like constipation, vomiting, and abdominal distension. Gastric ulcer (Option C) manifests with epigastric pain, not lower abdominal symptoms. Appendicitis (Option D) typically presents with right lower quadrant pain, fever, and rebound tenderness, not the symptoms described in the scenario.

Question 2: Correct Answer: A) Adding a short-acting opioid analgesic
Rationale: Breakthrough pain in cancer patients requires rapid relief, which is best achieved by adding a short-acting opioid to the existing long-acting opioid regimen. Increasing the long-acting opioid dose may lead to overdose. NSAIDs are not typically used for breakthrough cancer pain. Tricyclic antidepressants are more commonly used for neuropathic pain rather than breakthrough pain.

Question 3: Correct Answer: C) Colonoscopy every 5 years
Rationale: Due to his family history of colorectal cancer, Mr. Brown should undergo colonoscopy every 5 years for early detection and prevention. Annual prostate exams are more relevant for prostate cancer screening. Low-dose aspirin regimen may be considered for cardiovascular health but is not specific to colorectal cancer prevention. Lung cancer screening is recommended for individuals with a history of smoking or exposure to lung carcinogens.

Question 4: Correct Answer: B) Bowel obstruction
Rationale: Emily's symptoms of abdominal distension, nausea, vomiting, and a palpable mass in the lower abdomen are suggestive of bowel obstruction, a common complication in patients with advanced gynecologic cancers. Urinary incontinence (Option A) presents with involuntary loss of urine, not related to the symptoms described. Peptic ulcer disease (Option C) manifests with epigastric pain, not lower abdominal symptoms. Pelvic inflammatory disease (Option D) presents with pelvic pain, abnormal vaginal discharge, and fever, not the symptoms described in the scenario.

Question 5: Correct Answer: B) Pneumonitis
Rationale: Pneumonitis is characterized by lung inflammation, leading to symptoms such as cough, shortness of breath, and chest pain. Nephritis (A) involves kidney inflammation, thyroiditis (C) is thyroid gland inflammation, and arthritis (D) is joint inflammation, all distinct from pneumonitis in terms of affected organs and clinical presentation.

Question 6: Correct Answer: B) Bones
Rationale: Prostate cancer commonly metastasizes to bones, especially the spine and pelvis. Brain metastasis is more typical in lung cancer. Liver involvement is common in colorectal cancer. Colon metastasis is frequent in colorectal cancer.

Question 7: Correct Answer: B) Providing opportunities for Mr. Patel to reminisce about his life
Rationale: Allowing Mr. Patel to reminisce about his life can help him find meaning, process his emotions, and create a sense of closure. This intervention validates his experiences and provides him with a supportive outlet to express his feelings. Options A, C, and D are not recommended as they may hinder Mr. Patel's coping mechanisms and emotional well-being during this challenging time.

Question 8: Correct Answer: A) Oncology nurse
Rationale: Oncology nurses play a crucial role in coordinating follow-up care for cancer patients by monitoring their progress, educating them about self-care practices, addressing concerns, and facilitating communication between the healthcare team and the patient. Radiology technicians perform imaging tests, physical therapists focus on rehabilitation, and nutritionists provide dietary guidance.

Question 9: Correct Answer: C) Encouraging shared decision-making and addressing concerns
Rationale: Encouraging shared decision-making and addressing concerns (Option C) empowers Mark and his family to actively participate in the decision-making process, fostering trust and understanding. Avoiding discussions about end-of-life care (Option A) can lead to misunderstandings, including only medical jargon (Option B) may confuse the family, and providing limited information (Option D) can hinder informed decision-making and emotional support.

Question 10: Correct Answer: C) Recognizing and destroying cancer cells
Rationale: The immune system plays a crucial role in recognizing and destroying cancer cells through mechanisms like cytotoxic T cells and natural killer cells. Options A, B, and D are incorrect as the immune system's primary function is to identify and eliminate abnormal cells, including cancer cells, rather than promoting tumor growth, suppressing immune response, or enhancing cancer cell proliferation.

Question 11: Correct Answer: C) Develops months to years after treatment
Rationale: Late symptoms in oncology patients manifest long after the completion of treatment, often emerging months to years later. Unlike acute and chronic symptoms that are more closely linked to active treatment phases, late symptoms pose unique challenges as they can impact survivors' quality of life in the survivorship phase. The other options do not align with the characteristic timeline of late symptoms.

Question 12: Correct Answer: B) Allowing her to participate in treatment decisions
Rationale: Allowing the patient to participate in treatment decisions empowers them and restores a sense of control. Options A, C, and D undermine the patient's autonomy and exacerbate distress.

Question 13: Correct Answer: A) Expressing emotions through journaling
Rationale: Expressing emotions through journaling is a constructive coping strategy that can help individuals like Mark process and release pent-up emotions in a safe and reflective manner. It allows him to gain insights into his feelings, identify triggers, and explore coping solutions. In contrast, options B (Suppressing emotions), C (Engaging in risky behaviors), and D (Blaming others for the setback) are maladaptive coping mechanisms that can lead to emotional suppression, increased risk-taking, and strained relationships. Journaling promotes emotional awareness and self-expression, fostering emotional healing and resilience.

Question 14: Correct Answer: B) Enhancing the immune response
Rationale: Biotherapy works by enhancing the body's immune response against cancer cells. Unlike traditional treatments that directly target cancer cells, biotherapy focuses on boosting the immune system's ability to recognize and destroy cancer cells. Inhibiting cell division, blocking blood vessel formation, and inducing DNA damage are mechanisms associated with other types of cancer treatments, such as chemotherapy and targeted therapy.

Question 15: Correct Answer: A) Allopurinol
Rationale: Allopurinol is frequently used for prophylaxis against tumor lysis syndrome in high-risk patients by inhibiting xanthine oxidase and reducing the production of uric acid. Spironolactone, metoprolol, and ondansetron are not indicated for tumor lysis syndrome prophylaxis and do not target the underlying pathophysiology of this condition.

Question 16: Correct Answer: C) Facilitating access to spiritual support services and resources
Rationale: To promote spiritual well-being in patients facing distress, oncology nurses should facilitate access to spiritual support services and resources (option C). Disregarding beliefs

(option A) or encouraging emotional suppression (option B) can be detrimental. Minimizing the importance of spirituality (option D) neglects a crucial aspect of holistic care, hindering the patient's coping mechanisms.

Question 17: Correct Answer: C) Engaging in regular physical activity
Rationale: Engaging in regular physical activity is a key component of promoting healthy survivorship outcomes in cancer patients. Physical activity can help improve physical function, reduce fatigue, enhance quality of life, and lower the risk of cancer recurrence. Isolating oneself from social support, ignoring physical symptoms, and avoiding follow-up appointments can have negative impacts on survivorship outcomes by hindering early detection of issues and limiting access to necessary support and care.

Question 18: Correct Answer: A) Initiate supplemental oxygen therapy
Rationale: Supplemental oxygen therapy is the mainstay for managing dyspnea in palliative care for patients with advanced lung cancer. Diuretics are not indicated unless there is concurrent heart failure. High-dose chemotherapy is not appropriate in palliative care for symptom management.

Question 19: Correct Answer: B) Providing Sarah with information on local caregiver support groups
Rationale: Caregiver support is crucial in the care continuum, especially in end-of-life situations. Connecting Sarah with local caregiver support groups can offer her emotional support, practical advice, and a sense of community. Options A, C, and D are incorrect as they do not address Sarah's need for support and may further contribute to her feelings of overwhelm and exhaustion.

Question 20: Correct Answer: D) Ensuring airway patency and calling for immediate medical assistance
Rationale: In the scenario of sudden onset paralysis and loss of bowel/bladder control, the priority nursing action is to ensure airway patency and call for immediate medical assistance. Initiating range of motion exercises, applying heat packs, or elevating the legs are not appropriate actions in this emergent situation.

Question 21: Correct Answer: C) Acupuncture therapy
Rationale: Acupuncture therapy can help alleviate symptoms of peripheral neuropathy by stimulating specific points in the body. Topical capsaicin cream (option A) may provide relief but is more focused on localized pain. Administering pain medication (option B) may be necessary but is not a non-pharmacologic measure. Hot and cold therapy (option D) can help with pain management but may not address neuropathy as effectively as acupuncture.

Question 22: Correct Answer: B) Thiazide diuretics
Rationale: Thiazide diuretics can exacerbate hypercalcemia by enhancing renal calcium reabsorption. Therefore, they should be avoided in patients with hypercalcemia. Prednisone (option A) can be used to reduce calcium levels in some cases. Lithium (option C) can also contribute to hypercalcemia. Vitamin D supplements (option D) are not typically used in the management of hypercalcemia.

Question 23: Correct Answer: B) Hypothyroidism
Rationale: Checkpoint inhibitors can lead to immune-related adverse events, with hypothyroidism being a common side effect. Options A, C, and D are incorrect as they are not commonly associated with checkpoint inhibitors.

Question 24: Correct Answer: D) Psychologist
Rationale: A psychologist specializes in addressing mental health concerns such as anxiety and depression, providing counseling and support for patients like John. While an oncology nurse, palliative care team, and oncology pharmacist are essential in cancer care, they may not have the expertise to address John's specific psychosocial needs.

Question 25: Correct Answer: D) Chaplain
Rationale: The correct answer is D) Chaplain. Chaplains are essential members of the interdisciplinary team in end-of-life care, offering spiritual support, counseling, and guidance to patients and families during challenging times. While social workers provide emotional support, physical therapists focus on rehabilitation, and dietitians address nutritional needs, the chaplain specifically addresses spiritual well-being, making them the most appropriate choice in this scenario.

Question 26: Correct Answer: A) Skin care
Rationale: Skin care is vital for patients undergoing radiation therapy to prevent and manage skin reactions such as redness, itching, and peeling. Proper skincare can help alleviate discomfort and reduce the risk of infections. While dental hygiene is important for overall health, hearing tests and eye examinations are not typically specific considerations during radiation therapy.

Question 27: Correct Answer: C) Packing the wound with alginate dressing
Rationale: Alginate dressings are suitable for wounds with high exudate levels, like those seen in tumor-infiltrated wounds. Hydrocolloid dressings are more appropriate for low to moderate exudate levels. Transparent film dressings are used for superficial wounds, not for wounds with significant exudate. Topical antibiotics are not recommended for wound management in the absence of infection.

Question 28: Correct Answer: A) Asbestos
Rationale: Asbestos is a well-known carcinogen that has been linked to the development of lung cancer. Exposure to asbestos fibers increases the risk of developing lung cancer, particularly in individuals who smoke. Options B, C, and D are not carcinogens associated with lung cancer and are therefore incorrect.

Question 29: Correct Answer: C) Seeking counseling or therapy
Rationale: Seeking counseling or therapy is a proactive step for cancer survivors to address intimacy issues post-treatment. It allows them to explore their feelings, concerns, and communication strategies in a supportive environment. Avoiding open communication, ignoring emotional needs, and isolating oneself can exacerbate intimacy challenges, making counseling or therapy the most effective option for improvement.

Question 30: Correct Answer: B) Fear of rejection
Rationale: Fear of rejection is a common psychological aspect experienced by cancer patients facing intimacy challenges. This fear can stem from concerns about how their partner may perceive them post-treatment. While increased self-esteem, enhanced body image, and strong social support are beneficial, fear of rejection often plays a more significant role in impacting intimacy.

Question 31: Correct Answer: A) Initiating prophylactic antibiotics
Rationale: Febrile neutropenia is a serious complication of chemotherapy, requiring prompt initiation of broad-spectrum antibiotics to prevent sepsis. Administering erythropoietin is not indicated in the management of febrile neutropenia. Encouraging raw food consumption can increase the risk of infection. Hand hygiene is crucial in preventing infections in neutropenic patients.

Question 32: Correct Answer: C) Age
Rationale: Age is a non-modifiable risk factor for cancer as the risk of developing cancer increases with age due to accumulated genetic mutations and decreased immune function. Smoking, obesity, and physical inactivity are modifiable risk factors that individuals can work on to reduce their risk of cancer.

Question 33: Correct Answer: C) Popliteal vein
Rationale: The popliteal vein is a common site for VTE in cancer patients, along with other deep veins such as the iliac, femoral, and subclavian veins. VTE in cancer patients often presents as deep vein thrombosis (DVT) in the lower extremities, with the potential to embolize to the lungs, causing pulmonary embolism (PE). Arterial sites like the femoral and brachial arteries are not typical locations for VTE.

Question 34: Correct Answer: A) Psychological support resources
Rationale: Survivorship care plans in oncology include psychological support resources to address the emotional and mental well-being of cancer survivors, helping them cope with anxiety, depression, and other psychosocial challenges post-treatment. Surgical procedures, radiation therapy, and laboratory tests are not typically part of survivorship care plans but may be

included based on individual patient needs.
Question 35: Correct Answer: B) Fatigue and weakness
Rationale: Anemia is a common complication in patients with AML, leading to symptoms such as fatigue and weakness due to decreased oxygen-carrying capacity. While easy bruising and bleeding may occur due to low platelet count, bone pain is more commonly associated with leukemia infiltration into the bone marrow. Headaches and dizziness are not typical symptoms of anemia in AML.
Question 36: Correct Answer: B) Hair loss
Rationale: Hair loss, or alopecia, is a common side effect of radiation therapy in cancer patients. Radiation damages hair follicles, leading to temporary or permanent hair loss in the treated area. Hypertension, weight gain, and anemia are not typically associated with radiation therapy but may occur due to other factors such as certain medications or the cancer itself.
Question 37: Correct Answer: C) Smoking
Rationale: Smoking is not only a risk factor for developing cancer but also negatively impacts cancer treatment outcomes. Smoking can reduce the effectiveness of treatments like chemotherapy and increase the likelihood of cancer recurrence. Exercise, occupation, and diet can all play roles in cancer prevention and treatment but do not have the same negative impact as smoking.
Question 38: Correct Answer: A) Type I
Rationale: Mr. Smith is experiencing a Type I hypersensitivity reaction, also known as immediate hypersensitivity. This reaction occurs rapidly after exposure to an allergen, leading to the release of histamine and other inflammatory mediators. Symptoms include rash, itching, and respiratory distress. Type II hypersensitivity involves cytotoxic reactions, Type III involves immune complex deposition, and Type IV involves delayed-type hypersensitivity reactions, none of which match Mr. Smith's presentation.
Question 39: Correct Answer: D) Renal failure
Rationale: Cisplatin chemotherapy is known to cause nephrotoxicity, leading to renal failure as a potential genitourinary alteration. Urinary retention is not a common side effect of cisplatin. Polyuria and hematuria are not typically associated with cisplatin chemotherapy.
Question 40: Correct Answer: C) Interdisciplinary Collaboration
Rationale: Magnet Recognition emphasizes interdisciplinary collaboration in oncology nursing practice to enhance patient outcomes and promote a culture of teamwork. High patient mortality rates, empirical nursing practice, and limited staff training are not indicative of Magnet Recognition standards in oncology nursing.
Question 41: Correct Answer: B) Leukemia
Rationale: Leukemia is a hematologic disorder where there is an overproduction of abnormal white blood cells in the bone marrow. Thrombocytopenia refers to low platelet count, anemia is a decrease in red blood cells, and lymphoma is a cancer of the lymphatic system. Therefore, the correct answer is B) Leukemia as it specifically relates to the overproduction of abnormal white blood cells.
Question 42: Correct Answer: B) Ensuring the patient is well-hydrated
Rationale: Ensuring the patient is well-hydrated before surgery is essential for optimal perioperative care, reducing the risk of complications such as dehydration and electrolyte imbalances. Administering high-dose vitamin supplements, allowing heavy meals, and encouraging smoking are contraindicated preoperative practices that can increase surgical risks.
Question 43: Correct Answer: B) Financial burden due to treatment costs
Rationale: Cancer survivors often face financial challenges due to the high costs associated with treatment, which can impact their family and social support systems. This burden may lead to stress, anxiety, and strain on relationships. While emotional support, communication, and social networks are important, the financial aspect is a significant concern that can affect the overall well-being of survivors and their families.
Question 44: Correct Answer: A) FISH

Rationale: Fluorescence in situ hybridization (FISH) is the gold standard for detecting HER2 gene amplification in breast cancer. PCR, ELISA, and Western blot are not specific for HER2 amplification and are used for different purposes in molecular testing.
Question 45: Correct Answer: C) At any stage of life, especially during significant life events or changes in health status
Rationale: Advance care planning discussions should take place at any stage of life, particularly during significant life events or changes in health status. It is important for individuals to regularly review and update their advance directives to ensure that their preferences are accurately documented. Options A, B, and D are incorrect as they limit the timing of advance care planning discussions and do not reflect best practices in healthcare.
Question 46: Correct Answer: A) Administering loperamide for symptomatic relief
Rationale: Loperamide is an anti-diarrheal medication commonly used to manage chemotherapy-induced diarrhea by slowing down bowel movements. Increasing chemotherapy dose can exacerbate diarrhea. High-fiber foods can worsen symptoms, and withholding fluids can lead to dehydration, making option A the most appropriate choice for symptom management in this scenario.
Question 47: Correct Answer: A) Constipation
Rationale: Constipation is a prevalent symptom in cancer patients with gastrointestinal alterations due to factors such as tumor compression, side effects of medications, or decreased mobility. It can significantly impact the quality of life and requires appropriate management strategies. Hypertension, insomnia, and allergic reactions are not typically directly linked to gastrointestinal alterations in cancer patients, making them incorrect choices.
Question 48: Correct Answer: C) Immunotherapy
Rationale: Immunotherapy is a type of biotherapy that uses the body's immune system to fight cancer. Unlike chemotherapy, which involves the use of drugs to kill cancer cells, immunotherapy boosts the body's natural defenses to target and destroy cancer cells. Radiation therapy and surgery are conventional treatment modalities that do not fall under biotherapy. Immunotherapy has gained significant attention in recent years for its promising results in treating various types of cancer.
Question 49: Correct Answer: C) Prolonged and persistent yearning for the deceased
Rationale: Complicated grief is distinguished by prolonged and intense yearning for the deceased individual, leading to difficulties in accepting the loss and moving forward. Unlike normal grief where feelings of sadness gradually diminish over time, complicated grief is marked by persistent emotional distress and longing. Resuming daily activities, seeking social support, and expressing emotions openly are typical healthy coping mechanisms observed in individuals experiencing normal grief reactions.
Question 50: Correct Answer: B) Support David's interest in alternative healing and provide information on reputable practitioners.
Rationale: Supporting David's interest in alternative healing practices while ensuring access to reliable information demonstrates patient-centered care and respect for his preferences. Option B acknowledges David's autonomy and promotes a collaborative approach to his care. Options A, C, and D dismiss David's preferences and may hinder effective communication and trust-building in the nurse-patient relationship.
Question 51: Correct Answer: B) Refer John to a mental health professional for evaluation.
Rationale: John's expressions of hopelessness and feeling like a burden indicate suicidal ideation, which requires immediate attention. Referring John to a mental health professional ensures he receives appropriate support and intervention. Dismissing his feelings or advising secrecy can worsen his mental health.
Question 52: Correct Answer: C) Engage in regular physical

activity
Rationale: Engaging in regular physical activity can help reduce stress, improve mood, and increase energy levels, thus combating caregiver fatigue. Options A, B, and D are incorrect as avoiding help, neglecting self-care, and isolating oneself can exacerbate caregiver fatigue.

Question 53: Correct Answer: C) Encouraging open dialogue
Rationale: Encouraging open dialogue (Option C) allows John to express his concerns, fears, and preferences openly. Dismissing John's fears (Option A) can lead to increased anxiety, providing factual information only (Option B) may overlook John's emotional needs, and rushing through the conversation (Option D) can hinder effective communication and trust-building.

Question 54: Correct Answer: A) Acknowledge Mr. Patel's feelings and concerns
Rationale: Validating Mr. Patel's emotions and addressing his concerns is crucial in fostering trust and effective communication. Dismissing his claims or avoiding the topic would only exacerbate the situation. Referring him to another provider should be considered only after attempts to resolve the issue within the current healthcare setting.

Question 55: Correct Answer: D) Opt for citrus fruits and marinades
Rationale: Citrus fruits and marinades can help enhance the flavor of foods for patients experiencing taste changes. Spicy foods may exacerbate taste alterations, plastic utensils can sometimes alter taste, and extreme temperatures may not be well-tolerated by patients undergoing chemotherapy.

Question 56: Correct Answer: A) Transportation costs to and from medical appointments
Rationale: Transportation costs to and from medical appointments are a significant financial concern for cancer patients, as they may have to visit healthcare facilities frequently for treatments, leading to increased expenses. The other options are incorrect as cancer treatment often requires various medications that may not be free, can impact employment due to treatment schedules, and usually necessitate additional support services.

Question 57: Correct Answer: C) Survivorship Nurse
Rationale: Survivorship nurses specialize in providing long-term care plans, education, and support to cancer survivors like Emily. They address survivorship issues, lifestyle modifications, and follow-up care, ensuring continuity and quality of life post-treatment. While radiology technologists, genetic counselors, and occupational therapists have specific roles in cancer care, the survivorship nurse is uniquely positioned to assist survivors in their journey.

Question 58: Correct Answer: D) Hormonal contraception
Rationale: Hormonal contraception is not a method of fertility preservation. It is used for birth control and does not protect against the potential fertility-damaging effects of chemotherapy. Options A, B, and C are recommended methods for fertility preservation in female cancer patients.

Question 59: Correct Answer: A) Getting regular Pap smears
Rationale: Getting regular Pap smears is a vital preventive health practice for reducing the risk of cervical cancer. Pap smears can detect abnormal cervical cells early on, allowing for timely intervention and treatment to prevent the progression to cervical cancer. Avoiding HPV vaccination, engaging in unprotected sexual activity, and smoking cigarettes are high-risk behaviors that can increase the risk of developing cervical cancer.

Question 60: Correct Answer: B) Skin self-examination
Rationale: Skin self-examination is crucial for the early detection of skin cancer, especially in individuals with a family history of the disease. Colonoscopy is for colorectal cancer, mammography for breast cancer, and PSA test for prostate cancer.

Question 61: Correct Answer: C) Difficulty concentrating
Rationale: Anxiety in oncology patients often presents with symptoms such as difficulty concentrating due to worry and fear about their diagnosis, treatment, and prognosis. This can impact their ability to focus on tasks and make decisions. Increased appetite, decreased heart rate, and excessive sleepiness are not typical symptoms of anxiety and are more likely to be associated with other conditions or medications.

Question 62: Correct Answer: C) Emotional distress
Rationale: Emotional distress, such as anxiety and depression, is a common factor contributing to fatigue in cancer patients. This can be due to the psychological impact of the diagnosis, treatment side effects, or fear of the future. While physical activity, rest, and nutrition play essential roles in managing fatigue, emotional well-being is often a significant determinant. Therefore, addressing emotional distress through counseling, support groups, or therapy can help alleviate fatigue in cancer patients.

Question 63: Correct Answer: B) PSA blood test
Rationale: PSA (Prostate-Specific Antigen) blood test is the standard test for monitoring prostate cancer recurrence. CA-125 is used for ovarian cancer, thyroglobulin for thyroid cancer, and CEA for colorectal cancer.

Question 64: Correct Answer: A) Oncology social worker
Rationale: An oncology social worker can assist David in finding financial assistance programs, patient support foundations, and drug discount programs to help him afford his medications. While an oncology dietician, oncology navigator, and oncology genetic counselor are important in cancer care, they may not specialize in financial assistance for medications.

Question 65: Correct Answer: D) Destroy cancer cells while minimizing damage to healthy tissue
Rationale: Radiation therapy uses high-energy radiation to kill cancer cells and shrink tumors. The primary goal is to destroy cancer cells while minimizing damage to surrounding healthy tissues. It can be used with curative intent to remove the tumor completely or as palliative treatment to relieve symptoms such as pain and discomfort. Radiation therapy is not typically used to prevent cancer spread to other organs.

Question 66: Correct Answer: B) Educate the healthcare team on appropriate blood test frequency
Rationale: Educating the healthcare team on appropriate blood test frequency will help optimize resource utilization by reducing unnecessary blood sample collection. Implementing a new blood collection procedure without addressing the root cause may not be effective. Continuing with the current protocol or disregarding the excess samples will perpetuate inefficiencies and increase resource wastage.

Question 67: Correct Answer: B) Ensure access to 24/7 hospice support and guidance
Rationale: Providing access to 24/7 hospice support and guidance is essential when supporting a patient's wish for home-based care in hospice. This ensures that the patient and family have assistance and resources available round-the-clock to address any concerns or emergencies that may arise. While monitoring his condition is important, frequent hospital visits may not align with his preference for home care. Encouraging transfer to an inpatient facility goes against his expressed wish for home-based care. Family involvement should be encouraged and supported to enhance the patient's quality of life and well-being during this time.

Question 68: Correct Answer: C) Providing grief counseling and support groups
Rationale: Providing grief counseling and support groups is an effective strategy for healthcare professionals to help individuals cope with bereavement in the care continuum. Rushing the grieving process, encouraging avoidance of emotions, and minimizing acknowledgment of the loss can impede the individual's ability to process their grief and heal effectively.

Question 69: Correct Answer: C) Obtain the necessary certification before administering the drug.
Rationale: In oncology nursing practice, administering specialized treatments like chemotherapy requires specific certifications to ensure patient safety and legal compliance. Proceeding without the required certification can jeopardize patient care and violate legal standards. Asking a colleague to administer the drug does not address the issue of lacking certification. Documenting the administration without the

necessary certification is unethical and can lead to legal consequences.

Question 70: Correct Answer: D) Team coordinator
Rationale: The oncology nurse acts as the team coordinator when collaborating with the interdisciplinary team, ensuring effective communication, coordination of care plans, and continuity of patient care. While the nurse provides valuable input and support, the role is focused on facilitating collaboration among team members rather than making sole decisions or prescribing treatments.

Question 71: Correct Answer: A) Resistance development by cancer cells
Rationale: One challenge of targeted therapies is the potential for cancer cells to develop resistance to these treatments over time. Cancer cells can adapt and find ways to bypass the targeted mechanism, leading to treatment resistance and disease progression. This highlights the importance of ongoing research to overcome resistance mechanisms and improve the effectiveness of targeted therapies in cancer care.

Question 72: Correct Answer: B) Visual disturbances
Rationale: Visual disturbances are a common neurological symptom in cancer patients with brain metastases due to the impact on the optic nerve or visual pathways. Muscle weakness may be more indicative of spinal cord compression. Hearing loss is not typically associated with brain metastases, and skin rash is not a neurological symptom.

Question 73: Correct Answer: C) Fatigue severity scale
Rationale: The fatigue severity scale is a validated tool used by healthcare providers to assess the severity of fatigue in cancer patients. This scale helps quantify the level of fatigue experienced by the patient, enabling healthcare teams to tailor interventions accordingly. Blood pressure measurement and X-ray imaging are not specific assessments for fatigue, while physical fitness tests may provide information on overall physical health but do not directly measure fatigue levels.

Question 74: Correct Answer: C) Acquired immunity
Rationale: Bone marrow transplant primarily restores acquired immunity, which involves the immune system's ability to adapt and remember specific pathogens. Options A, B, and D are incorrect as they do not directly relate to the type of immunity primarily restored through a bone marrow transplant.

Question 75: Correct Answer: A) Activation of the immune system to target cancer cells
Rationale: Immunotherapy works by activating the patient's immune system to recognize and attack cancer cells. Option B is incorrect as immunotherapy does not directly inhibit cancer cell division. Option C is incorrect as immunotherapy aims to inhibit angiogenesis. Option D is incorrect as immunotherapy does not induce cancer cell apoptosis.

Question 76: Correct Answer: A) Fatigue
Rationale: Fatigue is a common side effect of checkpoint inhibitor immunotherapy due to the activation of the immune system. Options B, C, and D are incorrect as hair loss, nausea, and muscle pain are not typically associated with checkpoint inhibitors.

Question 77: Correct Answer: B) Double-check the medication order with another nurse
Rationale: In oncology nursing practice, ensuring the accuracy of medication administration is crucial for patient safety. Double-checking the medication order with another nurse helps in verifying the dosage and prevents errors. Consulting the physician or informing the patient should be done after confirming the discrepancy with another healthcare professional.

Question 78: Correct Answer: B) Encouraging independence in decision-making
Rationale: Encouraging independence in decision-making can help support cognitive function by promoting autonomy and critical thinking skills. Providing excessive choices can overwhelm the patient and worsen decision-making abilities. Limiting social interactions can lead to isolation and cognitive decline. Minimizing cognitive stimulation may further impair problem-solving skills and cognitive function.

Question 79: Correct Answer: A) Health Maintenance Organization (HMO)
Rationale: HMOs mandate the selection of a primary care physician and necessitate referrals for specialist consultations. This option is correct as it highlights the key features of HMO plans, distinguishing them from PPOs, EPOs, and HDHPs, which do not typically require referrals for specialist visits.

Question 80: Correct Answer: B) Encourage open communication and exploration of alternative forms of intimacy
Rationale: Encouraging open communication and exploration of alternative forms of intimacy fosters understanding and support between James and his partner. Avoiding discussion, prioritizing physical recovery, or discouraging professional support may hinder James' emotional well-being and relationship dynamics.

Question 81: Correct Answer: C) Depression
Rationale: Depression is a frequent psychological effect of sexual dysfunction in cancer survivors, stemming from issues like body image changes, relationship strain, or loss of sexual function. Decreased anxiety, enhanced self-esteem, and improved body image are less commonly linked to sexual dysfunction in this population, making them incorrect choices.

Question 82: Correct Answer: A) Providing emotional support can improve work performance
Rationale: Emotional support plays a crucial role in helping oncology patients cope with their diagnosis, which in turn can positively impact their ability to work. Social isolation, lack of communication skills, and avoiding stress can all hinder work productivity and overall well-being.

Question 83: Correct Answer: D) Hyponatremia
Rationale: SIADH leads to water retention and dilutional hyponatremia due to the excessive release of antidiuretic hormone (ADH), causing the kidneys to retain water.

Question 84: Correct Answer: C) Environmental Manipulation
Rationale: Environmental Manipulation involves creating a calming and soothing environment for the patient through the use of soft music, dim lighting, and aromatherapy. This approach aims to enhance the patient's comfort and well-being. Acupuncture, massage therapy, and radiation therapy are not focused on creating a soothing environment but rather involve specific interventions for symptom management in cancer care.

Question 85: Correct Answer: C) Evaluate for any underlying causes of restlessness
Rationale: Restlessness and agitation in hospice patients can be caused by various factors such as pain, medication side effects, anxiety, or unmet needs. It is crucial to evaluate the underlying cause before considering changes in medication or introducing new interventions. While music therapy can be beneficial, addressing the root cause is essential for effective management. Changing the diet is unlikely to directly impact restlessness in this context.

Question 86: Correct Answer: C) Offering empathetic listening and emotional support to validate John's feelings
Rationale: Validating John's feelings through empathetic listening can help build trust, enhance communication, and provide emotional support. It acknowledges John's concerns and fosters a therapeutic relationship, which is essential in addressing anxiety effectively. Options A, B, and D are inappropriate as they may invalidate John's emotions, increase distress, and hinder open communication.

Question 87: Correct Answer: D) Regular physical activity and maintaining a healthy weight
Rationale: Primary prevention aims to prevent the occurrence of a disease before it ever occurs. In the context of breast cancer, promoting regular physical activity and maintaining a healthy weight are key strategies in reducing the risk of developing breast cancer. Mammography screening (option A) falls under secondary prevention, genetic testing (option B) is more relevant to high-risk individuals for early detection, and smoking cessation programs (option C) are important for reducing the risk of lung cancer, not breast cancer.

Question 88: Correct Answer: B) Thyroiditis
Rationale: Thyroiditis is a common immune-related adverse event characterized by hypothyroidism. Hypophysitis involves pituitary gland inflammation, adrenal insufficiency involves

adrenal gland dysfunction, and nephritis involves kidney inflammation, which are less likely in this scenario.

Question 89: Correct Answer: D) Clinical breast exam every 6-12 months
Rationale: Regular clinical breast exams every 6-12 months are crucial for breast cancer survivors to detect any signs of recurrence or new primary cancers. Mammograms are typically done annually, bone density scans are recommended based on individual risk factors, and routine blood tests are not necessary for follow-up care in breast cancer survivors.

Question 90: Correct Answer: B) Validating James' emotions and acknowledging his unique experience
Rationale: Disenfranchised grief occurs when individuals experience loss that is not openly acknowledged by society. Validating James' emotions and recognizing his unique experience can provide him with a sense of validation and support. Ignoring his feelings, encouraging conformity, or minimizing societal impact can exacerbate feelings of isolation and distress.

Question 91: Correct Answer: B) Adding a short-acting opioid for breakthrough pain
Rationale: In this scenario, Sarah's severe breakthrough pain warrants the addition of a short-acting opioid for better pain control during peak pain episodes. Increasing the around-the-clock opioid dose may lead to excessive sedation or respiratory depression. Switching to a different class of analgesic should be considered if there are contraindications or intolerable side effects. Non-pharmacological techniques alone may not provide adequate relief for Sarah's level of pain intensity.

Question 92: Correct Answer: A) Pneumonitis
Rationale: Pneumonitis is a common immune-related adverse event characterized by lung inflammation. Myocarditis involves heart inflammation, arthritis involves joint inflammation, and encephalitis involves brain inflammation, which are less likely in this scenario.

Question 93: Correct Answer: C) Graft-versus-host disease
Rationale: Graft-versus-host disease is a common complication of allogeneic transplants where the donor cells attack the recipient's tissues, leading to various symptoms and complications.

Question 94: Correct Answer: D) Hematuria
Rationale: Pneumonitis in oncology patients typically presents with symptoms such as cough, shortness of breath, and chest pain due to inflammation of lung tissue. Hematuria, which is blood in the urine, is not a characteristic symptom of pneumonitis. It is important for oncology nurses to recognize the hallmark signs of pneumonitis to promptly intervene and prevent further complications.

Question 95: Correct Answer: C) Diarrhea
Rationale: Mr. Patel's symptoms of persistent diarrhea and abdominal cramping are characteristic of radiation-induced gastrointestinal toxicity, a common chronic side effect of radiation therapy. While fatigue, nausea, and anemia can also occur as chronic side effects of cancer treatment, they are not typically associated with these specific gastrointestinal symptoms.

Question 96: Correct Answer: A) Inhibiting angiogenesis
Rationale: Targeted therapies can work through various mechanisms, one of which is inhibiting angiogenesis, the process of forming new blood vessels that tumors need to grow. By blocking this process, targeted therapies can cut off the tumor's blood supply, starving it of nutrients and oxygen needed for growth.

Question 97: Correct Answer: C) Acknowledging and validating diverse identities and experiences
Rationale: Acknowledging and validating diverse identities and experiences (option C) is essential in creating an inclusive and supportive environment for sexual and gender minorities. Providing standardized care without customization (option A) overlooks individual needs. Offering support groups exclusively for heterosexual patients (option B) excludes the specific needs of sexual and gender minorities. Avoiding discussions about sexual health (option D) can hinder open communication and tailored care.

Question 98: Correct Answer: B) Engaging in continuous education to stay updated on best practices
Rationale: Engaging in continuous education (Option B) is a proactive way for OCNs to enhance their knowledge and skills, leading to more informed and efficient resource utilization. Ignoring patient preferences (Option A) undermines patient-centered care. Stockpiling supplies (Option C) is unethical and can lead to shortages for others. Disregarding institutional policies (Option D) jeopardizes standard practices. Therefore, the correct answer is B as it promotes professional growth and effective resource management in oncology nursing practice.

Question 99: Correct Answer: A) Elevating the head of the bed
Rationale: Elevating the head of the bed can help improve lung expansion and ease breathing for patients experiencing dyspnea. Options B, C, and D do not directly address the comfort and respiratory needs of a patient with dyspnea in end-of-life care.

Question 100: Correct Answer: B) Pneumonitis
Rationale: Mrs. Thompson's symptoms of shortness of breath and persistent cough are suggestive of pneumonitis, a potential chronic side effect of immunotherapy that can affect the lungs. While fatigue, mucositis, and cardiomyopathy can also occur as chronic side effects of cancer treatment, they do not typically present with these specific respiratory symptoms.

Question 101: Correct Answer: A) Genetic predisposition
Rationale: Genetic predisposition plays a significant role in the development of site-specific cancers. While factors like regular physical exercise, high intake of antioxidants, and low exposure to environmental toxins can influence overall cancer risk, they are not as directly linked to the development of site-specific cancers as genetic predisposition.

Question 102: Correct Answer: C) Facilitate a family meeting to address concerns and promote understanding of James' treatment choices.
Rationale: A family meeting can provide a platform for open communication, mutual understanding, and collaboration in decision-making, ultimately fostering support for James during his treatment journey. Options A, B, and D are incorrect as they do not promote constructive dialogue or address the underlying issues within the family dynamic.

Question 103: Correct Answer: B) Trastuzumab
Rationale: Trastuzumab is a targeted therapy commonly used in the treatment of HER2-positive breast cancer. It works by targeting the HER2 protein, which is overexpressed in these cancer cells. Options A, C, and D are traditional chemotherapy agents and do not fall under the category of targeted therapies. Therefore, they are incorrect choices in this context.

Question 104: Correct Answer: C) "Personalized treatment in precision medicine is guided by genetic testing and research evidence."
Rationale: Evidence-based practice in precision medicine involves utilizing genetic testing and research evidence to tailor treatment based on individual genetic variations. Option C aligns with this principle by emphasizing the role of genetic information and research evidence in guiding personalized treatment decisions. Options A, B, and D present misconceptions or inaccuracies regarding the application of evidence-based practice in precision medicine.

Question 105: Correct Answer: B) To identify areas for improvement in patient care
Rationale: Professional practice evaluation in oncology nursing aims to enhance patient care by identifying areas that require improvement. Options A, C, and D are incorrect as they do not align with the purpose of professional practice evaluation. Increasing workload, discouraging professional growth, and limiting scope of practice are not the objectives of this evaluation process.

Question 106: Correct Answer: B) Ensuring patient confidentiality in oncology care
Rationale: The correct answer is B because ensuring patient confidentiality in oncology care is a fundamental Standard of Practice for an OCN. Options A, C, and D are incorrect as they

involve tasks that are not typically within the scope of practice for an OCN.

Question 107: Correct Answer: B) Document the deviation and report it to the appropriate personnel
Rationale: When a deviation from standards of care is observed during a professional practice evaluation, the correct action is to document the deviation and report it to the appropriate personnel for further investigation and resolution. Ignoring, confronting, or covering up the deviation are not appropriate actions and can compromise patient care and professional integrity.

Question 108: Correct Answer: A) Promoting physical activity and exercise
Rationale: Rehabilitation in cancer survivorship aims to enhance physical well-being, promote functional independence, and improve quality of life. Encouraging physical activity and exercise helps survivors regain strength, manage fatigue, and improve overall health. Smoking cessation, limiting support groups, and discouraging emotional expression are not primary goals of cancer rehabilitation and survivorship care.

Question 109: Correct Answer: C) Providing him with a quiet environment to process his emotions.
Rationale: Providing Mr. Patel with a quiet environment to process his emotions allows him the space and time to reflect on his diagnosis and express his feelings. Scheduling additional tests may increase his anxiety levels. Encouraging physical activities may not address his immediate emotional needs. Ignoring his emotional cues can lead to feelings of isolation and distress.

Question 110: Correct Answer: C) Avoid dairy products
Rationale: Dairy products can exacerbate diarrhea in some patients. Limiting fluid intake can lead to dehydration, high-fiber foods may worsen diarrhea, and high-fat foods can be harder to digest during this time.

Question 111: Correct Answer: A) Fatigue
Rationale: Fatigue is a prevalent side effect of radiation therapy due to its impact on healthy cells in addition to cancerous cells. This can lead to feelings of tiredness and low energy levels. Hair loss, not hair growth stimulation, is a common side effect of radiation therapy. Weight loss or maintenance, not weight gain, is often observed during radiation therapy due to potential appetite changes and nausea.

Question 112: Correct Answer: A) Providing a safe environment
Rationale: When managing a patient experiencing suicidal ideation, the priority intervention is to provide a safe environment. This involves removing any potential means of self-harm, closely monitoring the patient, and ensuring constant supervision. Ignoring the patient's statements or leaving them alone can increase the risk of harm. Encouraging isolation may further exacerbate feelings of loneliness and hopelessness, potentially escalating the situation.

Question 113: Correct Answer: C) Collaborate with community resources to arrange transportation assistance for Emily.
Rationale: Collaborating with community resources to arrange transportation assistance for Emily addresses the barrier she faces in accessing supportive care services, promoting effective navigation and coordination of care. Providing a list of services or relying on family members may not address the transportation issue effectively. Telehealth consultations, while beneficial, may not fully address Emily's need for in-person supportive care services.

Question 114: Correct Answer: C) Immunotherapy boosts the body's immune system to fight cancer
Rationale: The correct answer is C as immunotherapy works by enhancing the immune system's ability to recognize and destroy cancer cells. Options A, B, and D are incorrect as immunotherapy can target both cancer cells and the immune system, involves the use of specific drugs, and has shown effectiveness in treating advanced cancers.

Question 115: Correct Answer: A) MSI-high tumors are associated with a better response to immunotherapy.
Rationale: MSI-high status in colorectal cancer indicates a higher likelihood of responding to immunotherapy, making it a crucial test for treatment decisions. Options B, C, and D are incorrect as MSI testing is not related to hormone receptor status, MSI status significantly impacts treatment choices, and MSI-high tumors have a lower mutation burden compared to MSI-low tumors.

Question 116: Correct Answer: B) The number of new cases of lung cancer diagnosed in a specific population over a defined period
Rationale: Incidence rate refers to the rate of new cases of a disease occurring in a specific population over a defined period. It is a key measure in epidemiology to understand the risk of developing a particular disease. Options A, C, and D do not directly relate to the concept of incidence rate and are therefore incorrect.

Question 117: Correct Answer: A) Encouraging caregivers to prioritize their own needs
Rationale: Encouraging caregivers to prioritize their own needs is essential in preventing burnout and ensuring they can provide effective care. Options B, C, and D are incorrect as they hinder effective caregiver support. Open communication, respite care, and detailed information are vital components in caregiver support, enhancing the quality of care provided to patients.

Question 118: Correct Answer: B) Cardiac tamponade
Rationale: The combination of hypotension, jugular venous distention, and pulsus paradoxus in a patient with advanced cancer and recent chemotherapy is highly suggestive of cardiac tamponade. This oncologic emergency requires prompt recognition and intervention. Sepsis, anaphylaxis, and hypovolemic shock may also cause hemodynamic instability but do not typically present with pulsus paradoxus and jugular venous distention as seen in cardiac tamponade.

Question 119: Correct Answer: B) Provide resources for family counseling to facilitate open communication and support.
Rationale: Encouraging open communication and providing support through family counseling can help address Ms. Johnson's concerns and strengthen family relationships during this challenging time. Options A, C, and D are incorrect as they do not promote healthy communication or support within the family, which are essential for coping with the psychosocial impact of cancer.

Question 120: Correct Answer: A) Provide Ms. Johnson with resources on legal rights for cancer survivors
Rationale: It is essential to empower cancer survivors like Ms. Johnson by providing them with information on their legal rights in the workplace. This enables them to make informed decisions and take necessary steps to protect themselves against discrimination. Options B and C are not appropriate as they do not address the root cause of discrimination concerns, while option D disregards the patient's valid fears.

Question 121: Correct Answer: B) Tadalafil (Cialis)
Rationale: Tadalafil (Cialis) is commonly used to manage erectile dysfunction in cancer survivors like Mr. Patel. It works by increasing blood flow to the penis during sexual stimulation. Options A, C, and D are not indicated for the management of erectile dysfunction. Finasteride is used for benign prostatic hyperplasia, Sertraline is an antidepressant, and Gabapentin is used for neuropathic pain.

Question 122: Correct Answer: D) Scarff-Bloom-Richardson Grading System
Rationale: The Scarff-Bloom-Richardson Grading System, also known as the Nottingham Grading System, is used to grade breast cancers based on tumor differentiation, nuclear pleomorphism, and mitotic count. It helps in predicting the aggressiveness of the tumor. The other options mentioned, such as the Gleason Score, are used for grading prostate cancer, not breast cancer.

Question 123: Correct Answer: C) Isolating oneself from colleagues and friends
Rationale: Isolating oneself from colleagues and friends can exacerbate feelings of loneliness and increase the risk of burnout. It is crucial for oncology nurses to maintain social connections for emotional support and to share experiences. Engaging in regular physical exercise, seeking professional counseling or therapy, and practicing mindfulness and

meditation are all effective strategies to manage compassion fatigue by promoting physical, emotional, and mental well-being.

Question 124: Correct Answer: C) Providing resources for sexual health
Rationale: Healthcare providers play a crucial role in supporting intimacy by providing resources for sexual health, addressing concerns, and offering guidance on maintaining intimacy during and after cancer treatment. Encouraging isolation, avoiding discussions, and disregarding emotional needs can hinder the patient's ability to cope with intimacy issues, making option C the most appropriate choice.

Question 125: Correct Answer: C) Swelling and pain
Rationale: Swelling and pain (Option C) are common signs of extravasation indicating tissue damage. Numbness or tingling (Option A) may occur but are not as specific. Redness and warmth (Option B) can be signs of infection. Normal blood return upon aspiration (Option D) is expected in a non-extravasated site.

Question 126: Correct Answer: B) Stop the infusion immediately
Rationale: The correct initial step in managing an extravasation injury is to stop the infusion immediately to prevent further damage. Applying an ice pack (Option A) may be used later but is not the primary step. Administering an antidote (Option C) is specific to certain extravasation cases and not the first action. Continuing the infusion (Option D) can exacerbate tissue damage and should be avoided.

Question 127: Correct Answer: D) Monitoring for fever and signs of infection
Rationale: Monitoring for fever and signs of infection is crucial in patients undergoing chemotherapy-induced myelosuppression to ensure early detection and prompt treatment of infections. Encouraging raw vegetable consumption, avoiding hand hygiene, and placing a potted plant in the room can increase the risk of infection and should be avoided.

Question 128: Correct Answer: B) Experiencing a crisis of faith or loss of meaning and purpose
Rationale: Spiritual distress in oncology refers to a profound inner turmoil involving a crisis of faith, loss of meaning, or questioning one's purpose in life due to the cancer diagnosis. While feeling sad or anxious (option A) is common, spiritual distress goes beyond emotional reactions. Difficulty in managing treatment side effects (option C) and fear of disease progression (option D) are more related to physical and psychological aspects, not specifically spiritual distress.

Question 129: Correct Answer: C) Scheduling rest periods throughout the day
Rationale: Managing radiation-induced fatigue involves scheduling rest periods throughout the day to conserve energy. High-intensity exercise can exacerbate fatigue, limiting fluid intake can lead to dehydration and worsen fatigue, and caffeine-rich beverages can disrupt sleep patterns, aggravating fatigue.

Question 130: Correct Answer: D) Short-acting opioids
Rationale: Short-acting opioids are frequently used to manage breakthrough cancer pain in patients with advanced cancer due to their rapid onset and short duration of action. NSAIDs (Option A) are used for pain and inflammation, muscle relaxants (Option B) are used for muscle spasms, and anticonvulsants (Option C) are used for seizures and neuropathic pain, but they are not the first-line treatment for breakthrough cancer pain.

Question 131: Correct Answer: C) Encouraging patient participation in care planning
Rationale: Encouraging patient participation in care planning empowers them to regain a sense of control and autonomy in their treatment journey. Options A and B involve restricting patient autonomy, while option D hinders informed decision-making, all of which are counterproductive in helping patients regain control.

Question 132: Correct Answer: D) Evaluation
Rationale: Evaluation is the phase where the nurse determines the effectiveness of the care plan by reassessing the patient and modifying the plan as needed. This phase ensures that the goals set during the planning phase have been met and that the care provided was effective. Assessment involves data collection, planning sets goals, and implementation carries out the plan.

Question 133: Correct Answer: C) Chemotherapy side effects
Rationale: Chemotherapy side effects, such as hormonal changes, fatigue, and neuropathy, can contribute to sexual dysfunction in cancer survivors. These treatment-related factors may impact libido, arousal, and overall sexual function. Options A, B, and D are incorrect as while exercise, diet, and social support are beneficial for overall health, they may not directly address the specific sexual concerns related to chemotherapy.

Question 134: Correct Answer: B) Ensuring seamless communication among healthcare providers
Rationale: The main objective of care coordination in oncology is to facilitate effective communication among the multidisciplinary team involved in a patient's care. This ensures that all providers are informed, working together, and aligned with the treatment plan. Options A, C, and D are contrary to the principles of care coordination and patient-centered care.

Question 135: Correct Answer: B) Cognitive-Behavioral Therapy (CBT)
Rationale: CBT is a evidence-based psychotherapy approach that helps patients identify and modify negative thought patterns and behaviors contributing to their distress. It equips patients with coping strategies and problem-solving skills to manage emotional challenges effectively. Relaxation techniques, massage therapy, and acupuncture can provide relaxation and comfort but may not address the underlying cognitive and behavioral aspects of emotional distress.

Question 136: Correct Answer: C) It may result in treatment delays or discontinuation
Rationale: Psychosocial distress can lead to treatment delays or discontinuation as patients may struggle to cope with the emotional burden of cancer, impacting their ability to adhere to treatment regimens. While psychosocial support can improve quality of life, untreated distress can have negative implications on treatment outcomes.

Question 137: Correct Answer: D) Secondary malignancy
Rationale: The liver tumor in Michael is considered a secondary malignancy, as it arises as a consequence of his previous lung cancer treatment. Distinguishing between metastatic lesions and secondary malignancies is essential for determining appropriate treatment strategies and providing comprehensive care for cancer survivors.

Question 138: Correct Answer: B) Active listening
Rationale: Active listening is crucial for an OCN when communicating with patients and families as it involves fully concentrating, understanding, responding, and remembering what is being said. This skill helps build trust, shows empathy, and ensures accurate information exchange. Options A, C, and D are incorrect as using medical jargon may confuse patients, interrupting can hinder effective communication, and avoiding eye contact can convey disinterest or lack of empathy, all of which are counterproductive in oncology nursing communication.

Question 139: Correct Answer: D) Cancer Financial Assistance
Rationale: Cancer Financial Assistance programs are specifically tailored to help cancer patients cover various expenses that may not be covered by insurance, such as transportation costs, home care, and certain treatments. While Medicaid and Medicare provide health coverage for eligible individuals, they may not cover all cancer-related expenses. Social Security Disability Insurance provides income support for individuals unable to work due to a disability, but it does not directly cover cancer-related costs. Therefore, Cancer Financial Assistance is the most suitable option for addressing non-insurance medical expenses for cancer patients.

Question 140: Correct Answer: D) Stop the infusion and assess vital signs
Rationale: In the scenario described, the patient is exhibiting signs and symptoms of a possible anaphylactic reaction. The priority nursing action is to stop the infusion and assess the patient's vital signs to determine the severity of the reaction. Administering oxygen therapy, notifying the healthcare provider, and administering intravenous fluids are important interventions but should follow the immediate action of stopping the infusion to

prevent further exposure to the allergen and assess the patient's condition.

Question 141: Correct Answer: A) Peripherally Inserted Central Catheter (PICC)
Rationale: A Peripherally Inserted Central Catheter (PICC) is the preferred VAD for long-term chemotherapy due to its ability to stay in place for an extended period, reducing the need for frequent insertions. Midline catheters are not ideal for long-term use, intraosseous catheters are typically used in emergency situations, and peripheral intravenous catheters are suitable for short-term treatment.

Question 142: Correct Answer: C) Spine
Rationale: Breast cancer often metastasizes to the spine, leading to symptoms like back pain. Lung metastasis is more common in sarcomas. Pancreatic metastasis is typical in pancreatic cancer. Kidney involvement is frequent in renal cell carcinoma.

Question 143: Correct Answer: C) Advance Directive
Rationale: An Advance Directive allows Ms. Garcia to document her values, beliefs, and preferences for care. It guides her family and healthcare providers in making decisions that align with her goals. POLST is a medical order form, Medical Power of Attorney designates a decision-maker, and DNI order is specific to intubation preferences.

Question 144: Correct Answer: C) Hair Loss
Rationale: Hair loss, also known as alopecia, is a common side effect of certain cancer treatments like chemotherapy, but it is not typically a symptom that requires palliative care. Palliative care focuses on managing symptoms that affect the quality of life and overall well-being of the patient. Fatigue, nausea and vomiting, and pain are common symptoms in cancer patients that may require palliative care interventions to improve comfort and quality of life.

Question 145: Correct Answer: C) Educate John about the importance of survivorship care and involve him in developing a follow-up plan.
Rationale: Educating John about survivorship care and involving him in developing a follow-up plan empowers him to actively participate in his care, promoting effective navigation and coordination. Providing general information or scheduling appointments without his input may not address John's specific needs and preferences. Recommending alternative therapies may not align with evidence-based survivorship care guidelines.

Question 146: Correct Answer: A) MRI
Rationale: MRI is the imaging modality of choice for diagnosing spinal cord compression in oncology patients as it provides detailed images of the spinal cord and surrounding structures. X-ray, CT scan, and ultrasound are not as effective in visualizing soft tissues like the spinal cord.

Question 147: Correct Answer: C) Headache
Rationale: Headache is a common symptom of increased intracranial pressure in oncologic emergencies due to the compression of brain tissues. Hypotension and bradycardia are not typical symptoms of increased intracranial pressure. Low-grade fever is also not directly associated with increased intracranial pressure.

Question 148: Correct Answer: C) Engaging in role-playing scenarios
Rationale: Sarah's preference for hands-on activities indicates a kinesthetic learning style. Engaging in role-playing scenarios allows her to actively participate and apply knowledge, catering to her learning preference. Watching videos (option A), group discussions (option B), and audio recordings (option D) may not provide the hands-on experience she prefers.

Question 149: Correct Answer: C) Provide the patient with detailed information about the drug's side effects and the trial process.
Rationale: Informed consent is a crucial ethical principle in clinical trials. Emily should provide the patient with comprehensive information about the drug's side effects and the trial process to ensure the patient can make an informed decision. Encouraging withdrawal without addressing the patient's concerns or minimizing risks would not uphold ethical standards of patient advocacy.

Question 150: Correct Answer: C) Increased risk of depression and anxiety
Rationale: Inadequate family and social support can significantly increase the risk of depression and anxiety among cancer survivors. Lack of support systems may lead to feelings of isolation, loneliness, and emotional distress. Strong family and social networks are essential for providing comfort, encouragement, and practical assistance during the survivorship phase, contributing to better mental health outcomes.

OCN Exam Practice Questions [SET 2]

Question 1: What role does the oncology nurse play in addressing psychosocial distress in cancer patients?
A) Administering medications
B) Providing emotional support and education
C) Performing surgical procedures
D) Analyzing lab results

Question 2: Which of the following is a common complication associated with site-specific radiation therapy in oncology patients?
A) Neuropathy
B) Alopecia
C) Mucositis
D) Anemia

Question 3: Sarah, a 30-year-old female, is concerned about her family history of skin cancer. Which non-modifiable risk factor should she be particularly mindful of?
A) Genetics
B) Stress levels
C) Fast food consumption
D) Regular medical check-ups

Question 4: Scenario: David, a 50-year-old male, is scheduled for a prostate biopsy following an abnormal prostate-specific antigen (PSA) test result. Which diagnostic measure involves the removal of small tissue samples from the prostate gland for analysis?
A) Colonoscopy
B) Bone marrow biopsy
C) Prostate biopsy
D) Skin biopsy

Question 5: Which factor can contribute to sexual dysfunction in cancer survivors?
A) Open communication with partner
B) Regular physical exercise
C) Emotional support from healthcare team
D) Psychological distress related to cancer experience

Question 6: Mr. Patel, a 45-year-old patient, is experiencing significant fatigue and deconditioning after completing radiation therapy for lung cancer. Which of the following interventions would be most beneficial for improving his energy levels and physical function?
A) Pulmonary rehabilitation
B) Mindfulness-based stress reduction
C) Tai Chi
D) Art therapy

Question 7: Mrs. Lee, a 60-year-old breast cancer survivor, is concerned about cancer recurrence. What preventive health practice should the nurse recommend to reduce the risk of cancer recurrence?
A) Annual skin cancer screening
B) Genetic testing for cancer risk
C) Regular exercise routine
D) Adherence to hormonal therapy

Question 8: Which palliative care intervention is important for managing pain in patients with hematologic disorders?
A) Physical therapy
B) Music therapy
C) Pharmacological interventions
D) Surgery

Question 9: Ms. Brown, a 60-year-old patient with pancreatic cancer, is experiencing severe diarrhea as a side effect of chemotherapy. Which pharmacologic intervention is recommended for managing chemotherapy-induced diarrhea in cancer patients?
A) Loperamide
B) Ondansetron
C) Dexamethasone
D) Prochlorperazine

Question 10: Scenario: John, a 60-year-old prostate cancer survivor, complains of abdominal pain and weight loss. Further evaluation reveals a new tumor in his colon. What is the most likely cause of this new tumor?
A) Genetic predisposition
B) Environmental factors
C) Radiation therapy
D) Hormonal imbalance

Question 11: Mr. Patel, a 70-year-old patient with terminal cancer, is experiencing severe pain despite medication. Which nursing action is a priority in managing Mr. Patel's pain effectively?
A) Administering pain medication only when requested by the patient
B) Assessing the pain intensity using a standardized pain scale
C) Encouraging distraction techniques to divert attention from pain
D) Limiting the frequency of pain medication administration

Question 12: Mr. Patel, a 60-year-old patient with prostate cancer, is starting hormone therapy. Which of the following assessments should the nurse prioritize to monitor treatment effectiveness?
A) Checking blood pressure
B) Monitoring PSA levels
C) Assessing lung sounds
D) Measuring blood glucose levels

Question 13: Which of the following is a common subsequent malignancy following treatment with alkylating agents and radiation therapy in oncology patients?
A) Thyroid cancer
B) Melanoma
C) Ovarian cancer
D) Prostate cancer

Question 14: Mr. Garcia, a 45-year-old patient with prostate cancer, is scheduled to undergo brachytherapy. Which precaution is essential for Mr. Garcia to follow post-brachytherapy?
A) Avoiding close contact with others
B) Swimming in chlorinated pools
C) Exercising vigorously
D) Applying heating pads to the treatment site

Question 15: How should oncology nurses educate patients at risk for anaphylaxis?
A) Provide written materials in complex medical terminology
B) Avoid discussing potential triggers to prevent anxiety
C) Encourage patients to self-monitor for symptoms and seek immediate help
D) Minimize the importance of carrying an epinephrine auto-injector

Question 16: Which contraceptive method is contraindicated for a patient with a history of estrogen receptor-positive breast cancer?
A) Combined oral contraceptives
B) Barrier methods

C) Progestin-only pills
D) Implant

Question 17: Which of the following is a common physical effect of sexual dysfunction in cancer patients?
A) Increased libido
B) Erectile dysfunction
C) Heightened sexual pleasure
D) Improved sexual performance

Question 18: What is a critical aspect of providing culturally competent care to sexual and gender minorities in oncology?
A) Making assumptions based on stereotypes
B) Respecting and embracing diversity
C) Using conversion therapy techniques
D) Excluding family involvement in care decisions

Question 19: Scenario: Mark, a 60-year-old male, is diagnosed with prostate cancer. He has a history of working in construction for over 30 years. Which modifiable risk factor is most likely contributing to his condition?
A) Smoking
B) High intake of red meat
C) Sedentary lifestyle
D) Occupational exposure to chemicals

Question 20: Scenario: Sarah, a 30-year-old Muslim patient, is receiving radiation therapy for cervical cancer. She requests a quiet space for daily prayers during her treatment sessions. How should the oncology nurse best address Sarah's request?
A) Deny Sarah's request as it may disrupt the treatment schedule.
B) Ignore Sarah's request as prayer is not essential for her treatment.
C) Provide Sarah with a designated quiet space for prayer during her treatment.
D) Advise Sarah to pray at home before coming for treatment.

Question 21: Mr. Patel, a 65-year-old patient with lung cancer, complains of persistent cough, shortness of breath, and chest pain. Which of the following patterns of symptoms is characteristic of chronic symptoms in cancer patients?
A) Sudden onset of severe headache
B) Acute abdominal pain and vomiting
C) Chronic cough with hemoptysis
D) Acute confusion and disorientation

Question 22: Which molecular alteration is targeted by tyrosine kinase inhibitors in the treatment of chronic myeloid leukemia (CML)?
A) BCR-ABL fusion gene
B) JAK2 mutation
C) FLT3-ITD
D) NTRK gene fusion

Question 23: Mrs. Lee, an 80-year-old patient with advanced pancreatic cancer, has been under hospice care for two weeks. She is experiencing significant shortness of breath, especially with minimal exertion. The hospice team decides to initiate oxygen therapy to alleviate her symptoms. What is an important consideration when providing oxygen therapy to hospice patients?
A) Administer oxygen at the highest flow rate possible
B) Use oxygen continuously, even during sleep
C) Monitor oxygen saturation levels regularly
D) Encourage the patient to self-adjust the oxygen flow

Question 24: Which diagnostic measure is commonly used to confirm a diagnosis of breast cancer?
A) Colonoscopy
B) Mammogram
C) Electrocardiogram
D) Pulmonary function test

Question 25: Ms. Brown, a 60-year-old female patient with ovarian cancer, is experiencing chemotherapy-induced peripheral neuropathy. Which of the following interventions is most appropriate for managing her neuropathic pain?
A) Topical capsaicin cream
B) Gabapentin
C) Aspirin
D) Muscle relaxants

Question 26: Scenario: Emily, a 40-year-old cancer survivor, visits the oncology clinic for a follow-up appointment. During the assessment, she discloses feelings of anxiety and fear of cancer recurrence. What is the nurse's best course of action?
A) Minimize Emily's concerns to prevent unnecessary worry.
B) Provide Emily with information on coping strategies and support services.
C) Ignore Emily's fears as they are common among cancer survivors.
D) Tell Emily to avoid thinking about cancer recurrence to reduce anxiety.

Question 27: Mrs. Smith, a 50-year-old patient with metastatic breast cancer, is experiencing severe nausea and vomiting despite receiving standard antiemetic therapy. Which pharmacologic intervention is recommended for refractory nausea and vomiting in cancer patients?
A) Haloperidol
B) Lorazepam
C) Ondansetron
D) Metoclopramide

Question 28: Ms. Johnson, a 45-year-old breast cancer survivor, expresses concerns about her sexual health post-treatment. Which of the following interventions would be most appropriate for addressing her sexuality concerns?
A) Referring her to a sex therapist for counseling
B) Prescribing hormone replacement therapy
C) Suggesting mindfulness-based stress reduction techniques
D) Recommending herbal supplements for libido enhancement

Question 29: Mrs. Lee, a 45-year-old lymphoma survivor, is attending her follow-up appointment. Which of the following screenings is recommended as part of survivorship care for lymphoma survivors?
A) Colonoscopy every 10 years
B) Skin cancer screening annually
C) Prostate exam every 2 years
D) PET-CT scan as clinically indicated

Question 30: How can healthcare providers support cancer patients experiencing altered body image?
A) Ignoring the topic to avoid discomfort
B) Providing education on body changes
C) Minimizing the importance of body image
D) Discouraging patients from expressing their feelings

Question 31: Scenario: During a peer review process as part of professional practice evaluation, the oncology nurse receives constructive feedback on communication skills. What is the most appropriate response by the nurse?
A) Disregard the feedback
B) Seek additional training to improve communication skills
C) Argue with the peers providing feedback
D) Blame others for communication shortcomings

Question 32: Which pharmacologic intervention is commonly used for managing breakthrough cancer pain in palliative care?

A) Acetaminophen
B) Ibuprofen
C) Morphine immediate-release
D) Amitriptyline

Question 33: What is the primary goal of end-of-life care for cancer patients?
A) Prolonging life at all costs
B) Ensuring a peaceful and comfortable death
C) Aggressive treatment to cure cancer
D) Avoiding discussions about prognosis

Question 34: Mrs. Johnson, a 70-year-old female with ovarian cancer, is admitted to the oncology unit with signs of septic shock. Which of the following clinical findings is most indicative of septic shock?
A) Fever and leukocytosis
B) Hypotension refractory to fluid resuscitation
C) Elevated C-reactive protein levels
D) Positive blood cultures for a bacterial pathogen

Question 35: Mrs. Lee, a 70-year-old patient with a history of melanoma, reports severe pruritus (itching) on her back. Which nursing intervention is most appropriate for managing her pruritus?
A) Applying a warm compress to the itchy area
B) Administering antihistamines as prescribed
C) Massaging the area with scented lotion
D) Encouraging frequent scratching to relieve itching

Question 36: What is the purpose of professional practice evaluation in oncology nursing?
A) To increase hospital revenue
B) To monitor patient outcomes
C) To ensure compliance with billing regulations
D) To assess and improve the quality of care provided

Question 37: How can healthcare providers support cancer survivors with sexuality concerns?
A) Avoid discussing sexuality altogether
B) Provide resources for sexual health education
C) Dismiss survivors' concerns as insignificant
D) Discourage survivors from seeking counseling

Question 38: Scenario: Sarah, a 45-year-old patient with breast cancer, is feeling overwhelmed by her recent diagnosis and treatment options. As an Oncology Certified Nurse, what is the most appropriate communication technique to use when providing emotional support to Sarah?
A) Offering unsolicited advice
B) Using therapeutic communication
C) Minimizing Sarah's feelings
D) Avoiding eye contact

Question 39: What does the 'N' represent in the TNM staging system for cancer?
A) Metastasis
B) Tumor size and invasion
C) Lymph node involvement
D) Histological grade

Question 40: What is an important psychosocial consideration when providing care to sexual and gender minorities with cancer?
A) Respecting confidentiality and privacy
B) Sharing patient information without consent
C) Using discriminatory language
D) Ignoring mental health concerns

Question 41: Scenario: John, a 60-year-old African American patient, is scheduled for a bone marrow biopsy. He expresses fear and anxiety about the procedure due to cultural beliefs. What is the most appropriate action for the nurse to take?
A) Provide John with detailed medical information to alleviate his fears.
B) Disregard John's cultural beliefs and proceed with the biopsy as planned.
C) Involve a spiritual leader from John's community to provide support.
D) Acknowledge John's fears and explore alternative coping strategies.

Question 42: Which of the following is a common psychological response to bereavement in the context of end-of-life care?
A) Denial
B) Hope
C) Acceptance
D) Joy

Question 43: Which statement best describes disenfranchised grief?
A) Grief experienced after the loss of a pet
B) Grief that is openly acknowledged and supported by society
C) Grief that is not socially recognized or validated
D) Grief that occurs due to a sudden loss

Question 44: Scenario: Sarah, a 45-year-old patient, has been recently diagnosed with advanced breast cancer. She expresses feelings of fear and uncertainty about the future. Which coping mechanism would be most appropriate for the nurse to suggest to Sarah?
A) Avoidance
B) Denial
C) Seeking social support
D) Substance abuse

Question 45: Which site-specific cancer is most commonly associated with asbestos exposure?
A) Lung
B) Breast
C) Prostate
D) Colon

Question 46: Mrs. Patel, a 70-year-old female with a history of ovarian cancer, experiences ascites and abdominal distension. Further evaluation shows metastasis to the peritoneum. Which site is a common location for ovarian cancer metastasis?
A) Lungs
B) Peritoneum
C) Skin
D) Thyroid

Question 47: Which hematologic condition is characterized by a deficiency in red blood cells, leading to fatigue and weakness?
A) Thrombocytopenia
B) Leukemia
C) Anemia
D) Lymphoma

Question 48: Scenario: Sarah, a 45-year-old breast cancer patient, is concerned about the financial burden of her treatment. She is worried about how she will manage the costs of chemotherapy and radiation therapy. Which resource can best assist Sarah with her financial concerns?
A) Social worker
B) Nutritionist
C) Physical therapist
D) Chaplain

Question 49: Which of the following is a common symptom of Syndrome of Inappropriate Antidiuretic Hormone

Secretion (SIADH)?
A) Polyuria
B) Hypertension
C) Thirst
D) Confusion

Question 50: Which of the following best describes the role of tumor suppressor genes in site-specific cancer development?
A) They promote uncontrolled cell growth.
B) They inhibit cell division.
C) They enhance angiogenesis.
D) They induce metastasis.

Question 51: Which nursing intervention is essential in the care of a cancer patient experiencing a seizure?
A) Administering a sedative
B) Placing a padded tongue blade
C) Restraining the patient
D) Ensuring a patent airway

Question 52: Mrs. Smith, a 55-year-old ovarian cancer survivor, expresses body image concerns after undergoing a hysterectomy. Which intervention would be most appropriate to support Mrs. Smith in coping with these concerns?
A) Referring her to a support group for cancer survivors
B) Suggesting cosmetic surgery to alter her appearance
C) Providing education on the benefits of exercise
D) Recommending mindfulness-based stress reduction techniques

Question 53: Which intervention is commonly used to manage cognitive symptoms in cancer patients receiving chemotherapy?
A) High-dose vitamin C supplementation
B) Cognitive behavioral therapy
C) Physical exercise regimen
D) Mindfulness meditation

Question 54: Scenario: David, a 50-year-old colon cancer patient, is prescribed oral chemotherapy medication. The nurse observes that many patients are non-adherent to their medication schedule, leading to wastage of medications. What intervention should the nurse implement to enhance resource utilization?
A) Disregard patient adherence as it is beyond the nurse's control
B) Provide education on the importance of medication adherence
C) Continue with the current practice despite the wastage
D) Increase the medication dosage to compensate for non-adherence

Question 55: Mrs. Lee, a 45-year-old patient receiving chemotherapy for breast cancer, develops increased intracranial pressure. Which intervention is a priority in the management of increased intracranial pressure?
A) Administering high-flow oxygen
B) Initiating hyperventilation
C) Elevating the head of the bed
D) Administering corticosteroids

Question 56: Which staging system is commonly used for solid tumors to determine the extent of cancer spread?
A) TNM staging
B) Gleason score
C) Bloom-Richardson grading
D) Fuhrman grade

Question 57: Which genetic mutation is commonly associated with non-small cell lung cancer (NSCLC)?
A) KRAS
B) BRCA1
C) APC
D) HER2

Question 58: Scenario: Sarah, a 65-year-old cancer patient receiving end-of-life care, is experiencing severe pain despite medication adjustments. The interdisciplinary team meets to discuss her case. Who among the following team members is primarily responsible for coordinating Sarah's pain management plan?
A) Social Worker
B) Nurse Practitioner
C) Physical Therapist
D) Chaplain

Question 59: Which of the following is a measure of disease frequency that represents the proportion of individuals in a population who have a particular disease at a specific point in time?
A) Incidence
B) Prevalence
C) Mortality rate
D) Case-fatality rate

Question 60: Ms. Lee, a 45-year-old patient with spinal cord compression, is experiencing severe back pain and weakness in her lower extremities. Which assessment finding should the nurse prioritize?
A) Skin integrity over bony prominences
B) Range of motion in upper extremities
C) Sensation in lower extremities
D) Bowel and bladder function

Question 61: Which of the following non-modifiable risk factors is associated with an increased risk of developing cancer due to inherited genetic mutations?
A) Pollution exposure
B) Genetics
C) Physical inactivity
D) Vaccination history

Question 62: Ms. Garcia, a 45-year-old female with ovarian cancer, develops a pulmonary embolism (PE) while undergoing chemotherapy. What is the recommended duration of anticoagulation therapy for a patient with cancer-associated VTE?
A) 3 months
B) 6 months
C) Indefinite
D) 1 year

Question 63: Which site is a common location for prostate cancer metastasis?
A) Bone
B) Lymph nodes
C) Skin
D) Stomach

Question 64: What is a common characteristic of oncogenes in the context of site-specific cancer considerations?
A) They promote cell growth and division.
B) They repair damaged DNA.
C) They induce programmed cell death.
D) They inhibit angiogenesis.

Question 65: Scenario: Sarah, a 45-year-old female, has a family history of breast cancer. She is concerned about her risk of developing cancer and asks the nurse about the process of carcinogenesis. Which of the following best describes carcinogenesis?
A) The formation of benign tumors
B) The spread of cancer to distant organs
C) The process of normal cells transforming into cancer cells

D) The development of cancer symptoms

Question 66: During a routine chemotherapy infusion, Mr. Lee, a 60-year-old patient with colon cancer, develops sudden onset shortness of breath, wheezing, and hypotension. Which type of hypersensitivity reaction is most likely occurring in this patient?
A) Type I
B) Type II
C) Type III
D) Type IV

Question 67: How can healthcare providers best support caregivers in the end-of-life care setting?
A) Withhold information about the patient's condition from caregivers
B) Offer education, resources, and emotional support to caregivers
C) Discourage caregivers from seeking external support
D) Minimize communication with caregivers regarding care plans

Question 68: Which coping mechanism involves an individual consciously avoiding situations or thoughts that are reminders of a stressful experience?
A) Suppression
B) Avoidance
C) Projection
D) Acceptance

Question 69: Which of the following is a key consideration for providing care to sexual and gender minorities in oncology settings?
A) Using gender-affirming language and communication
B) Avoiding discussions about sexual orientation
C) Assuming all patients are heterosexual
D) Excluding partners from discussions

Question 70: Mr. Johnson, a 65-year-old patient with advanced lung cancer, is experiencing cognitive decline. Which intervention is most appropriate for managing his altered cognition?
A) Administering high-dose opioids
B) Implementing a structured daily routine
C) Increasing chemotherapy dosage
D) Encouraging isolation from family and friends

Question 71: What is the purpose of a port-a-cath in cancer patients receiving chemotherapy?
A) To administer oral medications
B) To monitor blood pressure
C) To access the bloodstream for chemotherapy
D) To assist with breathing

Question 72: Scenario: Mr. Johnson, a 70-year-old patient with advanced lung cancer, is considering completing an advance directive. He wants a document that provides clear instructions to guide his healthcare team in making decisions about his care. Which option best fits Mr. Johnson's needs?
A) Physician Orders for Life-Sustaining Treatment (POLST)
B) Medical Power of Attorney
C) Living Will
D) Do Not Resuscitate (DNR) Order

Question 73: Ms. Johnson, a 55-year-old patient diagnosed with breast cancer, prefers visual aids during education sessions. Which of the following strategies would be most effective in meeting her learning preference?
A) Providing written handouts
B) Using diagrams and charts
C) Conducting verbal discussions
D) Demonstrating procedures

Question 74: Which of the following is a key component of professional practice evaluation for Oncology Certified Nurses (OCNs)?
A) Patient satisfaction surveys
B) Peer review
C) Financial performance analysis
D) Equipment maintenance logs

Question 75: Scenario: Mark, a 50-year-old lung cancer patient, is considering enrolling in a new insurance plan to better manage his treatment costs. Which insurance feature allows Mark to see specialists without referrals and has a moderate premium cost?
A) Health Savings Account (HSA)
B) Catastrophic Health Insurance
C) Medicare Advantage Plan
D) Point of Service (POS) Plan

Question 76: Mr. Patel, a 60-year-old prostate cancer survivor, is experiencing feelings of isolation and loneliness since completing his treatment. Which support intervention would be most effective in addressing his psychosocial needs?
A) Encouraging him to volunteer at a local charity
B) Arranging individual counseling sessions
C) Organizing regular check-in calls with a nurse
D) Connecting him with a survivorship program

Question 77: Scenario: Sarah, an oncology nurse, is caring for a terminally ill patient who expresses a desire to discontinue aggressive treatment and opt for palliative care. The patient's family insists on continuing aggressive treatment against the patient's wishes. What should Sarah do?
A) Respect the patient's autonomy and advocate for the patient's wishes.
B) Follow the family's wishes as they are the primary decision-makers.
C) Seek guidance from the hospital administration before taking any action.
D) Convince the patient to continue aggressive treatment for the family's sake.

Question 78: Mr. Lee, a 70-year-old patient with multiple myeloma, is at risk for pathological fractures due to bone involvement. Which nursing intervention is crucial to prevent fractures in this patient?
A) Encourage weight-bearing exercises
B) Administer corticosteroids for pain management
C) Monitor serum calcium levels regularly
D) Provide a safe environment to prevent falls

Question 79: Which of the following is a key characteristic of carcinogenesis?
A) Rapid cell differentiation
B) Controlled cell growth
C) Loss of normal cell function
D) Maintenance of cellular homeostasis

Question 80: How does adherence to the Scope and Standards of Practice contribute to quality of practice in oncology nursing?
A) It limits nurses' autonomy in decision-making
B) It ensures consistency and accountability in care delivery
C) It hinders innovation and creativity in patient care
D) It increases the risk of medical errors

Question 81: Scenario: John, an OCN, is reviewing the Standards of Practice for Oncology Nursing. Which of the following is an essential component of the Standards of Practice for an OCN?
A) Providing legal advice to oncology patients
B) Participating in research studies related to oncology care

C) Performing financial assessments for oncology treatment
D) Offering spiritual counseling to oncology patients

Question 82: Scenario: David, a terminally ill cancer patient, expresses spiritual distress and the need for existential support. Which team member is trained to provide spiritual care and address David's existential concerns at this critical juncture?
A) Pharmacist
B) Palliative Care Physician
C) Music Therapist
D) Chaplain

Question 83: Which cancer classification system is commonly used for staging lymphomas and classifies the disease based on the involvement of lymph nodes and extralymphatic organs?
A) FIGO Staging System
B) Dukes' Staging System
C) Lugano Classification
D) Breslow Depth Classification

Question 84: Scenario: Mark, a caregiver for his mother with advanced cancer, has been neglecting his own needs, experiencing sleep disturbances, and feeling detached from his emotions. Which intervention is most appropriate to address Mark's symptoms of caregiver fatigue?
A) Encouraging Mark to increase caregiving responsibilities
B) Suggesting Mark attend a support group for caregivers
C) Advising Mark to ignore his own needs and focus solely on his mother
D) Recommending Mark take on additional work to distract himself

Question 85: During a support group session, a patient expresses worries about being discriminated against by their insurance company due to their cancer diagnosis. How can the Oncology Certified Nurse best support this patient?
A) Encourage the patient to switch to a different insurance provider
B) Provide information on patient rights and resources for advocacy
C) Minimize the patient's concerns to alleviate anxiety
D) Advise the patient to hide their cancer diagnosis from the insurance company

Question 86: Scenario: David, a 50-year-old male, is diagnosed with prostate cancer. The biopsy results show poorly differentiated tumor cells with marked variation in size and shape. Which histological grade is most likely assigned to this type of tumor?
A) Grade I
B) Grade II
C) Grade III
D) Grade IV

Question 87: What is the primary goal of early recognition and treatment of sepsis in oncology patients?
A) Preventing fever
B) Avoiding antibiotic therapy
C) Preventing organ dysfunction
D) Limiting fluid intake

Question 88: Which statement best describes the concept of cancer surveillance in survivorship care?
A) It involves regular screening tests to detect cancer recurrence early.
B) It focuses solely on managing treatment side effects.
C) It is not necessary once the patient completes cancer treatment.
D) It is only applicable to certain types of cancer.

Question 89: What is a common nursing intervention for managing cardiovascular symptoms in cancer patients receiving palliative care?
A) Administering Chemotherapy
B) Monitoring Electrolyte Levels
C) Encouraging Physical Activity
D) Providing Comfort Measures

Question 90: How can cancer survivors address body image issues affecting their sexuality?
A) Avoid discussing body image concerns
B) Engage in open communication with partners
C) Ignore the impact of body image on sexuality
D) Compare themselves to unrealistic standards

Question 91: Which healthcare professionals are typically involved in providing palliative care to cancer patients?
A) Oncologists only
B) Surgeons only
C) Palliative care specialists, oncologists, nurses, and social workers
D) Primary care physicians only

Question 92: Mr. Patel, a 50-year-old patient with a brain tumor, is at risk for increased intracranial pressure. Which nursing intervention is essential in preventing complications associated with increased intracranial pressure?
A) Encouraging the patient to perform Valsalva maneuver
B) Administering IV fluids rapidly
C) Monitoring and maintaining adequate oxygenation
D) Keeping the patient in a supine position

Question 93: Sarah, a 30-year-old leukemia patient, is struggling with the financial burden of her chemotherapy treatments. What support can the Oncology Certified Nurse offer to help Sarah address her financial concerns?
A) Encourage her to forego essential tests and procedures to save money
B) Provide information on patient assistance programs offered by pharmaceutical companies
C) Advise her to discontinue treatment to reduce costs
D) Recommend she seek treatment at a more expensive facility

Question 94: How can a nurse enhance cultural competence in oncology nursing practice?
A) Continuing education on cultural stereotypes
B) Stereotyping patients based on their cultural background
C) Engaging in self-reflection and seeking cultural knowledge
D) Avoiding interactions with patients from diverse backgrounds

Question 95: Which intervention is recommended for managing dyspnea in a patient with advanced cancer?
A) Administering high-flow oxygen
B) Prescribing benzodiazepines
C) Positioning the patient upright
D) Initiating non-invasive ventilation

Question 96: Scenario: Alex, a caregiver for his sibling with cancer, has been experiencing physical symptoms such as headaches, muscle tension, and gastrointestinal issues. Which coping strategy is most appropriate for Alex to manage his caregiver fatigue?
A) Ignoring his physical symptoms and pushing through caregiving duties
B) Engaging in regular physical exercise and relaxation techniques
C) Increasing caffeine intake to boost energy levels
D) Avoiding seeking professional help for his symptoms

Question 97: Mr. Patel, a 55-year-old prostate cancer patient, is worried about the financial implications of his ongoing treatment. What intervention can the Oncology Certified Nurse recommend to help Mr. Patel manage his financial

concerns?
A) Encourage him to skip follow-up appointments to save money
B) Refer him to a financial counselor to discuss budgeting and cost-saving strategies
C) Advise him to stop taking prescribed medications to cut costs
D) Suggest he borrow money from friends and family to cover expenses

Question 98: In the context of oncology nursing practice, collaboration with which healthcare professional is essential for ensuring comprehensive patient care?
A) Radiology technician
B) Physical therapist
C) Social worker
D) Nutritionist

Question 99: Which of the following is a common symptom of caregiver fatigue?
A) Increased energy levels
B) Improved sleep patterns
C) Decreased motivation
D) Enhanced concentration

Question 100: Mrs. Wong, a 70-year-old female with metastatic breast cancer, presents with DIC. Which of the following statements regarding DIC is true?
A) DIC is characterized by isolated thrombocytopenia.
B) DIC always presents with excessive clotting and thrombosis.
C) DIC is a self-limiting condition that resolves spontaneously.
D) DIC can lead to microvascular thrombosis and organ failure.

Question 101: Which type of clinical trial is designed to assess whether a new treatment is more effective than the current standard treatment?
A) Randomized controlled trial
B) Observational trial
C) Cross-sectional study
D) Case-control study

Question 102: Which of the following is a potential cause of spinal cord compression in oncology patients?
A) Benign tumor
B) Osteoporosis
C) Metastatic cancer
D) Muscle strain

Question 103: Mr. Lee, a 60-year-old patient with renal cell carcinoma, presents with pruritus, rash, and elevated liver enzymes after receiving immunotherapy. Which immune-related adverse event is he most likely experiencing?
A) Dermatitis
B) Hepatitis
C) Nephritis
D) Pancreatitis

Question 104: Mrs. Lee, a 60-year-old patient, is experiencing peripheral neuropathy as a side effect of chemotherapy for ovarian cancer. Which of the following interventions would be most effective in managing her neuropathic symptoms?
A) Acupuncture
B) Transcutaneous electrical nerve stimulation (TENS)
C) Hot and cold therapy
D) Aromatherapy

Question 105: Scenario: John, an oncology nurse, is working with a social worker, nutritionist, and oncologist to coordinate care for a patient undergoing chemotherapy. Which activity exemplifies effective collaboration?
A) John makes treatment decisions without consulting other team members.
B) John communicates only with the oncologist regarding the patient's care.
C) John actively engages with all team members to address the patient's holistic needs.
D) John ignores input from the social worker and nutritionist.

Question 106: Which accreditation program recognizes nursing excellence and high-quality patient care across various healthcare settings, including oncology units?
A) The Joint Commission
B) QOPI
C) ANCC Magnet Recognition Program
D) National Cancer Institute (NCI)

Question 107: How can an Oncology Certified Nurse contribute to improving care continuity for cancer patients?
A) Disregarding patient preferences in treatment decisions
B) Focusing solely on physical health without considering psychosocial needs
C) Providing comprehensive discharge instructions
D) Avoiding collaboration with other healthcare team members

Question 108: Which of the following statements regarding venous thromboembolism (VTE) in cancer patients is true?
A) VTE is less common in cancer patients compared to the general population.
B) VTE in cancer patients is primarily provoked by immobility.
C) Cancer patients with VTE have a lower risk of mortality.
D) VTE in cancer patients is associated with a higher risk of recurrence.

Question 109: Mrs. Smith, a 55-year-old colorectal cancer survivor, experiences persistent fear of cancer recurrence and struggles with insomnia. Which intervention by the oncology nurse is most appropriate to address Mrs. Smith's psychosocial distress?
A) Encouraging Mrs. Smith to avoid discussing her fears
B) Providing education on relaxation techniques and sleep hygiene
C) Administering sedatives to manage insomnia
D) Discharging Mrs. Smith from follow-up care

Question 110: Which site-specific cancer is characterized by the presence of Reed-Sternberg cells?
A) Hodgkin lymphoma
B) Pancreatic cancer
C) Ovarian cancer
D) Brain cancer

Question 111: Ms. Johnson, a 45-year-old breast cancer patient, expresses feelings of anxiety and fear about her upcoming chemotherapy sessions. Which nursing intervention would be most appropriate to address her psychosocial needs?
A) Provide her with detailed medical information about chemotherapy.
B) Encourage her to join a support group for cancer patients.
C) Administer anti-anxiety medication without consulting the healthcare team.
D) Advise her to avoid discussing her feelings to prevent emotional distress.

Question 112: Mr. Patel, a 50-year-old prostate cancer patient, expresses feelings of guilt and worthlessness due to his inability to work during treatment. Which therapeutic communication technique should the oncology nurse utilize to support Mr. Patel's psychosocial well-being?
A) Minimizing Mr. Patel's feelings to maintain a positive outlook
B) Acknowledging Mr. Patel's emotions and providing empathy
C) Avoiding discussions about work-related concerns
D) Criticizing Mr. Patel for not coping well with his situation

Question 113: Mr. Patel, a 65-year-old prostate cancer survivor, is concerned about the possibility of cancer recurrence. During the consultation, he asks about the

signs and symptoms that may indicate cancer recurrence. Which of the following symptoms should Mr. Patel be educated to report to his healthcare provider promptly?
A) Fatigue and weight loss
B) Hair loss and skin changes
C) Nausea and vomiting
D) Joint pain and muscle aches

Question 114: Which phase of the nursing process involves setting priorities and determining interventions?
A) Assessment
B) Planning
C) Implementation
D) Evaluation

Question 115: Mr. Patel, a 28-year-old male with testicular cancer, is interested in fertility preservation options. Which of the following interventions is a standard approach for sperm preservation in male cancer patients?
A) Testicular shielding during radiation therapy
B) Testicular biopsy for sperm extraction
C) Testicular self-examination
D) Testicular prosthesis implantation

Question 116: Scenario: Alex, a 28-year-old gay man, is scheduled for a prostate cancer screening. He expresses discomfort with the procedure due to fear of discrimination. What is the most appropriate nursing intervention?
A) Proceed with the screening without addressing Alex's concerns.
B) Provide a safe and nonjudgmental environment for the screening.
C) Cancel the screening to avoid causing further distress to Alex.
D) Refer Alex to a different healthcare facility for the screening.

Question 117: Mrs. Patel, a 70-year-old lung cancer patient, is experiencing anxiety and insomnia. Which complementary modality is most suitable to address her symptoms?
A) Aromatherapy
B) Reflexology
C) Chiropractic care
D) Hypnotherapy

Question 118: Scenario: Jamie, a 50-year-old non-binary individual, is receiving palliative care for advanced lung cancer. They express distress about the lack of gender-neutral facilities in the hospital. What should the nurse prioritize in this situation?
A) Advocate for the immediate establishment of gender-neutral facilities.
B) Ignore Jamie's concerns as they are receiving end-of-life care.
C) Offer emotional support and explore alternative solutions.
D) Transfer Jamie to a different healthcare facility with gender-neutral facilities.

Question 119: Scenario: Emily, a 70-year-old patient receiving palliative care, is experiencing difficulty sleeping. Which non-pharmacologic comfort measure would be most appropriate for Emily?
A) Warm milk before bedtime
B) Administering sedative medication
C) Creating a calming bedtime routine
D) Progressive muscle relaxation

Question 120: Scenario: Sarah, a 45-year-old patient with breast cancer, requires long-term chemotherapy. The healthcare provider decides to insert a central venous catheter for her treatment. Which of the following is a type of central venous catheter that can be used for Sarah's treatment?
A) Peripherally Inserted Central Catheter (PICC)
B) Midline Catheter
C) Arteriovenous Fistula
D) Tunneled Central Venous Catheter

Question 121: Which process describes the spread of cancer cells from the primary tumor to distant sites?
A) Metaplasia
B) Hyperplasia
C) Metastasis
D) Dysplasia

Question 122: Mrs. Lee, a 55-year-old gynecologic cancer survivor, is concerned about vaginal dryness affecting her sexual health. Which of the following interventions can help alleviate vaginal dryness in cancer survivors?
A) Regular use of scented soaps for hygiene
B) Avoiding water-based lubricants during intercourse
C) Hormone replacement therapy
D) Wearing tight-fitting synthetic underwear

Question 123: Scenario: Michael, a 60-year-old patient with advanced cancer, is experiencing severe breakthrough pain despite being on long-acting opioids. The healthcare provider decides to prescribe a medication for rapid pain relief during these episodes. Which pharmacologic comfort measure is most appropriate for Michael's breakthrough pain?
A) Ibuprofen
B) Oxycodone
C) Hydromorphone
D) Prednisone

Question 124: Scenario: Mark, a 60-year-old prostate cancer survivor, is struggling with sexual dysfunction and urinary incontinence following his treatment. Which healthcare professional is best suited to address Mark's concerns?
A) Oncologist
B) Primary Care Physician
C) Urologist
D) Gynecologist

Question 125: Which surgical procedure involves the removal of a part of the colon affected by cancer along with nearby lymph nodes?
A) Colectomy
B) Cholecystectomy
C) Nephrectomy
D) Thyroidectomy

Question 126: Sarah, a 45-year-old patient with terminal pancreatic cancer, expresses fear of dying and worries about what will happen to her family after she's gone. She mentions feeling a loss of hope and purpose. What intervention by the nurse is most appropriate to address Sarah's spiritual distress?
A) Providing her with information on funeral arrangements
B) Encouraging her to avoid discussing her fears
C) Connecting her with a palliative care team for symptom management
D) Facilitating a conversation with a spiritual counselor

Question 127: What is a crucial aspect of providing support to family caregivers of oncology patients?
A) Ignoring their emotional needs
B) Minimizing communication
C) Providing education and resources
D) Isolating them from the patient

Question 128: Which symptom is characteristic of cardiac tamponade?
A) Hypertension
B) Bradycardia
C) Muffled heart sounds

D) Increased pulse pressure

Question 129: Mr. Lee, a 50-year-old male, is a heavy smoker with a 30 pack-year smoking history. Which screening test is most appropriate for Mr. Lee to detect early signs of lung cancer?
A) Prostate-specific antigen (PSA) test
B) Mammography
C) Colonoscopy
D) Low-dose computed tomography (LDCT)

Question 130: Mr. Lee, a 60-year-old patient with prostate cancer, is considering undergoing a radical prostatectomy. What is the primary purpose of a radical prostatectomy?
A) To remove the testicles.
B) To remove the entire prostate gland.
C) To perform radiation therapy.
D) To administer hormone therapy.

Question 131: What is a recommended nursing intervention for managing anxiety in oncology patients?
A) Encouraging isolation
B) Limiting communication with healthcare team
C) Providing relaxation techniques
D) Avoiding discussing emotions

Question 132: Mr. Johnson, a 65-year-old patient with advanced lung cancer, presents with dyspnea, chest pain, and lower extremity edema. On assessment, you note jugular venous distention, crackles in the lungs, and pedal edema. Which of the following conditions is most likely contributing to his symptoms?
A) Pericardial effusion
B) Atrial fibrillation
C) Hypertension
D) Pulmonary embolism

Question 133: Mr. Lee, a 60-year-old patient with non-small cell lung cancer, presents with fever, chills, and productive cough with purulent sputum. His recent chemotherapy regimen included docetaxel. What is the most likely cause of his symptoms?
A) Pulmonary embolism
B) Pneumonitis
C) Pneumonia
D) Lung abscess

Question 134: When leading a multidisciplinary oncology team, what is a key aspect of effective leadership for an OCN?
A) Micromanagement
B) Delegating tasks appropriately
C) Avoiding team meetings
D) Imposing decisions without input

Question 135: Mr. Smith, a 58-year-old patient with metastatic lung cancer, presents with sudden onset of dyspnea, non-productive cough, and low-grade fever. His recent treatment included immunotherapy. What is the most likely cause of his symptoms?
A) Pulmonary embolism
B) Pneumonitis
C) Pneumonia
D) Acute respiratory distress syndrome

Question 136: Ms. Johnson, a 55-year-old breast cancer patient undergoing chemotherapy, expresses interest in trying acupuncture to alleviate her treatment-related nausea. Which statement regarding acupuncture is true?
A) Acupuncture involves the insertion of thin needles into specific points on the body to help restore the flow of energy.
B) Acupuncture is a form of massage therapy that focuses on muscle relaxation.
C) Acupuncture primarily uses herbal supplements to promote healing.
D) Acupuncture is a high-risk intervention with no proven benefits for cancer patients.

Question 137: Ms. Patel, a 45-year-old female with advanced ovarian cancer, develops DIC. Which of the following is a common trigger for DIC in cancer patients?
A) Hypertension
B) Sepsis
C) Hypothyroidism
D) Peptic Ulcer Disease

Question 138: Scenario: Sarah, a 45-year-old female patient with breast cancer, is scheduled to start chemotherapy. Which of the following is a common side effect of chemotherapy that Sarah should be educated about?
A) Hypertension
B) Peripheral neuropathy
C) Constipation
D) Hyperthyroidism

Question 139: Which of the following best describes the primary goal of hospice care?
A) To provide curative treatment
B) To prolong life at all costs
C) To focus on comfort and quality of life
D) To administer aggressive medical interventions

Question 140: John, a 50-year-old male, is found to have a genetic mutation associated with an increased risk of colorectal cancer. Which non-modifiable risk factor is evident in this case?
A) Genetics
B) High cholesterol levels
C) Occupational exposure
D) Vegetarian diet

Question 141: How does professional practice evaluation benefit oncology nursing practice?
A) By increasing administrative workload
B) By promoting evidence-based care
C) By reducing staff morale
D) By limiting professional growth opportunities

Question 142: Which of the following immune-related adverse events is characterized by inflammation of the colon and diarrhea in patients receiving immunotherapy?
A) Pneumonitis
B) Hepatitis
C) Colitis
D) Nephritis

Question 143: Which financial concern is commonly faced by cancer patients due to the loss of income during treatment?
A) Transportation Costs
B) Housing Expenses
C) Childcare Fees
D) Reduced Work Hours

Question 144: Which leadership skill is essential for an Oncology Certified Nurse (OCN) to demonstrate when advocating for patients' rights and access to quality care?
A) Conflict resolution
B) Emotional intelligence
C) Time management
D) Technical proficiency

Question 145: Which of the following best describes the role of a support group in oncology care?
A) Providing medical treatment to cancer patients
B) Offering emotional support and shared experiences to

individuals facing similar challenges
C) Conducting research on new cancer treatments
D) Coordinating appointments for cancer patients

Question 146: Scenario: John, a 60-year-old male patient with lung cancer, is receiving combination chemotherapy. Which laboratory parameter should the nurse monitor closely during John's treatment?
A) Serum potassium levels
B) White blood cell count
C) Serum albumin levels
D) Blood urea nitrogen (BUN)

Question 147: Ms. Johnson, an Oncology Nurse, has been feeling emotionally drained and overwhelmed lately due to the constant exposure to patients' suffering. Which self-care strategy is most appropriate for her to manage compassion fatigue?
A) Ignoring her feelings and focusing solely on work tasks.
B) Engaging in regular physical exercise and maintaining a healthy diet.
C) Increasing her workload to keep her mind occupied.
D) Avoiding social interactions outside of work to prevent emotional stress.

Question 148: How can a nurse support a patient's religious beliefs during cancer treatment?
A) Disregarding religious practices during care
B) Encouraging patients to abandon religious beliefs
C) Accommodating religious practices in care plans
D) Imposing the nurse's religious beliefs on patients

Question 149: Which alteration in functioning is commonly seen in oncology patients undergoing radiation therapy to the head and neck region?
A) Xerostomia
B) Hypotension
C) Increased visual acuity
D) Enhanced olfactory senses

Question 150: Mr. Smith, a 55-year-old patient with metastatic lung cancer, is scheduled to start immunotherapy. Which of the following mechanisms is utilized by immunotherapy to treat cancer?
A) Activation of oncogenes
B) Inhibition of tumor suppressor genes
C) Enhancement of the immune system to target cancer cells
D) Suppression of the immune response

ANSWER WITH DETAILED EXPLANATION SET [2]

Question 1: Correct Answer: B) Providing emotional support and education
Rationale: Oncology nurses play a crucial role in addressing psychosocial distress by providing emotional support, education on coping strategies, and facilitating access to psychosocial resources. Administering medications and analyzing lab results are part of their clinical responsibilities, while surgical procedures are typically performed by surgeons.

Question 2: Correct Answer: C) Mucositis
Rationale: Mucositis is a common side effect of site-specific radiation therapy, characterized by inflammation and ulceration of the mucous membranes. Neuropathy is more commonly associated with certain chemotherapy drugs, alopecia with systemic chemotherapy, and anemia can be a side effect of various cancer treatments but is not specific to site-specific radiation therapy.

Question 3: Correct Answer: A) Genetics
Rationale: Genetics is a non-modifiable risk factor as family history of skin cancer can increase an individual's susceptibility to the condition. Stress levels, fast food consumption, and regular medical check-ups are modifiable factors and do not directly impact the genetic predisposition to skin cancer.

Question 4: Correct Answer: C) Prostate biopsy
Rationale: A prostate biopsy is a procedure where small tissue samples are taken from the prostate gland using a needle to determine if cancer cells are present. Colonoscopy is used to examine the colon, bone marrow biopsy for bone marrow evaluation, and skin biopsy for skin lesions, not for prostate tissue sampling.

Question 5: Correct Answer: D) Psychological distress related to cancer experience
Rationale: Psychological distress, such as anxiety, depression, and post-traumatic stress related to the cancer experience, can significantly contribute to sexual dysfunction in cancer survivors. These emotional factors can impact libido, arousal, and overall sexual satisfaction. While open communication, physical exercise, and emotional support are essential for holistic care, addressing psychological distress is paramount in managing sexual dysfunction in cancer survivors.

Question 6: Correct Answer: A) Pulmonary rehabilitation
Rationale: Pulmonary rehabilitation is a comprehensive program that includes exercise training, education, and breathing techniques to improve lung function, endurance, and overall quality of life. While mindfulness-based stress reduction, Tai Chi, and art therapy can be beneficial for emotional well-being, they may not directly address the physical deconditioning and fatigue experienced by Mr. Patel.

Question 7: Correct Answer: D) Adherence to hormonal therapy
Rationale: Adherence to hormonal therapy is crucial for hormone receptor-positive breast cancer survivors like Mrs. Lee to reduce the risk of cancer recurrence. While regular exercise is beneficial, hormonal therapy adherence directly impacts cancer recurrence risk. Annual skin cancer screening is important but not specific to breast cancer survivors. Genetic testing may be considered but is not the primary preventive measure in this case.

Question 8: Correct Answer: C) Pharmacological interventions
Rationale: Pharmacological interventions, such as analgesics and opioids, play a crucial role in managing pain in patients with hematologic disorders. Physical therapy may help with mobility, music therapy for emotional support, and surgery for specific cases, but pharmacological interventions are the primary approach for pain management in palliative care for hematologic disorders.

Question 9: Correct Answer: A) Loperamide
Rationale: Loperamide is the preferred agent for managing chemotherapy-induced diarrhea in cancer patients as it helps to reduce stool frequency and improve symptoms. Ondansetron is an antiemetic and not indicated for diarrhea. Dexamethasone and prochlorperazine are not first-line treatments for chemotherapy-induced diarrhea.

Question 10: Correct Answer: C) Radiation therapy
Rationale: Radiation therapy is a known risk factor for developing secondary malignancies, particularly in the area that received radiation. In John's case, the colon tumor is likely a consequence of his previous prostate cancer treatment. Understanding the relationship between treatment modalities and subsequent malignancies is essential for long-term survivorship care.

Question 11: Correct Answer: B) Assessing the pain intensity using a standardized pain scale
Rationale: Effective pain management in end-of-life care requires regular pain assessment using a standardized scale to determine the intensity and adjust medication accordingly. Options A, C, and D may lead to inadequate pain control and are not recommended in managing severe pain in terminally ill patients.

Question 12: Correct Answer: B) Monitoring PSA levels
Rationale: Monitoring PSA levels is essential during hormone therapy for prostate cancer to assess treatment response and disease progression. Checking blood pressure, assessing lung sounds, and measuring blood glucose levels are important assessments but are not specific to monitoring the effectiveness of hormone therapy in prostate cancer.

Question 13: Correct Answer: A) Thyroid cancer
Rationale: Alkylating agents and radiation therapy are known to increase the risk of developing secondary malignancies, with thyroid cancer being one of the most common subsequent malignancies in this context. Thyroid cancer arises due to the exposure of the thyroid gland to radiation during treatment. Melanoma, ovarian cancer, and prostate cancer are not typically associated with alkylating agents and radiation therapy, making them less likely as subsequent malignancies in this scenario.

Question 14: Correct Answer: A) Avoiding close contact with others
Rationale: After brachytherapy, patients should avoid close contact with pregnant women and young children due to radiation exposure. Swimming in chlorinated pools can increase skin irritation. Vigorous exercise may cause discomfort at the treatment site. Applying heating pads can exacerbate skin reactions post-brachytherapy.

Question 15: Correct Answer: C) Encourage patients to self-monitor for symptoms and seek immediate help
Rationale: Educating patients to self-monitor for symptoms of anaphylaxis and seek immediate medical assistance is crucial in preventing severe outcomes. Providing clear, simple instructions and emphasizing the importance of carrying an epinephrine auto-injector can empower patients to take control of their health and safety. It is essential to avoid complex medical jargon, address potential triggers openly, and stress the significance of having an epinephrine auto-injector at all times.

Question 16: Correct Answer: A) Combined oral contraceptives
Rationale: Combined oral contraceptives containing estrogen are contraindicated in patients with a history of estrogen receptor-positive breast cancer due to the potential for estrogen to stimulate cancer growth. Options B, C, and D are safer alternatives in this case.

Question 17: Correct Answer: B) Erectile dysfunction
Rationale: Erectile dysfunction is a prevalent physical effect of sexual dysfunction in cancer patients due to factors such as surgery, radiation, or chemotherapy affecting blood flow or nerve function. Increased libido, heightened sexual pleasure, and improved sexual performance are less likely in the context of cancer-related sexual dysfunction, making them incorrect options.

Question 18: Correct Answer: B) Respecting and embracing diversity
Rationale: Respecting and embracing diversity (option B) is fundamental in providing culturally competent care to sexual and gender minorities, fostering trust and understanding. Making assumptions based on stereotypes (option A) can lead to biased care. Using conversion therapy techniques (option C) is harmful

and unethical. Excluding family involvement in care decisions (option D) can impact the support system crucial for patients' well-being.

Question 19: Correct Answer: D) Occupational exposure to chemicals
Rationale: Mark's occupational exposure to chemicals in the construction industry is a significant modifiable risk factor for his prostate cancer. While smoking, high intake of red meat, and sedentary lifestyle are risk factors for various health conditions, in Mark's case, his work environment plays a more direct role in his cancer diagnosis.

Question 20: Correct Answer: C) Provide Sarah with a designated quiet space for prayer during her treatment.
Rationale: Accommodating Sarah's religious practices, such as providing a quiet space for prayer, is essential in respecting her cultural and spiritual needs. Option C demonstrates cultural sensitivity and supports Sarah's well-being during treatment. Options A, B, and D do not prioritize Sarah's cultural and religious diversity, which is crucial in psychosocial care.

Question 21: Correct Answer: C) Chronic cough with hemoptysis
Rationale: Chronic symptoms in cancer patients often include persistent issues such as chronic cough with hemoptysis (coughing up blood). Sudden onset of severe headache is more indicative of an acute issue, such as intracranial bleeding. Acute abdominal pain and vomiting may suggest an acute gastrointestinal problem. Acute confusion and disorientation are more likely related to metabolic disturbances or central nervous system issues.

Question 22: Correct Answer: A) BCR-ABL fusion gene
Rationale: Tyrosine kinase inhibitors like imatinib target the BCR-ABL fusion gene in CML. JAK2 mutation is seen in myeloproliferative neoplasms, FLT3-ITD in acute myeloid leukemia, and NTRK gene fusion in various solid tumors, making them incorrect for CML treatment.

Question 23: Correct Answer: C) Monitor oxygen saturation levels regularly
Rationale: Regular monitoring of oxygen saturation levels is crucial when providing oxygen therapy to hospice patients to ensure that the prescribed flow rate is appropriate and to prevent potential complications such as oxygen toxicity. Administering oxygen at the highest flow rate possible is unnecessary and can be harmful. Oxygen therapy should be used based on the patient's needs, including during sleep if indicated, but continuous use may not always be necessary. Patients should not self-adjust the oxygen flow without proper guidance to prevent adverse effects.

Question 24: Correct Answer: B) Mammogram
Rationale: A mammogram is the appropriate diagnostic measure for breast cancer screening and diagnosis. It is a low-dose X-ray of the breast that can detect abnormalities such as lumps or tumors. Colonoscopy is used to examine the colon, while an electrocardiogram assesses heart function, and a pulmonary function test evaluates lung health. Therefore, the correct option is B.

Question 25: Correct Answer: B) Gabapentin
Rationale: Gabapentin is a first-line medication for managing neuropathic pain, including chemotherapy-induced peripheral neuropathy. Topical capsaicin cream is more commonly used for localized pain, while aspirin and muscle relaxants are not typically indicated for neuropathic pain.

Question 26: Correct Answer: B) Provide Emily with information on coping strategies and support services.
Rationale: Acknowledging Emily's fears and providing her with coping strategies and support services can help her manage anxiety effectively. Minimizing or ignoring her concerns may invalidate her feelings and hinder her emotional well-being.

Question 27: Correct Answer: A) Haloperidol
Rationale: Haloperidol is often used for refractory nausea and vomiting in cancer patients due to its potent antiemetic properties. Lorazepam is more commonly used for anxiety and anticipatory nausea. Ondansetron and metoclopramide are standard antiemetics but may not be effective for refractory cases.

Question 28: Correct Answer: A) Referring her to a sex therapist for counseling
Rationale: Referring Ms. Johnson to a sex therapist for counseling is the most appropriate intervention to address her sexuality concerns as sex therapists are trained to help individuals navigate sexual issues post-cancer treatment. Options B, C, and D are not the first-line interventions for addressing sexuality concerns in cancer survivors. Hormone replacement therapy may not be suitable for all survivors, mindfulness-based stress reduction techniques may not directly address sexual issues, and herbal supplements lack evidence-based support for efficacy in improving sexual health post-cancer treatment.

Question 29: Correct Answer: B) Skin cancer screening annually
Rationale: Lymphoma survivors are at increased risk of developing skin cancers due to treatments and compromised immune systems. Therefore, annual skin cancer screenings are recommended. Colonoscopy is more relevant for colorectal cancer survivors, prostate exam for prostate cancer survivors, and PET-CT scans are done based on clinical indications in lymphoma survivors.

Question 30: Correct Answer: B) Providing education on body changes
Rationale: Healthcare providers can support cancer patients with altered body image by providing education on the expected body changes during treatment, offering resources for coping strategies, and encouraging open communication about their feelings. Ignoring the topic, minimizing its importance, or discouraging patients from expressing their feelings can further isolate the patient and hinder their ability to address and cope with altered body image effectively.

Question 31: Correct Answer: B) Seek additional training to improve communication skills
Rationale: Constructive feedback during a peer review process is an opportunity for professional growth. The nurse should respond by seeking additional training to enhance communication skills. Disregarding, arguing, or blaming others for shortcomings will hinder professional development and impact patient care negatively.

Question 32: Correct Answer: C) Morphine immediate-release
Rationale: Morphine immediate-release is the preferred pharmacologic intervention for managing breakthrough cancer pain due to its rapid onset of action and effectiveness in providing quick relief. Acetaminophen and ibuprofen are not typically used for severe cancer pain management. Amitriptyline is more commonly indicated for neuropathic pain rather than breakthrough cancer pain.

Question 33: Correct Answer: B) Ensuring a peaceful and comfortable death
Rationale: The primary goal of end-of-life care for cancer patients is to ensure a peaceful and comfortable death, focusing on quality of life, symptom management, and emotional support. Prolonging life at all costs or aggressive treatment may not be appropriate in the terminal phase, while avoiding discussions about prognosis can hinder effective communication and shared decision-making.

Question 34: Correct Answer: B) Hypotension refractory to fluid resuscitation
Rationale: Septic shock is characterized by hypotension that persists despite adequate fluid resuscitation. While fever, leukocytosis, elevated inflammatory markers, and positive blood cultures are important in the diagnosis of sepsis, the presence of refractory hypotension is a hallmark of septic shock.

Question 35: Correct Answer: B) Administering antihistamines as prescribed
Rationale: Antihistamines help alleviate itching by blocking histamine receptors. Warm compresses may exacerbate itching. Massaging with scented lotion can irritate the skin further. Frequent scratching can lead to skin damage and infection.

Question 36: Correct Answer: D) To assess and improve the quality of care provided

Rationale: Professional practice evaluation in oncology nursing aims to assess and enhance the quality of care delivered to patients. It involves ongoing review, analysis, and feedback mechanisms to identify areas for improvement and ensure best practices. While monitoring patient outcomes is part of this process, the primary goal is to elevate the standard of care rather than focusing on financial aspects or billing compliance.

Question 37: Correct Answer: B) Provide resources for sexual health education
Rationale: Healthcare providers should offer resources for sexual health education to support cancer survivors in addressing their sexuality concerns. Open communication and access to information can help survivors navigate changes and seek appropriate support. Options A, C, and D are incorrect as avoiding the topic, dismissing concerns, or discouraging counseling can hinder survivors' well-being and quality of life.

Question 38: Correct Answer: B) Using therapeutic communication
Rationale: Using therapeutic communication involves active listening, empathy, and providing emotional support without judgment. Offering unsolicited advice (Option A) may come across as dismissive, minimizing Sarah's feelings (Option C) is not supportive, and avoiding eye contact (Option D) can signal disinterest. Therapeutic communication fosters trust and allows patients like Sarah to express their emotions freely.

Question 39: Correct Answer: C) Lymph node involvement
Rationale: In the TNM staging system, 'N' signifies the extent of lymph node involvement by cancer cells. This parameter is crucial in determining the spread of the disease beyond the primary tumor site. Options A, B, and D are incorrect as they represent metastasis, tumor size, and histological grade, respectively, which are categorized under 'T,' 'M,' and histological grading in the TNM system.

Question 40: Correct Answer: A) Respecting confidentiality and privacy
Rationale: Respecting confidentiality and privacy (option A) is crucial in building trust and ensuring the emotional well-being of sexual and gender minorities. Sharing patient information without consent (option B) violates ethical standards. Using discriminatory language (option C) can cause harm and distress. Ignoring mental health concerns (option D) neglects a vital aspect of comprehensive care for this population.

Question 41: Correct Answer: D) Acknowledge John's fears and explore alternative coping strategies.
Rationale: Culturally congruent care involves acknowledging and addressing patients' cultural beliefs and emotions. By acknowledging John's fears and exploring alternative coping strategies, the nurse demonstrates sensitivity to his cultural background and promotes patient-centered care. Providing medical information alone may not address John's emotional needs, and disregarding his beliefs can lead to mistrust.

Question 42: Correct Answer: A) Denial
Rationale: Denial is a common initial psychological response to bereavement where the individual may refuse to accept the reality of the loss. Hope, acceptance, and joy are emotions that may come later in the grieving process. Denial serves as a defense mechanism to protect the individual from overwhelming emotions initially.

Question 43: Correct Answer: C) Grief that is not socially recognized or validated
Rationale: Disenfranchised grief refers to a type of grief that is not openly acknowledged or socially supported, often leading to feelings of isolation and lack of validation. Options A, B, and D do not capture the essence of disenfranchised grief, making option C the correct choice.

Question 44: Correct Answer: C) Seeking social support
Rationale: Seeking social support is a healthy coping mechanism that can help individuals like Sarah navigate through the emotional challenges of a cancer diagnosis. It allows her to share her feelings, receive empathy, and gain practical advice from others who may have gone through similar experiences. In contrast, options A and B (Avoidance and Denial) involve avoiding or suppressing emotions, which can be detrimental to Sarah's emotional well-being. Option D (Substance abuse) is a maladaptive coping mechanism that can lead to further complications.

Question 45: Correct Answer: A) Lung
Rationale: Asbestos exposure is strongly linked to lung cancer development. The mineral fibers in asbestos, when inhaled, can cause genetic mutations leading to lung cancer. Breast, prostate, and colon cancers are not primarily associated with asbestos exposure, making them incorrect choices.

Question 46: Correct Answer: B) Peritoneum
Rationale: Ovarian cancer often metastasizes to the peritoneum, leading to symptoms like ascites. Lung metastasis is more common in breast cancer. Skin involvement is typical in melanoma. Thyroid metastasis is frequent in thyroid cancer.

Question 47: Correct Answer: C) Anemia
Rationale: Anemia is a hematologic condition characterized by a deficiency in red blood cells, resulting in symptoms such as fatigue and weakness. Thrombocytopenia is a low platelet count, leukemia is an overproduction of abnormal white blood cells, and lymphoma is a cancer of the lymphatic system. Therefore, the correct answer is C) Anemia as it specifically relates to red blood cell deficiency and associated symptoms.

Question 48: Correct Answer: A) Social worker
Rationale: A social worker can help Sarah navigate financial resources such as assistance programs, grants, and support services to alleviate the financial burden of her treatment. While a nutritionist, physical therapist, and chaplain play important roles in cancer care, they do not directly address financial concerns.

Question 49: Correct Answer: D) Confusion
Rationale: Confusion is a common neurological symptom in patients with SIADH due to the cerebral edema resulting from hyponatremia. Other symptoms include nausea, vomiting, and muscle cramps.

Question 50: Correct Answer: B) They inhibit cell division.
Rationale: Tumor suppressor genes are responsible for regulating cell division and preventing cells from growing and dividing uncontrollably. Inhibiting cell division is a crucial function of tumor suppressor genes in preventing the development of cancer. Options A, C, and D are incorrect as tumor suppressor genes do not promote uncontrolled cell growth, enhance angiogenesis, or induce metastasis.

Question 51: Correct Answer: D) Ensuring a patent airway
Rationale: Ensuring a patent airway is crucial in the care of a patient experiencing a seizure to prevent hypoxia and maintain adequate oxygenation. Administering a sedative, placing a padded tongue blade, and restraining the patient are not recommended interventions during a seizure as they can pose risks to the patient's safety and well-being.

Question 52: Correct Answer: A) Referring her to a support group for cancer survivors
Rationale: Referring Mrs. Smith to a support group for cancer survivors can provide her with a safe space to share experiences and receive emotional support related to body image concerns. Suggesting cosmetic surgery may not address the underlying emotional issues. Exercise and mindfulness techniques can be beneficial but may not directly address Mrs. Smith's specific concerns.

Question 53: Correct Answer: B) Cognitive behavioral therapy
Rationale: Cognitive behavioral therapy (CBT) is a proven intervention for managing cognitive symptoms in cancer patients undergoing chemotherapy. CBT helps patients identify and change negative thought patterns and behaviors that may contribute to cognitive difficulties. While physical exercise and mindfulness meditation have overall health benefits, they are not specifically tailored to address cognitive symptoms in the same way CBT is.

Question 54: Correct Answer: B) Provide education on the importance of medication adherence
Rationale: Providing education on the importance of medication adherence is crucial to enhance resource utilization by reducing medication wastage. Disregarding patient adherence will perpetuate the issue and impact treatment outcomes. Increasing

medication dosage or continuing with the current practice without addressing non-adherence will not optimize resource utilization effectively.

Question 55: Correct Answer: C) Elevating the head of the bed
Rationale: Elevating the head of the bed at a 30-45 degree angle is a priority intervention in the management of increased intracranial pressure as it helps promote venous drainage from the brain, reducing intracranial pressure. Administering high-flow oxygen, initiating hyperventilation, and administering corticosteroids are not first-line interventions for increased intracranial pressure.

Question 56: Correct Answer: A) TNM staging
Rationale: TNM staging system is widely utilized to classify the extent of cancer spread based on T (tumor size and invasion), N (lymph node involvement), and M (metastasis). This system provides crucial information for treatment planning and prognosis prediction. Gleason score is specific to prostate cancer, Bloom-Richardson grading is for breast cancer, and Fuhrman grade is used for renal cell carcinoma, making them incorrect options in the context of general solid tumors.

Question 57: Correct Answer: A) KRAS
Rationale: KRAS mutation is frequently found in NSCLC, leading to uncontrolled cell growth. BRCA1 is linked to breast and ovarian cancers, APC to colorectal cancer, and HER2 to breast and gastric cancers, making them incorrect choices for NSCLC.

Question 58: Correct Answer: B) Nurse Practitioner
Rationale: In end-of-life care, the nurse practitioner plays a crucial role in coordinating pain management plans for patients like Sarah. They have the expertise to assess, prescribe medications, and adjust treatment regimens to ensure optimal pain control. While other team members such as social workers, physical therapists, and chaplains provide valuable support, the nurse practitioner is at the forefront of managing complex pain issues in palliative care.

Question 59: Correct Answer: B) Prevalence
Rationale: Prevalence is the number of existing cases of a disease in a defined population at a specific time. Incidence, on the other hand, refers to the number of new cases of a disease that develop in a population at risk during a specified time period. Mortality rate is the number of deaths in a given population due to a specific cause, while case-fatality rate is the proportion of individuals with a particular condition who die from that condition.

Question 60: Correct Answer: D) Bowel and bladder function
Rationale: In a patient with spinal cord compression, the nurse should prioritize assessing bowel and bladder function. Changes in bowel and bladder function can indicate spinal cord compromise and require immediate intervention to prevent complications. While assessing skin integrity, range of motion, and sensation are important, bowel and bladder function take precedence due to the risk of neurologic impairment.

Question 61: Correct Answer: B) Genetics
Rationale: Genetics is a non-modifiable risk factor that can predispose individuals to certain types of cancer, such as BRCA gene mutations increasing the risk of breast and ovarian cancer. Pollution exposure, physical inactivity, and vaccination history are modifiable risk factors not directly linked to inherited genetic mutations.

Question 62: Correct Answer: C) Indefinite
Rationale: Patients with cancer-associated VTE are recommended to receive indefinite anticoagulation therapy due to the high risk of recurrent VTE. Limited duration of therapy (3-6 months) is not sufficient in this population, and long-term anticoagulation is necessary to prevent VTE recurrence.

Question 63: Correct Answer: A) Bone
Rationale: Prostate cancer frequently metastasizes to the bone, particularly the spine, pelvis, and femur. The affinity of prostate cancer cells for bone tissue contributes to this pattern. Lymph nodes, skin, and stomach are not primary sites for prostate cancer metastasis, making them incorrect options.

Question 64: Correct Answer: A) They promote cell growth and division.
Rationale: Oncogenes are genes that have the potential to cause normal cells to become cancerous. They promote cell growth and division by encoding proteins that regulate these processes. Options B, C, and D are incorrect as oncogenes do not repair damaged DNA, induce programmed cell death, or inhibit angiogenesis.

Question 65: Correct Answer: C) The process of normal cells transforming into cancer cells
Rationale: Carcinogenesis is the process by which normal cells are transformed into cancer cells. This involves a series of genetic changes that lead to uncontrolled cell growth and the formation of tumors. Options A and B are incorrect as they do not accurately describe carcinogenesis. Option D is incorrect as carcinogenesis refers to the initiation and progression of cancer at a cellular level, not the development of symptoms.

Question 66: Correct Answer: A) Type I
Rationale: Mr. Lee is experiencing a Type I hypersensitivity reaction, also known as anaphylaxis or immediate hypersensitivity. Symptoms such as shortness of breath, wheezing, and hypotension are indicative of a systemic allergic response. Type II involves cytotoxic reactions, Type III involves immune complex deposition, and Type IV involves delayed hypersensitivity, none of which match Mr. Lee's acute presentation.

Question 67: Correct Answer: B) Offer education, resources, and emotional support to caregivers
Rationale: Healthcare providers can best support caregivers by offering education, resources, and emotional support, empowering caregivers with the knowledge and tools needed to provide optimal care. Options A, C, and D are incorrect as they hinder effective caregiver support by limiting communication, resources, and emotional assistance, which are vital in enhancing caregiver well-being and patient care outcomes.

Question 68: Correct Answer: B) Avoidance
Rationale: Avoidance coping is when individuals deliberately steer clear of triggers that remind them of distressing events. This differs from suppression (A), which is a conscious effort to push thoughts away, projection (C), which involves attributing one's thoughts or feelings to others, and acceptance (D), which involves acknowledging and coming to terms with the situation.

Question 69: Correct Answer: A) Using gender-affirming language and communication
Rationale: It is essential to use gender-affirming language and communication when caring for sexual and gender minorities to create a safe and inclusive environment. Avoiding discussions about sexual orientation (option B) can hinder effective care and support. Assuming all patients are heterosexual (option C) can lead to misunderstandings and inadequate care. Excluding partners from discussions (option D) can impact the holistic care approach and patient support, which is crucial in oncology care.

Question 70: Correct Answer: B) Implementing a structured daily routine
Rationale: Implementing a structured daily routine can help patients with altered cognition maintain a sense of normalcy and reduce confusion. This intervention provides predictability and stability, which can enhance cognitive function. Administering high-dose opioids may worsen cognitive decline, while increasing chemotherapy dosage is not indicated for managing altered cognition. Encouraging isolation from family and friends can lead to social withdrawal and exacerbate cognitive symptoms.

Question 71: Correct Answer: C) To access the bloodstream for chemotherapy
Rationale: A port-a-cath, or port, is a device implanted under the skin that provides direct access to the bloodstream. It is used in cancer patients receiving chemotherapy to administer medications, draw blood for tests, and avoid repeated needle sticks. Ports are not used for administering oral medications, monitoring blood pressure, or assisting with breathing.

Question 72: Correct Answer: C) Living Will
Rationale: A Living Will is a legal document that outlines a person's preferences regarding end-of-life medical care. It provides clear instructions to healthcare providers about the

treatments Mr. Johnson would want or refuse in specific situations. POLST is a medical order form, Medical Power of Attorney designates a decision-maker, and DNR order is specific to resuscitation preferences.

Question 73: Correct Answer: B) Using diagrams and charts
Rationale: Ms. Johnson's preference for visual aids indicates a visual learning style. Using diagrams and charts aligns with this preference by providing her with visual representations that can enhance her understanding. Written handouts (option A) may not be as effective for visual learners. Verbal discussions (option C) and demonstrating procedures (option D) may not cater directly to her visual learning preference.

Question 74: Correct Answer: B) Peer review
Rationale: Professional practice evaluation for OCNs involves peer review, where colleagues assess each other's practice to ensure adherence to standards and guidelines. This process promotes accountability, quality improvement, and professional development. Patient satisfaction surveys, financial performance analysis, and equipment maintenance logs are important but not direct components of professional practice evaluation in oncology nursing.

Question 75: Correct Answer: D) Point of Service (POS) Plan
Rationale: POS plans offer flexibility to see specialists without referrals, similar to PPOs, but with a balance of cost and coverage. HSAs are savings accounts for medical expenses, Catastrophic Health Insurance provides coverage for major medical expenses, and Medicare Advantage Plans are for Medicare beneficiaries, not suitable for Mark's situation.

Question 76: Correct Answer: D) Connecting him with a survivorship program
Rationale: Connecting Mr. Patel with a survivorship program would be the most effective intervention to address his feelings of isolation and loneliness. Survivorship programs provide ongoing support, resources, and opportunities for social connection with other cancer survivors, which can help alleviate these psychosocial challenges. While volunteering, counseling, and check-in calls are valuable interventions, they may not offer the same level of peer support and understanding as a survivorship program.

Question 77: Correct Answer: A) Respect the patient's autonomy and advocate for the patient's wishes.
Rationale: In this scenario, the nurse's primary ethical responsibility is to respect the patient's autonomy and advocate for their wishes, even if it conflicts with the family's desires. Patient advocacy involves supporting the patient's right to make informed decisions about their care. While family input is important, the patient's autonomy should be prioritized in end-of-life care decisions.

Question 78: Correct Answer: D) Provide a safe environment to prevent falls
Rationale: Patients with multiple myeloma are at risk for pathological fractures, and preventing falls is essential to reduce this risk. Options A, B, and C focus on other aspects of care but do not directly address the risk of fractures in this scenario.

Question 79: Correct Answer: C) Loss of normal cell function
Rationale: Carcinogenesis involves the transformation of normal cells into cancer cells, leading to the loss of normal cellular function. This process disrupts the regulation of cell growth and differentiation, resulting in uncontrolled proliferation. Options A, B, and D are incorrect as rapid cell differentiation, controlled cell growth, and maintenance of cellular homeostasis are not indicative of the changes seen in carcinogenesis.

Question 80: Correct Answer: B) It ensures consistency and accountability in care delivery
Rationale: Adherence to the Scope and Standards of Practice in oncology nursing plays a crucial role in maintaining quality of practice by ensuring consistency and accountability in care delivery. These guidelines provide a framework for safe and effective nursing practice, promoting standardized approaches that enhance quality and patient outcomes. Options A, C, and D are incorrect as adherence to standards supports, rather than limits, nurses' ability to provide high-quality, safe care through established best practices.

Question 81: Correct Answer: B) Participating in research studies related to oncology care
Rationale: The correct answer is B because participating in research studies related to oncology care is a key component of the Standards of Practice for an OCN. Options A, C, and D are incorrect as they involve tasks that are outside the scope of practice for an OCN.

Question 82: Correct Answer: D) Chaplain
Rationale: Chaplains are integral members of the interdisciplinary team who specialize in providing spiritual care, emotional support, and addressing existential concerns for patients like David nearing the end of life. While pharmacists focus on medications, palliative care physicians manage medical aspects, and music therapists offer therapeutic interventions, chaplains cater to the spiritual and emotional needs of patients and their families during this challenging phase.

Question 83: Correct Answer: C) Lugano Classification
Rationale: The Lugano Classification is specifically designed for staging lymphomas, including Hodgkin and non-Hodgkin lymphomas. It categorizes the disease based on the involvement of lymph nodes and extralymphatic organs. The other options mentioned, such as the FIGO Staging System, are used for gynecological cancers, not lymphomas.

Question 84: Correct Answer: B) Suggesting Mark attend a support group for caregivers
Rationale: Attending a support group for caregivers (Option B) can provide Mark with emotional support, coping strategies, and a sense of community, which can help alleviate his symptoms of caregiver fatigue. Encouraging Mark to increase caregiving responsibilities (Option A) and ignore his own needs (Option C) can exacerbate his fatigue. Taking on additional work (Option D) as a distraction does not address the root cause of his symptoms.

Question 85: Correct Answer: B) Provide information on patient rights and resources for advocacy
Rationale: Empowering the patient with knowledge about their rights and available support services is essential in addressing discrimination concerns. Encouraging the patient to switch insurance or conceal their diagnosis does not address the systemic issue of discrimination and may have negative consequences in the long run.

Question 86: Correct Answer: D) Grade IV
Rationale: Grade IV tumors are poorly differentiated with marked variation in cell size and shape, indicating a higher risk of aggressive behavior. Grades I, II, and III represent progressively more differentiated tumor cells, making Grade IV the appropriate choice for David's case.

Question 87: Correct Answer: C) Preventing organ dysfunction
Rationale: The primary goal of early recognition and treatment of sepsis in oncology patients is to prevent organ dysfunction by promptly addressing the underlying infection and supporting vital organ function. Fever is a common symptom of sepsis, antibiotic therapy is essential for treating the infection, and fluid intake should be managed judiciously based on the patient's hemodynamic status.

Question 88: Correct Answer: A) It involves regular screening tests to detect cancer recurrence early.
Rationale: Cancer surveillance in survivorship care entails the ongoing monitoring of patients through regular screening tests to detect any signs of cancer recurrence at an early stage. This proactive approach helps in timely intervention and management if cancer does return. It is a crucial aspect of survivorship care to ensure the best possible outcomes for cancer survivors. Managing treatment side effects is important but not the sole focus of cancer surveillance, and it is generally applicable to all types of cancer, emphasizing the need for continuous monitoring.

Question 89: Correct Answer: D) Providing Comfort Measures
Rationale: Providing comfort measures such as pain management, positioning for comfort, and emotional support is crucial in managing cardiovascular symptoms in cancer patients under palliative care. Administering chemotherapy, monitoring electrolyte levels, and encouraging physical activity are not

primary interventions for managing cardiovascular symptoms in this context.

Question 90: Correct Answer: B) Engage in open communication with partners
Rationale: Engaging in open communication with partners can help cancer survivors address body image issues affecting their sexuality. Sharing feelings, concerns, and needs can foster understanding and intimacy in relationships. Options A, C, and D are incorrect as avoiding discussions, ignoring impacts, or comparing to unrealistic standards can exacerbate body image issues and hinder sexual well-being.

Question 91: Correct Answer: C) Palliative care specialists, oncologists, nurses, and social workers
Rationale: Palliative care in cancer patients is a multidisciplinary approach involving a team of healthcare professionals, including palliative care specialists, oncologists, nurses, social workers, and other specialists. This team works together to address the physical, emotional, and psychosocial needs of the patient, providing comprehensive care throughout the cancer journey.

Question 92: Correct Answer: C) Monitoring and maintaining adequate oxygenation
Rationale: Monitoring and maintaining adequate oxygenation is essential in preventing complications associated with increased intracranial pressure as hypoxia can exacerbate brain edema. Encouraging the Valsalva maneuver, administering IV fluids rapidly, and keeping the patient in a supine position can increase intracranial pressure and worsen the condition.

Question 93: Correct Answer: B) Provide information on patient assistance programs offered by pharmaceutical companies
Rationale: Offering information on patient assistance programs provided by pharmaceutical companies can help Sarah access financial support for her treatment. These programs often offer discounts, rebates, or free medications to eligible patients, easing the financial burden associated with chemotherapy. Options A, C, and D are not appropriate as they suggest actions that may compromise Sarah's treatment and well-being.

Question 94: Correct Answer: C) Engaging in self-reflection and seeking cultural knowledge
Rationale: Enhancing cultural competence in oncology nursing practice involves engaging in self-reflection, seeking cultural knowledge, and understanding the impact of culture on healthcare. Continuing education, avoiding interactions with diverse patients, or stereotyping based on cultural backgrounds can hinder the development of cultural competence and impede the delivery of quality care.

Question 95: Correct Answer: C) Positioning the patient upright
Rationale: Positioning the patient upright is a non-pharmacological intervention that can help improve dyspnea in patients with advanced cancer by optimizing lung expansion and ventilation. Administering high-flow oxygen may not always be beneficial and can even be harmful in certain cases. Benzodiazepines are not first-line for dyspnea in cancer patients. Non-invasive ventilation may be considered in specific situations but is not the initial intervention.

Question 96: Correct Answer: B) Engaging in regular physical exercise and relaxation techniques
Rationale: Engaging in regular physical exercise and relaxation techniques (Option B) can help alleviate physical symptoms of stress and improve overall well-being for caregivers like Alex. Ignoring physical symptoms (Option A), increasing caffeine intake (Option C), and avoiding seeking professional help (Option D) can worsen his condition and lead to further caregiver fatigue.

Question 97: Correct Answer: B) Refer him to a financial counselor to discuss budgeting and cost-saving strategies
Rationale: Referring Mr. Patel to a financial counselor can help him explore budgeting options, cost-saving strategies, and potential financial assistance programs. This intervention can empower the patient to make informed decisions about managing his treatment expenses effectively. Options A, C, and D are not recommended as they propose actions that may compromise Mr. Patel's health and treatment outcomes.

Question 98: Correct Answer: C) Social worker
Rationale: Collaboration with a social worker is crucial in oncology nursing practice as they provide vital support to patients and families in coping with emotional, financial, and social challenges that arise during cancer treatment. While other healthcare professionals play important roles, the social worker specifically addresses the psychosocial aspects of care, making them the most essential collaborator in this context.

Question 99: Correct Answer: C) Decreased motivation
Rationale: Caregiver fatigue often manifests as decreased motivation due to the physical, emotional, and mental strain of providing care. This can lead to feelings of burnout and exhaustion. Options A, B, and D are incorrect as caregiver fatigue typically results in decreased energy levels, disrupted sleep patterns, and difficulty concentrating.

Question 100: Correct Answer: D) DIC can lead to microvascular thrombosis and organ failure.
Rationale: DIC is characterized by both bleeding and thrombosis, with microvascular thrombosis contributing to organ dysfunction and failure. Isolated thrombocytopenia is not typical of DIC, and the condition is not self-limiting but requires prompt management to prevent complications.

Question 101: Correct Answer: A) Randomized controlled trial
Rationale: Randomized controlled trials (RCTs) are considered the gold standard in clinical research as they randomly assign participants to either the new treatment or standard treatment group, minimizing bias and providing reliable evidence on treatment effectiveness. Observational, cross-sectional, and case-control studies have different objectives and methodologies.

Question 102: Correct Answer: C) Metastatic cancer
Rationale: Metastatic cancer is a common cause of spinal cord compression in oncology patients as cancer cells can spread to the spine and exert pressure on the spinal cord. Benign tumors, osteoporosis, and muscle strain are less likely to cause spinal cord compression.

Question 103: Correct Answer: B) Hepatitis
Rationale: Hepatitis is a common immune-related adverse event associated with immunotherapy, presenting with symptoms such as elevated liver enzymes. Dermatitis involves skin inflammation, nephritis involves kidney inflammation, and pancreatitis involves pancreas inflammation, which are less likely in this scenario.

Question 104: Correct Answer: B) Transcutaneous electrical nerve stimulation (TENS)
Rationale: TENS is a non-invasive treatment that can help relieve neuropathic pain by delivering electrical impulses to the affected area. Acupuncture may also provide pain relief, while hot and cold therapy and aromatherapy are more focused on relaxation and may not directly address neuropathic symptoms.

Question 105: Correct Answer: C) John actively engages with all team members to address the patient's holistic needs.
Rationale: Effective collaboration in oncology nursing involves actively engaging with all members of the multidisciplinary team to address the holistic needs of the patient. This approach ensures comprehensive care coordination and integration of diverse expertise for optimal patient care. Options A, B, and D represent actions that do not reflect effective collaboration as they involve working in silos or disregarding input from other team members.

Question 106: Correct Answer: C) ANCC Magnet Recognition Program
Rationale: The ANCC Magnet Recognition Program acknowledges nursing excellence and quality patient care in healthcare organizations. Achieving Magnet status demonstrates a commitment to providing exceptional nursing care, including in oncology units. Nurses in Magnet-recognized facilities are known for their high levels of expertise, professionalism, and dedication to improving patient outcomes.

Question 107: Correct Answer: C) Providing comprehensive discharge instructions
Rationale: By offering detailed and clear discharge instructions, an Oncology Certified Nurse can enhance care continuity for cancer patients transitioning between care settings. Options A, B, and D are counterproductive to promoting care continuity and

patient-centered care.
Question 108: Correct Answer: D) VTE in cancer patients is associated with a higher risk of recurrence.
Rationale: Cancer patients with VTE have a significantly higher risk of recurrence compared to non-cancer patients. Immobility, cancer-related pro-coagulant factors, and chemotherapy contribute to the increased risk of VTE in cancer patients. VTE is more common and carries a worse prognosis in cancer patients due to the underlying hypercoagulable state associated with malignancy.
Question 109: Correct Answer: B) Providing education on relaxation techniques and sleep hygiene
Rationale: Providing education on relaxation techniques and sleep hygiene can empower Mrs. Smith to manage her fear of recurrence and insomnia effectively. Encouraging avoidance, administering sedatives as the first-line treatment, or discharging her from follow-up care without addressing her concerns can worsen her psychosocial distress and compromise her well-being.
Question 110: Correct Answer: A) Hodgkin lymphoma
Rationale: Reed-Sternberg cells are unique to Hodgkin lymphoma, aiding in its diagnosis. Pancreatic, ovarian, and brain cancers do not exhibit Reed-Sternberg cells, differentiating them from Hodgkin lymphoma.
Question 111: Correct Answer: B) Encourage her to join a support group for cancer patients.
Rationale: Encouraging Ms. Johnson to join a support group for cancer patients is the most appropriate intervention as it provides her with a platform to share experiences, receive emotional support, and cope better with her anxiety and fear. Providing medical information alone may not address her emotional needs. Administering medication without consultation can be risky and may not address the underlying psychosocial concerns. Advising her to avoid discussing her feelings can lead to emotional suppression and hinder her coping mechanisms.
Question 112: Correct Answer: B) Acknowledging Mr. Patel's emotions and providing empathy
Rationale: Acknowledging Mr. Patel's feelings of guilt and worthlessness, and providing empathy, validates his emotions and fosters a trusting nurse-patient relationship. Minimizing his feelings, avoiding discussions, or criticizing him can invalidate his experiences, worsen his distress, and hinder effective psychosocial support.
Question 113: Correct Answer: A) Fatigue and weight loss
Rationale: Fatigue and unexplained weight loss are symptoms that may indicate cancer recurrence and should be reported to the healthcare provider promptly. Options B, C, and D are symptoms that are less likely to be directly associated with cancer recurrence in prostate cancer survivors.
Question 114: Correct Answer: B) Planning
Rationale: Planning is the phase where the nurse sets priorities based on the data collected during the assessment phase. Goals and outcomes are established, and interventions are determined in this phase. Assessment involves data collection, implementation carries out the plan, and evaluation determines the effectiveness of the care provided.
Question 115: Correct Answer: B) Testicular biopsy for sperm extraction
Rationale: Testicular biopsy for sperm extraction is a standard approach for sperm preservation in male cancer patients.
Options A, C, and D are not related to fertility preservation in this context.
Question 116: Correct Answer: B) Provide a safe and nonjudgmental environment for the screening.
Rationale: Creating a safe and supportive environment is essential for addressing the unique concerns of sexual and gender minority patients. By acknowledging and respecting Alex's fears, the nurse can build trust and ensure a positive healthcare experience. Options A, C, and D neglect the importance of sensitivity and inclusivity in providing care to LGBTQ+ individuals.
Question 117: Correct Answer: A) Aromatherapy
Rationale: Aromatherapy, the use of essential oils to promote relaxation and alleviate symptoms, is a suitable complementary modality for managing anxiety and insomnia in cancer patients. Reflexology focuses on pressure points in the feet, chiropractic care on spinal health, and hypnotherapy on altered states of consciousness, making them less appropriate for Mrs. Patel's symptoms.
Question 118: Correct Answer: C) Offer emotional support and explore alternative solutions.
Rationale: In palliative care settings, addressing the emotional needs of patients is paramount. The nurse should provide empathy, support, and work collaboratively with the healthcare team to find practical solutions that respect Jamie's gender identity. Options A, B, and D do not prioritize the holistic care approach needed in palliative care for gender-diverse individuals.
Question 119: Correct Answer: C) Creating a calming bedtime routine
Rationale: Creating a calming bedtime routine can help improve sleep quality by signaling to the body that it is time to rest. Warm milk before bedtime (option A) may have a soothing effect but is not as comprehensive as a bedtime routine. Administering sedative medication (option B) should be a last resort and is not a non-pharmacologic measure. Progressive muscle relaxation (option D) can help with relaxation but may not address the overall sleep routine.
Question 120: Correct Answer: D) Tunneled Central Venous Catheter
Rationale: A tunneled central venous catheter is a type of central venous access device that is suitable for long-term chemotherapy administration due to its durability and reduced risk of infection compared to other options. Options A and B are more suitable for short-term use, while option C is typically used for hemodialysis, not chemotherapy.
Question 121: Correct Answer: C) Metastasis
Rationale: Metastasis is the process by which cancer cells break away from the primary tumor, travel through the bloodstream or lymphatic system, and form secondary tumors in distant organs. Metaplasia (Option A) is the reversible change in cell type in response to stress or injury. Hyperplasia (Option B) is an increase in the number of cells in a tissue. Dysplasia (Option D) refers to abnormal changes in cell size, shape, and organization, which can be a precursor to cancer but is not the spread of cancer cells.
Question 122: Correct Answer: C) Hormone replacement therapy
Rationale: Hormone replacement therapy can help alleviate vaginal dryness in cancer survivors like Mrs. Lee by restoring estrogen levels. Options A, B, and D can exacerbate vaginal dryness. Scented soaps can irritate the vaginal area, water-based lubricants are recommended for intercourse, and tight-fitting synthetic underwear can worsen vaginal dryness by trapping moisture.
Question 123: Correct Answer: C) Hydromorphone
Rationale: Hydromorphone, a potent opioid analgesic, is commonly used for managing breakthrough cancer pain due to its rapid onset and short duration of action. Ibuprofen is not suitable for breakthrough pain. Oxycodone is a long-acting opioid and not ideal for rapid relief. Prednisone is a corticosteroid and not typically used for breakthrough pain management.
Question 124: Correct Answer: C) Urologist
Rationale: A urologist specializes in the diagnosis and treatment of conditions affecting the male reproductive system and urinary tract, making them the most appropriate healthcare provider to manage Mark's issues with sexual dysfunction and urinary incontinence. While an oncologist may oversee Mark's cancer follow-up, a primary care physician focuses on overall health maintenance, and a gynecologist specializes in female reproductive health.
Question 125: Correct Answer: A) Colectomy
Rationale: Colectomy is the surgical removal of a portion of the colon affected by cancer. This procedure aims to remove the tumor along with nearby lymph nodes to prevent the spread of cancer. Cholecystectomy involves removing the gallbladder,

nephrectomy is the removal of a kidney, and thyroidectomy is the removal of the thyroid gland, none of which are specific to colon cancer treatment.

Question 126: Correct Answer: D) Facilitating a conversation with a spiritual counselor
Rationale: A spiritual counselor can help Sarah explore her fears, find meaning in her situation, and address her existential concerns. This intervention focuses on supporting her spiritual well-being and can provide comfort and guidance during this challenging time. The other options do not directly address Sarah's spiritual distress and may not offer the same level of support and understanding.

Question 127: Correct Answer: C) Providing education and resources
Rationale: Offering education and resources to family caregivers helps empower them to provide better care, understand the patient's condition, and cope with the challenges they may face. Options A, B, and D are counterproductive and can lead to increased stress and isolation for the caregiver, making them incorrect choices.

Question 128: Correct Answer: C) Muffled heart sounds
Rationale: A key clinical feature of cardiac tamponade is muffled heart sounds due to the presence of fluid around the heart, which dampens the sound of cardiac contractions. Hypotension, tachycardia, and pulsus paradoxus (decrease in systolic blood pressure during inspiration) are more commonly associated with cardiac tamponade than hypertension, bradycardia, or increased pulse pressure.

Question 129: Correct Answer: D) Low-dose computed tomography (LDCT)
Rationale: LDCT is recommended for lung cancer screening in individuals with a significant smoking history. PSA test is for prostate cancer, mammography for breast cancer, and colonoscopy for colorectal cancer.

Question 130: Correct Answer: B) To remove the entire prostate gland.
Rationale: A radical prostatectomy is a surgical procedure that involves the complete removal of the prostate gland along with surrounding tissues. This intervention is aimed at treating localized prostate cancer and preventing its spread. Options A, C, and D are incorrect as radical prostatectomy does not involve removing the testicles, performing radiation therapy, or administering hormone therapy.

Question 131: Correct Answer: C) Providing relaxation techniques
Rationale: Providing relaxation techniques such as deep breathing exercises, guided imagery, and progressive muscle relaxation can help oncology patients manage their anxiety levels. Encouraging isolation and limiting communication with the healthcare team can exacerbate feelings of loneliness and distress. Avoiding discussing emotions can hinder the patient's ability to cope and seek support.

Question 132: Correct Answer: A) Pericardial effusion
Rationale: The scenario describes signs and symptoms suggestive of cardiac tamponade due to pericardial effusion, such as jugular venous distention, crackles, and pedal edema. Pericardial effusion can lead to impaired cardiac function, resulting in dyspnea, chest pain, and edema. Atrial fibrillation, hypertension, and pulmonary embolism may present with similar symptoms but are less likely in this context.

Question 133: Correct Answer: C) Pneumonia
Rationale: The patient's symptoms of fever, chills, and productive cough with purulent sputum following chemotherapy with docetaxel are more indicative of bacterial pneumonia rather than pneumonitis. While pneumonitis can occur as a side effect of chemotherapy, the presence of purulent sputum suggests an infectious etiology, making pneumonia the more likely diagnosis in this case. Pulmonary embolism, although a consideration, is less likely given the productive cough and purulent sputum.

Question 134: Correct Answer: B) Delegating tasks appropriately
Rationale: Effective leadership for an OCN leading a multidisciplinary team involves delegating tasks appropriately based on team members' strengths, fostering collaboration, and empowering team members. Micromanagement, avoiding team meetings, and imposing decisions without input can hinder team dynamics and overall effectiveness.

Question 135: Correct Answer: B) Pneumonitis
Rationale: In this scenario, the patient's symptoms of dyspnea, cough, and fever following immunotherapy are suggestive of pneumonitis, which is an inflammatory response in the lungs. While pulmonary embolism and pneumonia can present similarly, the temporal relationship with immunotherapy favors pneumonitis over other differential diagnoses. Acute respiratory distress syndrome (ARDS) typically presents with more severe respiratory distress and diffuse lung infiltrates on imaging.

Question 136: Correct Answer: A) Acupuncture involves the insertion of thin needles into specific points on the body to help restore the flow of energy.
Rationale: Acupuncture is a traditional Chinese medicine practice that involves the insertion of thin needles into specific points on the body to help restore the flow of energy, known as Qi. It is commonly used to manage symptoms such as nausea, pain, and fatigue in cancer patients. Options B, C, and D are incorrect as they do not accurately describe acupuncture, leading to the correct answer.

Question 137: Correct Answer: B) Sepsis
Rationale: Sepsis is a common trigger for DIC in cancer patients due to the release of pro-inflammatory cytokines and activation of the coagulation cascade. Hypertension, Hypothyroidism, and Peptic Ulcer Disease are not typically associated with triggering DIC in cancer patients.

Question 138: Correct Answer: B) Peripheral neuropathy
Rationale: Chemotherapy-induced peripheral neuropathy is a common side effect characterized by tingling, numbness, and pain in the hands and feet. It is crucial for nurses to educate patients like Sarah about this potential side effect to ensure early detection and management. Hypertension, constipation, and hyperthyroidism are not typically associated with chemotherapy.

Question 139: Correct Answer: C) To focus on comfort and quality of life
Rationale: Hospice care aims to enhance the quality of life for patients with terminal illnesses by focusing on pain management, symptom control, and emotional support rather than pursuing curative treatments. Providing comfort and dignity during the end-of-life phase is the central tenet of hospice care.

Question 140: Correct Answer: A) Genetics
Rationale: Genetics is a non-modifiable risk factor as certain genetic mutations can predispose individuals to colorectal cancer. High cholesterol levels, occupational exposure, and diet are modifiable risk factors and do not directly influence the genetic predisposition to colorectal cancer.

Question 141: Correct Answer: B) By promoting evidence-based care
Rationale: Professional practice evaluation in oncology nursing promotes evidence-based care by encouraging nurses to align their practice with the latest research and guidelines. This process enhances patient outcomes, fosters a culture of continuous learning, and elevates the quality of care provided. Contrary to increasing workload or limiting growth opportunities, professional practice evaluation empowers nurses to deliver high-quality, evidence-based care while supporting their professional development and job satisfaction.

Question 142: Correct Answer: C) Colitis
Rationale: Colitis is a common immune-related adverse event associated with immunotherapy, presenting as inflammation of the colon leading to symptoms such as diarrhea, abdominal pain, and sometimes blood in the stool. Pneumonitis (A) refers to lung inflammation, hepatitis (B) is liver inflammation, and nephritis (D) is kidney inflammation, which are distinct immune-related adverse events with different clinical manifestations compared to colitis.

Question 143: Correct Answer: D) Reduced Work Hours
Rationale: Reduced work hours or the inability to work during cancer treatment often leads to a loss of income for patients, creating a significant financial concern. While transportation

costs, housing expenses, and childcare fees are also important considerations, the loss of income due to reduced work hours can have a substantial impact on a patient's financial stability. Addressing this concern may require exploring options such as disability benefits, flexible work arrangements, or financial assistance programs.

Question 144: Correct Answer: B) Emotional intelligence
Rationale: Emotional intelligence is crucial for OCNs in leadership roles as it enables them to empathize with patients, communicate effectively, and navigate complex situations with sensitivity. Conflict resolution, time management, and technical proficiency are important skills but may not directly impact patient advocacy and quality care access as significantly as emotional intelligence does.

Question 145: Correct Answer: B) Offering emotional support and shared experiences to individuals facing similar challenges
Rationale: Support groups offer a platform for cancer patients to connect with others facing similar challenges, share experiences, and provide emotional support. While medical treatment, research, and appointment coordination are essential components of oncology care, the primary role of support groups is to address the psychosocial needs of patients.

Question 146: Correct Answer: B) White blood cell count
Rationale: Monitoring the white blood cell count is essential during chemotherapy to assess for myelosuppression and risk of infection. Changes in serum potassium levels, serum albumin levels, and BUN are not typically directly related to chemotherapy toxicity.

Question 147: Correct Answer: B) Engaging in regular physical exercise and maintaining a healthy diet.
Rationale: Engaging in regular physical exercise and maintaining a healthy diet are essential self-care strategies to combat compassion fatigue. These activities help in reducing stress, improving overall well-being, and boosting resilience. Options A, C, and D are incorrect as they promote avoidance of emotions, overworking, and isolation, which can exacerbate compassion fatigue rather than alleviate it.

Question 148: Correct Answer: C) Accommodating religious practices in care plans
Rationale: Respecting and accommodating patients' religious beliefs within care plans can enhance their coping mechanisms, emotional well-being, and overall treatment experience. Disregarding or pressuring patients to abandon their religious practices can lead to feelings of isolation and distress. By integrating religious considerations into care, nurses can provide holistic support tailored to individual needs.

Question 149: Correct Answer: A) Xerostomia
Rationale: Xerostomia (dry mouth) is a common alteration in functioning seen in oncology patients undergoing radiation therapy to the head and neck region due to damage to salivary glands. Hypotension (option B), increased visual acuity (option C), and enhanced olfactory senses (option D) are not typically associated with this type of radiation therapy.

Question 150: Correct Answer: C) Enhancement of the immune system to target cancer cells
Rationale: Immunotherapy works by enhancing the body's immune system to recognize and attack cancer cells. Options A and B are incorrect as they refer to mechanisms that promote cancer growth. Option D is incorrect as immunosuppression is not the goal of immunotherapy in cancer treatment.

OCN Exam Practice Questions [SET 3]

Question 1: Scenario: David, a 55-year-old colorectal cancer survivor, is interested in joining a support group to connect with others who have gone through similar experiences. Which benefit of survivorship support groups is David likely seeking?
A) Financial Assistance
B) Physical Rehabilitation
C) Emotional Support
D) Medication Management

Question 2: Scenario: John, a caregiver for his mother with terminal cancer, is experiencing burnout and emotional distress. What is the most appropriate action to support John in this situation?
A) Suggesting John to ignore his own well-being and focus solely on his mother
B) Encouraging John to take breaks and engage in self-care activities
C) Advising John to isolate himself from friends and family to focus on caregiving
D) Instructing John to avoid seeking professional help and manage everything independently

Question 3: Which non-pharmacologic comfort measure is commonly used in end-of-life care to alleviate pain and promote relaxation?
A) Therapeutic Touch
B) High-dose Opioids
C) Chemotherapy
D) Antibiotics

Question 4: Which modifiable risk factor is strongly associated with an increased risk of developing various types of cancers, including lung, throat, and bladder cancer?
A) Diet
B) Exercise
C) Smoking
D) Occupation

Question 5: Scenario: John, a 60-year-old male with lung cancer, is participating in a clinical trial comparing two different chemotherapy regimens. Which type of clinical trial compares the effectiveness of two or more treatments?
A) Phase I
B) Phase II
C) Phase III
D) Phase IV

Question 6: Which medication is commonly prescribed for chemotherapy-induced nausea and vomiting (CINV) prophylaxis?
A) Metoclopramide
B) Lorazepam
C) Ondansetron
D) Furosemide

Question 7: Sarah, a 30-year-old leukemia patient, is struggling with financial difficulties due to her cancer treatment expenses. Which support intervention would best address her psychosocial needs in this situation?
A) Providing information on financial assistance programs
B) Offering her complementary therapy sessions
C) Referring her to a social worker for financial counseling
D) Suggesting she start a crowdfunding campaign

Question 8: Which resource can help cancer patients understand their insurance coverage, rights, and options for financial assistance?
A) Hospital Billing Department
B) Online Medical Forums
C) Cancer Treatment Centers of America
D) Patient Advocacy Organizations

Question 9: How can family dynamics be affected by the long-term effects of cancer treatment?
A) Strengthening of family bonds
B) Decreased need for communication
C) Financial stability due to reduced treatment costs
D) Strain on relationships due to caregiving challenges

Question 10: Ms. Patel, a 45-year-old female with breast cancer, presents with edema of the face, neck, and upper extremities, along with headache and visual disturbances. What is the most likely diagnosis?
A) Lymphedema
B) Cushing's syndrome
C) Superior vena cava syndrome
D) Myasthenia gravis

Question 11: Which intervention is essential in the management of tumor lysis syndrome?
A) Hydration
B) Hyperventilation
C) Furosemide administration
D) Potassium supplementation

Question 12: Which of the following is a primary purpose of documentation in oncology nursing practice?
A) To increase workload for nurses
B) To ensure accurate communication among healthcare team members
C) To violate patient confidentiality
D) To avoid legal responsibilities

Question 13: Sarah, a 40-year-old patient, is struggling with complicated grief following the loss of her child to cancer. Which nursing approach would be most appropriate in supporting Sarah through this challenging time?
A) Suggesting Sarah move on and focus on the present
B) Encouraging Sarah to avoid reminders of her child
C) Providing a safe space for Sarah to express her emotions
D) Minimizing the significance of Sarah's loss

Question 14: Which of the following is a common cause of cardiac tamponade in oncology patients?
A) Pulmonary embolism
B) Pneumonia
C) Pericardial metastases
D) Gastric ulcer

Question 15: Which of the following is a primary function of the immune system in cancer patients?
A) Promoting tumor growth
B) Suppressing the immune response
C) Recognizing and destroying cancer cells
D) Inducing cancer metastasis

Question 16: Mr. Patel, a 60-year-old patient with lung cancer, experiences severe fatigue that impacts his ability to participate in social activities. Which approach should the nurse recommend to help Mr. Patel manage his fatigue?
A) Limiting fluid intake to reduce bathroom trips
B) Encouraging Mr. Patel to push through the fatigue
C) Scheduling activities during times of peak energy
D) Avoiding daytime naps to improve nighttime sleep

Question 17: Mr. Johnson, a 65-year-old patient with small cell lung cancer, presents with confusion, nausea, and hyponatremia. His serum osmolality is low, and urine osmolality is high. Which condition is most likely responsible for his symptoms?
A) Syndrome of inappropriate antidiuretic hormone secretion (SIADH)
B) Cerebral salt-wasting syndrome
C) Hypothyroidism
D) Diabetes insipidus

Question 18: Which factor can significantly impact intimacy in cancer patients?
A) Financial burden
B) Physical appearance changes
C) Increased emotional support
D) Improved communication skills

Question 19: What is the typical source of stem cells for an allogeneic blood and marrow transplant?
A) Patient's own stem cells
B) Identical twin's stem cells
C) Unrelated donor's stem cells
D) Animal donor's stem cells

Question 20: What is a common characteristic of anticipatory grief?
A) Occurs only after the actual loss
B) Involves emotional preparation for an impending loss
C) Resolves quickly once the loss happens
D) Is less intense than grief experienced post-loss

Question 21: Scenario: John, a cancer patient transitioning from active treatment to palliative care, requires assistance with symptom management and emotional support. Which team member is best suited to address John's holistic needs during this care continuum phase?
A) Oncologist
B) Psychologist
C) Dietitian
D) Case Manager

Question 22: What is an essential component of a caregiver support program for oncology patients?
A) Providing no information about the patient's treatment
B) Offering respite care services
C) Discouraging self-care activities
D) Avoiding communication with healthcare team

Question 23: James, a 50-year-old testicular cancer survivor, is experiencing loss of libido after treatment. Which of the following factors can contribute to sexual dysfunction in male cancer survivors?
A) Regular exercise
B) Hormonal changes
C) Healthy diet
D) Adequate sleep

Question 24: Which of the following is a key goal of palliative care in cancer patients?
A) Curing the cancer
B) Providing emotional support only
C) Managing symptoms and improving quality of life
D) Discontinuing all cancer treatments

Question 25: Ms. Patel, a 65-year-old patient with end-stage COPD, is experiencing severe shortness of breath at rest. Which of the following pharmacological interventions is most appropriate for managing her dyspnea?
A) Inhaled corticosteroids
B) Long-acting beta-agonists
C) Nebulized morphine
D) Oral antibiotics

Question 26: Ms. Johnson, a 65-year-old patient with advanced pancreatic cancer, is experiencing severe pain despite being on regular analgesics. Which of the following is the most appropriate intervention for her palliative care?
A) Initiate a trial of corticosteroids
B) Consider switching to a different opioid
C) Start low-dose methotrexate
D) Increase the dose of the current opioid

Question 27: How can healthcare professionals best support bereaved individuals in end-of-life care settings?
A) Disregarding cultural beliefs
B) Offering empathy and compassion
C) Avoiding discussions about the deceased
D) Providing generic responses

Question 28: As a leader in oncology nursing practice, what is a critical aspect for an OCN to prioritize when mentoring novice nurses?
A) Discouraging questions
B) Providing constructive feedback
C) Limiting exposure to diverse cases
D) Avoiding sharing experiences

Question 29: Which of the following is a key component of maintaining quality of practice in oncology nursing?
A) Ignoring patient feedback
B) Avoiding professional development opportunities
C) Engaging in continuous learning and skill development
D) Following outdated treatment protocols

Question 30: Which of the following is an essential component of personal protective equipment (PPE) for oncology nurses to ensure environmental health and safety?
A) Stethoscope
B) Safety goggles
C) Penlight
D) Watch

Question 31: Which organization focuses on accrediting healthcare organizations based on quality and safety standards, including those related to oncology care?
A) The Joint Commission
B) American Cancer Society
C) Centers for Medicare & Medicaid Services (CMS)
D) National Cancer Institute (NCI)

Question 32: Scenario: Emily, a 55-year-old female patient, is receiving treatment for colorectal cancer. She presents with diarrhea as a side effect of chemotherapy. What is a critical site-specific consideration for managing Emily's chemotherapy-induced diarrhea?
A) Encouraging a low-fiber diet
B) Administering antiemetics
C) Monitoring for mucositis
D) Providing oral rehydration solutions

Question 33: How can a nurse best address spiritual needs in a diverse oncology patient population?
A) Encouraging patients to adopt the nurse's spiritual beliefs
B) Providing a quiet space for prayer or meditation
C) Ignoring spiritual aspects of care
D) Suggesting patients abandon their spiritual practices

Question 34: Mr. Patel, a 70-year-old male, has a history of prostate cancer. Which of the following statements best describes the concept of prevalence in epidemiology?
A) The number of deaths due to prostate cancer in a specific population
B) The proportion of individuals with prostate cancer who are

currently alive
C) The likelihood of developing prostate cancer in a lifetime
D) The number of individuals diagnosed with prostate cancer at a specific point in time

Question 35: Which of the following is a common form of discrimination concerns faced by cancer survivors in the care continuum?
A) Ageism
B) Gender equality
C) Socioeconomic parity
D) Religious tolerance

Question 36: Which of the following activities can help oncology nurses prevent burnout and compassion fatigue?
A) Working overtime to stay on top of patient care
B) Setting boundaries between work and personal life
C) Avoiding taking breaks during shifts
D) Ignoring signs of stress and emotional exhaustion

Question 37: Which of the following is a common mechanism of carcinogenesis?
A) Apoptosis promotion
B) DNA repair enhancement
C) Angiogenesis inhibition
D) Genetic mutations

Question 38: Which intervention is commonly used to manage depression in cancer patients?
A) Avoid discussing emotions with patients
B) Prescribe antidepressant medication
C) Ignore signs of distress
D) Limit access to support services

Question 39: Mrs. Lee, a 45-year-old colorectal cancer survivor, is anxious about the risk of cancer recurrence. As part of survivorship care, which of the following strategies should be included in Mrs. Lee's follow-up plan to address her concerns about cancer recurrence?
A) Psychological support and counseling services
B) Herbal supplements and alternative therapies
C) Avoiding all types of physical activity
D) Smoking and alcohol consumption

Question 40: What is a key nursing intervention for managing lymphedema in oncology patients?
A) Application of heat packs
B) Avoiding limb movement
C) Compression therapy
D) Massaging the affected area

Question 41: Scenario: Taylor, a 40-year-old lesbian woman, is scheduled for a double mastectomy as part of her breast cancer treatment. She expresses concerns about body image and intimacy post-surgery. What is the most appropriate nursing response?
A) Dismiss Taylor's concerns as common post-surgery anxieties.
B) Provide resources on body image support groups for cancer survivors.
C) Avoid discussing intimacy issues to respect Taylor's privacy.
D) Recommend hormone therapy to address body image concerns.

Question 42: How can oncology nurses contribute to the advancement of evidence-based practice in cancer care?
A) By relying solely on tradition and past practices
B) By engaging in continuous learning and professional development
C) By avoiding involvement in research initiatives
D) By isolating themselves from interdisciplinary collaboration

Question 43: Sarah, a 45-year-old patient with metastatic ovarian cancer, is struggling with feelings of isolation and loneliness due to her diagnosis. Which nursing intervention would be most effective in addressing Sarah's psychosocial distress?
A) Ignoring Sarah's emotional needs
B) Encouraging Sarah to isolate herself further
C) Connecting Sarah with a counselor for emotional support
D) Dismissing Sarah's feelings as common in cancer patients

Question 44: Mrs. Patel, a 55-year-old patient with ovarian cancer, is receiving her first cycle of chemotherapy with cisplatin. She develops dyspnea, chest tightness, and hypotension. What is the priority nursing action for managing suspected anaphylaxis in this patient?
A) Administer corticosteroids intravenously
B) Administer a bolus of normal saline
C) Place the patient in Trendelenburg position
D) Stop the infusion and administer epinephrine

Question 45: Ms. Johnson, a 45-year-old female, presents to the clinic for her routine check-up. She has a family history of breast cancer. Which screening modality is recommended for Ms. Johnson based on her risk factors?
A) Colonoscopy
B) Mammography
C) Prostate-specific antigen (PSA) test
D) Pap smear

Question 46: Which of the following legal principles guides oncology nurses in protecting patient information?
A) Breaching patient confidentiality
B) HIPAA regulations
C) Sharing patient information without consent
D) Ignoring patient privacy concerns

Question 47: Mr. Smith, a 65-year-old male patient with metastatic prostate cancer, presents with severe bone pain. Which of the following pharmacological interventions is most appropriate for managing his pain?
A) NSAIDs
B) Acetaminophen
C) Opioids
D) Corticosteroids

Question 48: How can oncology nurses best support patients experiencing 'Loss of personal control' in their cancer journey?
A) Encouraging patients to research treatment options independently
B) Providing clear information and involving them in decision-making
C) Discouraging questions to prevent confusion
D) Minimizing discussions about prognosis

Question 49: Which immune checkpoint protein is commonly targeted in immunotherapy for cancer?
A) PD-1
B) HER2
C) EGFR
D) BCR-ABL

Question 50: Which of the following best describes the concept of cancer survivorship?
A) The period from diagnosis through the end of treatment
B) The time after cancer treatment ends
C) The time from symptom onset to diagnosis
D) The period of active cancer treatment

Question 51: Which type of insurance plan typically has the lowest monthly premium but higher out-of-pocket costs when care is needed?
A) Health Maintenance Organization (HMO)
B) Preferred Provider Organization (PPO)
C) Exclusive Provider Organization (EPO)

D) High Deductible Health Plan (HDHP)

Question 52: What is a critical aspect of providing culturally competent care to sexual and gender minorities in oncology?
A) Making assumptions based on stereotypes
B) Respecting and embracing diversity
C) Using conversion therapy techniques
D) Excluding family involvement in care decisions

Question 53: Mrs. Wong, a 70-year-old female with a history of non-Hodgkin lymphoma, presents with facial swelling, dilated veins over the chest wall, and difficulty breathing when lying flat. She also reports a persistent cough and chest pain. What is the most likely diagnosis?
A) Congestive heart failure
B) Chronic obstructive pulmonary disease (COPD) exacerbation
C) Superior vena cava syndrome
D) Pericarditis

Question 54: What is the impact of depression on cancer treatment outcomes?
A) Improves response to treatment
B) Has no effect on treatment outcomes
C) Increases risk of non-compliance with treatment
D) Reduces side effects of treatment

Question 55: Which of the following is a common risk factor for developing pneumonitis in oncology patients?
A) Hypertension
B) Smoking history
C) Diabetes mellitus
D) Osteoarthritis

Question 56: James, a 50-year-old patient with prostate cancer, mentions feeling overwhelmed by the amount of information provided during educational sessions. Which approach would be most effective in addressing his learning barrier?
A) Providing additional reading materials
B) Breaking down information into smaller segments
C) Increasing the pace of information delivery
D) Using technical medical terminology

Question 57: Which of the following is NOT a common cause of Syndrome of Inappropriate Antidiuretic Hormone Secretion (SIADH)?
A) Small cell lung cancer
B) Head injury
C) Ovarian cancer
D) Renal failure

Question 58: Scenario: Lisa, a 35-year-old leukemia patient, is worried about the financial implications of her treatment and the impact on her family. Which insurance option provides coverage for lost wages during her treatment period?
A) Disability Insurance
B) Long-Term Care Insurance
C) Vision Insurance
D) Dental Insurance

Question 59: Scenario: John, a 60-year-old male, has been diagnosed with colon cancer. The oncologist informs him that the cancer has spread to nearby lymph nodes but not to distant organs. Which stage of cancer is John most likely in based on this information?
A) Stage I
B) Stage II
C) Stage III
D) Stage IV

Question 60: Which laboratory finding is typically associated with septic shock in oncology patients?
A) Hypernatremia
B) Hypokalemia
C) Lactic acidosis
D) Hypoglycemia

Question 61: Scenario: Mark, a 60-year-old prostate cancer patient, is considering participating in a clinical trial for a new treatment. The nurse explains the importance of research ethics in oncology. Which statement best exemplifies ethical considerations in oncology research?
A) "Patients in clinical trials are not provided with full information to avoid bias."
B) "Informed consent is not necessary for oncology research involving experimental treatments."
C) "Research involving human subjects must prioritize participant safety and well-being."
D) "Oncology research ethics do not require transparency in reporting study outcomes."

Question 62: Which communication approach is recommended for an OCN when discussing treatment options with a patient?
A) Providing only one option
B) Using complex language to sound professional
C) Encouraging patient involvement in decision-making
D) Rushing through the discussion

Question 63: Ms. Johnson, a 45-year-old breast cancer patient, presents with progressive dyspnea, dry cough, and bilateral lung infiltrates on imaging. She is currently receiving radiation therapy to the chest. What is the most likely diagnosis?
A) Pulmonary embolism
B) Pneumonitis
C) Lung metastases
D) Pleural effusion

Question 64: Mr. Patel, a 60-year-old patient with colorectal cancer, is experiencing severe diarrhea as a side effect of chemotherapy. Which intervention should the nurse prioritize to address Mr. Patel's altered functioning?
A) Administering antidiarrheal medication
B) Increasing fluid intake
C) Recommending a high-fiber diet
D) Encouraging bed rest

Question 65: Mrs. Lee, a 70-year-old patient with chronic lymphocytic leukemia (CLL), presents with splenomegaly. Which of the following complications is commonly associated with splenomegaly in patients with CLL?
A) Thrombocytopenia
B) Hypertension
C) Hyperglycemia
D) Hypokalemia

Question 66: Which member of the interdisciplinary team is responsible for assessing and addressing the psychological and emotional needs of patients undergoing cancer treatment?
A) Occupational Therapist
B) Psychologist
C) Speech Therapist
D) Respiratory Therapist

Question 67: What is a key consideration for an OCN regarding resource utilization in oncology nursing practice?
A) Prioritizing cost over patient outcomes
B) Collaborating with interdisciplinary teams to optimize resource allocation
C) Hoarding supplies for personal use
D) Disregarding evidence-based practice guidelines

Question 68: Which of the following is an example of a psychosocial intervention for cancer patients?
A) Chemotherapy
B) Radiation therapy
C) Support groups
D) Surgery

Question 69: Which communication strategy is beneficial for an OCN when addressing end-of-life care discussions with a patient and their family?
A) Avoiding the topic to prevent distress
B) Using euphemisms to soften the conversation
C) Providing honest and clear information
D) Rushing through the discussion to save time

Question 70: Ms. Johnson, a 40-year-old female, is diagnosed with breast cancer. Which of the following statements best explains the pathophysiology of breast cancer?
A) Breast cancer is caused by a viral infection in the breast tissue.
B) Breast cancer is characterized by the presence of non-cancerous lumps in the breast.
C) Breast cancer originates in the milk ducts or lobules of the breast.
D) Breast cancer is a result of hormonal imbalance in the body.

Question 71: Which intervention is recommended for managing cancer-related fatigue?
A) Limiting fluid intake
B) Avoiding physical activity
C) Cognitive-behavioral therapy
D) Isolation from social interactions

Question 72: Which of the following strategies can help oncology nurses build resilience and cope with the emotional challenges of caring for cancer patients?
A) Suppressing emotions and avoiding self-reflection
B) Engaging in peer support groups and debriefing sessions
C) Taking on additional work responsibilities to stay busy
D) Relying solely on medication for stress management

Question 73: Which technology is commonly used to deliver precise radiation doses to tumors while minimizing exposure to surrounding healthy tissues?
A) Intensity-modulated radiation therapy (IMRT)
B) Magnetic resonance imaging (MRI)
C) Positron emission tomography (PET)
D) Computed tomography (CT)

Question 74: Mrs. Smith, a 50-year-old patient with metastatic breast cancer, is experiencing significant fatigue impacting her daily activities. What intervention should the nurse recommend to address Mrs. Smith's altered functioning?
A) Encouraging regular exercise
B) Increasing caffeine intake
C) Prescribing antidepressant medication
D) Suggesting frequent naps

Question 75: Scenario: Mark, an Oncology Nurse Leader, encourages open communication, collaboration, and shared decision-making among team members. Which leadership approach is Mark utilizing?
A) Democratic leadership
B) Servant leadership
C) Charismatic leadership
D) Situational leadership

Question 76: Ms. Smith, a 50-year-old patient with advanced breast cancer, is experiencing limited mobility due to bone metastases in her spine. Which nursing intervention is essential to prevent complications related to immobility?
A) Encourage active range of motion exercises
B) Administer intravenous bisphosphonates
C) Apply warm compresses to the affected areas
D) Initiate a turning schedule to prevent pressure ulcers

Question 77: Which member of the interdisciplinary team is responsible for managing pain and symptom control to ensure optimal comfort for patients receiving palliative care?
A) Radiologist
B) Oncology Nurse
C) Anesthesiologist
D) Palliative Care Physician

Question 78: Which of the following is a key role of an Oncology Certified Nurse (OCN) in the navigation and coordination of care for cancer patients?
A) Performing surgical procedures
B) Administering chemotherapy
C) Educating patients about treatment options
D) Managing hospital finances

Question 79: Which factor is crucial in determining the prognosis of cancer patients?
A) Family history of cancer
B) Socioeconomic status
C) Emotional well-being
D) Genetic mutations

Question 80: Which of the following is a recommended strategy for reducing the risk of subsequent malignancies in cancer survivors?
A) Avoiding regular screenings
B) Limiting physical activity
C) Smoking cessation
D) Excessive sun exposure

Question 81: During a chemotherapy session, a patient receiving treatment for breast cancer develops severe neutropenia. Which of the following cells is primarily affected in neutropenia?
A) Lymphocytes
B) Monocytes
C) Neutrophils
D) Eosinophils

Question 82: Which non-verbal communication cue is important for an OCN when providing emotional support to a patient?
A) Crossing arms
B) Maintaining a neutral facial expression
C) Leaning in attentively
D) Checking the time frequently

Question 83: Scenario: John, a 40-year-old African American patient, is undergoing chemotherapy for colon cancer. He mentions that he follows certain dietary restrictions based on his cultural beliefs. How should the oncology nurse best support John's cultural dietary practices?
A) Disregard John's dietary restrictions to ensure he receives proper nutrition.
B) Encourage John to abandon his cultural dietary practices during treatment.
C) Respect John's dietary restrictions and work with the healthcare team to accommodate them.
D) Inform John that cultural dietary practices have no impact on cancer treatment.

Question 84: What is the primary goal of patient advocacy in oncology nursing practice?
A) Making decisions on behalf of the patient
B) Respecting patient autonomy and preferences

C) Limiting patient access to treatment information
D) Prioritizing the nurse's opinions over the patient's choices

Question 85: Which of the following actions by an oncology nurse demonstrates professional accountability?
A) Blaming others for errors
B) Falsifying patient records
C) Seeking continuing education opportunities
D) Disregarding evidence-based practice

Question 86: Which aspect of collaboration is essential for promoting positive patient outcomes in oncology care?
A) Maintaining professional silos
B) Limited communication with team members
C) Sharing information openly and transparently
D) Avoiding interprofessional discussions

Question 87: Scenario: Sarah, a 45-year-old breast cancer survivor, presents with persistent cough and shortness of breath. She underwent chemotherapy and radiation therapy five years ago. Imaging reveals a new mass in her lung. Which term best describes this new mass?
A) Secondary malignancy
B) Recurrent cancer
C) Metastatic tumor
D) Benign growth

Question 88: Mr. Garcia, a 60-year-old patient with advanced prostate cancer, is experiencing intractable nausea and vomiting. Which of the following interventions is most appropriate for managing his symptoms in palliative care?
A) Initiate antiemetic therapy with a different mechanism of action
B) Increase the dose of the current antiemetic
C) Start high-dose radiation therapy
D) Perform a surgical procedure

Question 89: Which member of the interdisciplinary team is primarily responsible for coordinating the overall care plan and ensuring seamless transitions between different care settings in the care continuum?
A) Nurse Practitioner
B) Case Manager
C) Pharmacist
D) Radiology Technologist

Question 90: Which of the following is a common cause of Superior vena cava syndrome in oncology patients?
A) Lung Cancer
B) Breast Cancer
C) Prostate Cancer
D) Colorectal Cancer

Question 91: Scenario: Emily, a 30-year-old female, has a family history of ovarian cancer. She is considering genetic testing to assess her risk. Which gene mutation is commonly associated with hereditary breast and ovarian cancer syndrome?
A) BRCA1
B) KRAS
C) APC
D) PTEN

Question 92: Which medication is commonly used for managing mucositis in cancer patients undergoing chemotherapy?
A) Nystatin oral suspension
B) Cetirizine
C) Sucralfate mouthwash
D) Dexamethasone

Question 93: Mrs. Garcia, a 70-year-old patient with brain metastases, is experiencing seizures. Which nursing action is appropriate during a seizure episode?
A) Restraining the patient's movements
B) Placing a padded tongue blade in the patient's mouth
C) Turning the patient to the side
D) Administering anticoagulants immediately

Question 94: Scenario: John, a 50-year-old male, presents with colorectal cancer. He works in a chemical plant where he is exposed to various carcinogens. Which modifiable risk factor is most likely contributing to his condition?
A) Smoking
B) High intake of processed meats
C) Sedentary lifestyle
D) Occupational exposure to carcinogens

Question 95: Which lifestyle factor is NOT typically recommended to reduce the risk of cancer recurrence?
A) Regular physical activity
B) Healthy diet rich in fruits and vegetables
C) Smoking cessation
D) Excessive alcohol consumption

Question 96: Ms. Johnson, a 45-year-old female, is diagnosed with breast cancer. Which histologic classification system is commonly used to classify breast cancer based on the tumor's appearance under the microscope?
A) Gleason score
B) Bloom-Richardson grade
C) Ann Arbor staging
D) Lugano classification

Question 97: Scenario: A patient named Ms. Brown is receiving radiation therapy for breast cancer. What precaution should the oncology nurse take to ensure environmental health and safety during radiation therapy sessions?
A) Administering radiation therapy in a well-ventilated room
B) Allowing visitors to stay with the patient during radiation sessions
C) Wearing lead apron and thyroid shield when in the radiation therapy room
D) Using the same linens for multiple patients receiving radiation therapy

Question 98: Which type of cancer has shown significant responses to immunotherapy?
A) Breast cancer
B) Prostate cancer
C) Melanoma
D) Leukemia

Question 99: Mrs. Smith, a 60-year-old female, has a family history of ovarian cancer. Which screening test should be considered for Mrs. Smith to aid in the early detection of ovarian cancer?
A) Pap smear
B) Mammography
C) CA-125 blood test
D) Colonoscopy

Question 100: Which of the following is a common trigger for Disseminated Intravascular Coagulation (DIC) in oncology patients?
A) Hypocalcemia
B) Sepsis
C) Hypernatremia
D) Hypoalbuminemia

Question 101: What is a key component of providing culturally congruent care in oncology nursing?
A) Imposing the nurse's cultural values on the patient
B) Recognizing and respecting cultural differences

C) Avoiding discussions about cultural beliefs
D) Assuming all patients have the same cultural background

Question 102: Which medication is considered the first-line treatment for moderate to severe cancer pain?
A) Acetaminophen
B) Ibuprofen
C) Morphine
D) Gabapentin

Question 103: Who can help individuals complete an advance directive?
A) Only physicians
B) Only lawyers
C) Only family members
D) Healthcare providers, lawyers, or family members

Question 104: Scenario: Emily, a 45-year-old lung cancer patient, is interested in complementary therapies to manage treatment side effects. The nurse discusses the importance of evidence-based practice when considering complementary interventions. Which statement best reflects the nurse's explanation?
A) "Complementary therapies are always safe and effective for cancer patients."
B) "Evidence-based practice involves integrating complementary therapies without evaluation."
C) "It is essential to assess the scientific evidence supporting the use of complementary therapies."
D) "Complementary therapies should be used without considering research findings."

Question 105: Which screening method is commonly used for early detection of cervical cancer?
A) Colonoscopy
B) Mammography
C) Prostate-specific antigen (PSA) test
D) Pap smear

Question 106: How can a nurse best support a patient disclosing a history of domestic violence?
A) Minimizing the impact of the abuse
B) Offering resources and support
C) Dismissing the patient's experience
D) Avoiding the topic altogether

Question 107: What is the primary purpose of a blood and marrow transplant in cancer treatment?
A) To provide pain relief
B) To prevent infection
C) To replace damaged organs
D) To restore the body's ability to produce blood cells

Question 108: What nutritional guidance is appropriate for a patient with dysphagia?
A) Encourage large bites of food
B) Recommend thin liquids
C) Suggest using straws for drinking
D) Advise pureed or soft foods

Question 109: James, a 50-year-old patient with leukemia, expresses guilt over being a burden to his family and struggles with feelings of unworthiness. He mentions feeling disconnected from his faith and spiritual beliefs. What action by the nurse is most appropriate to address James's spiritual distress?
A) Encouraging him to focus on his physical symptoms
B) Providing him with information on financial assistance programs
C) Suggesting he spends more time alone to reflect on his feelings
D) Arranging for a visit from a hospital chaplain

Question 110: John, a 55-year-old lung cancer patient, is experiencing depression following his treatment. Which nursing intervention would be most beneficial in addressing John's psychosocial needs?
A) Encouraging John to suppress his emotions to focus on recovery.
B) Referring John to a mental health professional for counseling.
C) Avoiding discussions about his emotional well-being to prevent discomfort.
D) Providing John with a list of self-help books to manage his depression.

Question 111: Ms. Patel, a 50-year-old patient with multiple myeloma, is experiencing hypercalcemia. Which of the following interventions is most appropriate for managing hypercalcemia in patients with multiple myeloma?
A) Encouraging increased fluid intake
B) Administering furosemide
C) Limiting weight-bearing activities
D) Providing a high-calcium diet

Question 112: Which medication is commonly used for managing cancer-related fatigue in palliative care?
A) Methylphenidate
B) Alprazolam
C) Diphenhydramine
D) Sertraline

Question 113: Which medication is commonly used to reduce intracranial pressure in oncologic emergencies?
A) Insulin
B) Furosemide
C) Aspirin
D) Morphine

Question 114: Ms. Johnson, a 55-year-old patient with advanced breast cancer, has been experiencing profound sadness and hopelessness since her recent diagnosis. She expresses feelings of guilt and struggles to find meaning in her life. Which of the following interventions by the oncology nurse would be most appropriate in addressing Ms. Johnson's psychosocial distress?
A) Encouraging her to avoid discussing her feelings
B) Referring her to a support group for cancer survivors
C) Minimizing the importance of her emotional state
D) Dismissing her concerns as common in cancer patients

Question 115: What is the immediate management priority for a patient with suspected spinal cord compression in oncology?
A) Administer pain medication
B) Initiate radiation therapy
C) Perform surgery
D) Provide corticosteroids

Question 116: Mrs. Patel, a 70-year-old patient receiving chemotherapy for breast cancer, complains of palpitations, dizziness, and fatigue. Her ECG shows a rapid irregular rhythm with absent P waves. Which of the following interventions is the most appropriate for managing her symptoms?
A) Administering beta-blockers
B) Initiating anticoagulation therapy
C) Performing electrical cardioversion
D) Starting rate control with calcium channel blockers

Question 117: Which preventive health practice is recommended for reducing the risk of skin cancer?
A) Avoiding sunscreen
B) Tanning bed use
C) Wearing protective clothing and hats
D) Excessive sun exposure

Question 118: Which of the following activities is within the scope of practice for an Oncology Certified Nurse (OCN)?
A) Ordering diagnostic imaging tests
B) Developing individualized care plans for patients
C) Performing surgical procedures
D) Prescribing medications

Question 119: James, a 55-year-old lung cancer patient, is experiencing fatigue and low libido. Which intervention would be most appropriate to address James's concerns regarding intimacy?
A) Recommend engaging in vigorous physical exercise to boost energy levels.
B) Provide education on managing fatigue and its impact on intimacy.
C) Advise complete avoidance of any sexual activity to conserve energy.
D) Prescribe over-the-counter energy supplements without further assessment.

Question 120: Mrs. Lee, a 60-year-old patient with ovarian cancer, is diagnosed with SIADH. Which intervention is essential in the management of SIADH to increase serum sodium levels?
A) Fluid restriction
B) Administering hypotonic fluids
C) Increasing ADH levels
D) Encouraging free water intake

Question 121: Which classification system is used to stage melanoma based on the thickness of the primary tumor and the presence of ulceration?
A) Gleason Score
B) Breslow Thickness Classification
C) Clark's Level of Invasion
D) Ann Arbor Staging System

Question 122: Which intervention is a priority in providing end-of-life care to a terminally ill cancer patient?
A) Administering aggressive chemotherapy
B) Initiating palliative care services
C) Scheduling additional radiation therapy sessions
D) Performing a major surgical procedure

Question 123: Which of the following is a common side effect of biotherapy?
A) Hair loss
B) Nausea and vomiting
C) Fatigue
D) Immune-related adverse events

Question 124: James, a 55-year-old lung cancer patient, feels overwhelmed by his treatment side effects. How can the nurse best address James' loss of personal control?
A) Encouraging him to avoid asking questions about his treatment
B) Involving him in developing strategies to manage side effects
C) Making decisions about his care without his input
D) Minimizing discussions about treatment side effects

Question 125: How can urinary obstruction in oncology patients manifest clinically?
A) Bradycardia
B) Hemoptysis
C) Suprapubic pain
D) Vision changes

Question 126: Which of the following is a potential barrier to learning for oncology patients receiving chemotherapy?
A) Regular follow-up appointments
B) Adequate pain management
C) Chemotherapy side effects
D) Emotional support groups

Question 127: Mr. Johnson, a 55-year-old patient, recently completed his chemotherapy for prostate cancer. He is now experiencing fatigue, muscle weakness, and difficulty with balance. Which of the following rehabilitation interventions would be most appropriate for Mr. Johnson to address his symptoms?
A) Aerobic exercise program
B) Resistance training
C) Yoga and meditation
D) Massage therapy

Question 128: Which route of administration is preferred for rapid pain relief in a patient with breakthrough cancer pain?
A) Oral
B) Transdermal
C) Intravenous
D) Subcutaneous

Question 129: Mrs. Brown, a 70-year-old female, is diagnosed with colorectal cancer. What is the key pathophysiological feature of colorectal cancer?
A) Colorectal cancer is characterized by the formation of polyps in the colon.
B) Colorectal cancer is primarily caused by a deficiency of vitamin D.
C) Colorectal cancer is a type of skin cancer that affects the colon.
D) Colorectal cancer is a result of inflammation in the small intestine.

Question 130: Scenario: Sarah, a 45-year-old female with breast cancer, is considering enrolling in a clinical trial to explore a new targeted therapy. Which phase of a clinical trial focuses on assessing the safety and dosage of the new treatment?
A) Phase I
B) Phase II
C) Phase III
D) Phase IV

Question 131: Mr. Patel, a 60-year-old patient with head and neck cancer, experiences self-esteem issues due to changes in his appearance post-surgery. What nursing intervention would be most beneficial for Mr. Patel?
A) Discourage Mr. Patel from using mirrors
B) Offer supportive counseling and resources
C) Minimize discussions about body image concerns
D) Advise Mr. Patel to focus solely on physical recovery

Question 132: Scenario: Sarah, a 35-year-old breast cancer survivor, is concerned about returning to work after her treatment. She is worried about how her financial situation will be affected due to the time off work. What should the oncology nurse prioritize when discussing employment concerns with Sarah?
A) Providing information on disability insurance benefits
B) Suggesting Sarah to quit her job for a less stressful lifestyle
C) Advising Sarah to not disclose her cancer history to her employer
D) Recommending Sarah to avoid seeking financial assistance

Question 133: Ms. Johnson, a 58-year-old breast cancer survivor, completed her chemotherapy six months ago. She now presents with persistent numbness and tingling in her fingers and toes. Which chronic side effect is she likely experiencing?
A) Fatigue
B) Neuropathy
C) Lymphedema
D) Cognitive impairment

Question 134: Mr. Smith, a 65-year-old male, presents with a

family history of breast cancer. Which non-modifiable risk factor plays a significant role in his predisposition to cancer?
A) Gender
B) Smoking history
C) Physical activity level
D) Diet rich in fruits and vegetables

Question 135: Scenario: John, a 60-year-old male patient, is undergoing treatment for prostate cancer. He is experiencing urinary incontinence post-prostatectomy. What is a vital site-specific consideration for managing John's urinary incontinence?
A) Encouraging high fluid intake
B) Performing Kegel exercises
C) Administering laxatives
D) Recommending weight-bearing exercises

Question 136: Which of the following best describes the role of an Oncology Certified Nurse (OCN) in resource utilization?
A) Ordering excessive supplies to ensure availability
B) Minimizing waste by accurately assessing patient needs
C) Using outdated equipment to cut costs
D) Ignoring budget constraints for patient comfort

Question 137: Which chronic side effect is a potential complication of long-term use of corticosteroids in oncology patients?
A) Osteoporosis
B) Peripheral edema
C) Hyperglycemia
D) Hypertension

Question 138: Ms. Garcia, a 55-year-old patient with leukemia, presents with chest pain and shortness of breath. An echocardiogram reveals a reduced left ventricular ejection fraction of 40%. Which of the following medications is indicated for the management of chemotherapy-induced cardiomyopathy in this patient?
A) Digoxin
B) Amiodarone
C) Carvedilol
D) Furosemide

Question 139: Scenario: Emily, a 30-year-old lymphoma survivor, is concerned about her fertility after undergoing chemotherapy. Which option is NOT a fertility preservation method that could have been discussed with Emily before treatment?
A) Egg Freezing
B) Ovarian Transposition
C) Sperm Banking
D) Hormone Replacement Therapy

Question 140: Scenario: Emily, a 55-year-old patient with end-stage cancer, is experiencing severe nausea and vomiting despite antiemetic therapy. The healthcare provider decides to add another medication to help control Emily's symptoms. Which pharmacologic comfort measure is most appropriate for Emily's situation?
A) Ondansetron
B) Haloperidol
C) Diazepam
D) Prochlorperazine

Question 141: Scenario: John, a 60-year-old cancer patient, has recently lost his sister, who was his primary caregiver during his treatment. He is experiencing intense sadness and loneliness. What is an essential aspect to consider when providing bereavement support to John?
A) Minimize discussions about his sister to avoid triggering emotions.
B) Acknowledge John's grief and validate his feelings of loss.
C) Discourage John from seeking professional help for his grief.
D) Advise John to distract himself by focusing solely on his treatment.

Question 142: Which action is a part of the implementation phase of the nursing process?
A) Setting patient goals
B) Collecting patient data
C) Administering medication
D) Evaluating patient outcomes

Question 143: What is the mechanism of action of chemotherapy in targeting cancer cells?
A) Inducing apoptosis
B) Promoting cell division
C) Enhancing DNA repair
D) Inhibiting immune response

Question 144: Which of the following laboratory findings is characteristic of tumor lysis syndrome?
A) Hypercalcemia
B) Hypokalemia
C) Hyperphosphatemia
D) Hypouricemia

Question 145: Mr. Lee, a 60-year-old male with a history of testicular cancer, presents with facial plethora, dyspnea, and hoarseness. He reports a recent onset of chest pain and cough. What is the most likely cause of his symptoms?
A) Aortic dissection
B) Superior vena cava syndrome
C) Esophageal cancer
D) Thyroid storm

Question 146: Which intervention is a priority in managing increased intracranial pressure in oncologic emergencies?
A) Administering antibiotics
B) Providing oxygen therapy
C) Initiating chemotherapy
D) Elevating the head of the bed

Question 147: Which action by the nurse best demonstrates culturally congruent care in oncology nursing practice?
A) Providing printed materials in English only
B) Using medical jargon to explain treatment options
C) Respecting the patient's cultural beliefs and practices
D) Disregarding the patient's family preferences

Question 148: Which integrative modality is known for its potential to reduce chemotherapy-induced nausea and vomiting?
A) Acupuncture
B) Reiki
C) Tai Chi
D) Homeopathy

Question 149: How can healthcare providers support cancer patients experiencing sexual dysfunction?
A) Dismissing the importance of sexual health
B) Providing resources for sexual counseling
C) Encouraging avoidance of intimacy
D) Minimizing the impact of cancer treatment on sexual function

Question 150: Scenario: You are preparing to administer chemotherapy to a patient named Mr. Lee. Which of the following actions demonstrates safe handling practices to promote environmental health and safety in the oncology setting?
A) Crushing chemotherapy tablets without wearing gloves
B) Using a needle and syringe to transfer chemotherapy drugs between vials
C) Spiking IV bags containing chemotherapy drugs in the

patient's room
D) Wearing a disposable gown when handling chemotherapy drugs

ANSWER WITH DETAILED EXPLANATION SET [3]

Question 1: Correct Answer: C) Emotional Support
Rationale: Survivorship support groups offer emotional support, camaraderie, and a sense of community for individuals navigating life after cancer. While financial assistance, physical rehabilitation, and medication management are essential aspects of survivorship care, emotional support through shared experiences and peer connections is often a primary motivation for joining support groups like the one David is considering.

Question 2: Correct Answer: B) Encouraging John to take breaks and engage in self-care activities
Rationale: Self-care is essential for caregivers to prevent burnout and maintain their well-being. Encouraging John to take breaks and engage in activities that bring him joy can help alleviate emotional distress. Options A, C, and D are incorrect as they neglect John's need for self-care and may exacerbate his burnout.

Question 3: Correct Answer: A) Therapeutic Touch
Rationale: Therapeutic Touch involves the use of gentle hand movements around the patient's body to promote relaxation and alleviate pain. This technique is often used in end-of-life care to provide comfort and support. High-dose opioids, chemotherapy, and antibiotics are not non-pharmacologic comfort measures and are typically used for different purposes in cancer care.

Question 4: Correct Answer: C) Smoking
Rationale: Smoking is a well-established modifiable risk factor for cancer. It contains carcinogens that can damage cells in the body, leading to the development of cancer. Diet and exercise play important roles in overall health but are not as directly linked to cancer development as smoking. Occupation may expose individuals to certain carcinogens, but smoking has a more significant and direct impact on cancer risk.

Question 5: Correct Answer: C) Phase III
Rationale: Phase III trials compare the effectiveness of different treatments, often against the current standard of care. These trials involve a larger number of participants and are crucial in determining which treatment option is superior. Options A, B, and D do not specifically focus on comparing treatments, making them incorrect choices.

Question 6: Correct Answer: C) Ondansetron
Rationale: Ondansetron is a first-line antiemetic medication for CINV prophylaxis due to its high efficacy and minimal side effects. Metoclopramide is more commonly used for gastroparesis. Lorazepam may be used for anxiety-related nausea but is not a primary choice for CINV prophylaxis. Furosemide is a diuretic and not indicated for CINV.

Question 7: Correct Answer: C) Referring her to a social worker for financial counseling
Rationale: Referring Sarah to a social worker for financial counseling would be the most appropriate intervention to address her psychosocial needs related to financial difficulties. Social workers can provide valuable support in navigating financial assistance programs, managing expenses, and accessing resources to alleviate the burden of treatment costs. While complementary therapy, crowdfunding, and information on financial assistance programs are helpful, direct financial counseling from a social worker would offer Sarah personalized support and guidance.

Question 8: Correct Answer: D) Patient Advocacy Organizations
Rationale: Patient Advocacy Organizations specialize in helping individuals navigate the healthcare system, understand their insurance coverage, and explore options for financial assistance. These organizations provide valuable support and resources to empower patients in making informed decisions about their care. While the Hospital Billing Department can offer information on billing and payments, they may not provide comprehensive guidance on insurance coverage and financial assistance. Online Medical Forums and Cancer Treatment Centers of America focus more on medical treatment rather than insurance and financial aspects, making Patient Advocacy Organizations the most suitable resource for addressing these specific needs.

Question 9: Correct Answer: D) Strain on relationships due to caregiving challenges
Rationale: The long-term effects of cancer treatment can strain family dynamics, particularly when caregiving challenges persist. Financial burdens, changes in roles, and emotional stress can impact relationships within the family. While some families may experience strengthened bonds through adversity, the overall impact tends to involve increased strain on relationships as they navigate the ongoing challenges associated with cancer treatment. It is essential for families to communicate openly, seek support, and address caregiving challenges to maintain healthy family dynamics.

Question 10: Correct Answer: C) Superior vena cava syndrome
Rationale: The constellation of symptoms described is classic for superior vena cava syndrome, which can occur due to compression or invasion of the superior vena cava by a tumor, such as in patients with breast cancer. Lymphedema typically presents with localized swelling, while Cushing's syndrome is characterized by specific signs such as central obesity and moon face. Myasthenia gravis presents with muscle weakness and fatigue, not edema and visual disturbances.

Question 11: Correct Answer: A) Hydration
Rationale: Adequate hydration is crucial in managing tumor lysis syndrome to prevent renal damage by promoting the excretion of uric acid and other waste products. Hydration helps maintain renal perfusion and urine output. Hyperventilation, furosemide administration, and potassium supplementation are not primary interventions for tumor lysis syndrome and may not address the underlying pathophysiology.

Question 12: Correct Answer: B) To ensure accurate communication among healthcare team members
Rationale: Documentation in oncology nursing serves as a crucial tool for ensuring accurate communication among healthcare team members, promoting continuity of care, and enhancing patient safety. It is not intended to increase workload unnecessarily, violate patient confidentiality, or avoid legal responsibilities. Proper documentation helps in tracking patient progress, treatment plans, and outcomes, thereby supporting effective decision-making and quality care delivery.

Question 13: Correct Answer: C) Providing a safe space for Sarah to express her emotions
Rationale: Complicated grief requires a supportive environment for emotional expression. By providing a safe space, Sarah can process her feelings of loss, guilt, and sadness. Encouraging avoidance, minimizing the loss, or suggesting moving on can invalidate Sarah's emotions and impede the healing process.

Question 14: Correct Answer: C) Pericardial metastases
Rationale: Pericardial metastases, the spread of cancer to the pericardium, are a common cause of cardiac tamponade in oncology patients. This condition leads to the accumulation of fluid in the pericardial sac, compressing the heart and impairing its function. Pulmonary embolism, pneumonia, and gastric ulcer are not typically associated with cardiac tamponade in oncology patients.

Question 15: Correct Answer: C) Recognizing and destroying cancer cells
Rationale: The correct answer is C because one of the crucial roles of the immune system in cancer patients is to recognize and eliminate cancer cells. Options A, B, and D are incorrect as the immune system's main function is to identify and target abnormal cells, including cancer cells, for destruction. This process is essential in preventing the progression and spread of cancer within the body.

Question 16: Correct Answer: C) Scheduling activities during times of peak energy
Rationale: Limiting fluid intake can lead to dehydration. Pushing through fatigue can worsen symptoms. Scheduling activities during times of peak energy allows patients to engage in

meaningful tasks when they feel most energetic, optimizing their participation in social activities.

Question 17: Correct Answer: A) Syndrome of inappropriate antidiuretic hormone secretion (SIADH)
Rationale: SIADH is characterized by the excessive release of antidiuretic hormone (ADH), leading to water retention, dilutional hyponatremia, and concentrated urine. In contrast, cerebral salt-wasting syndrome presents with hyponatremia and dehydration due to renal salt loss. Hypothyroidism and diabetes insipidus do not typically cause the same pattern of hyponatremia seen in SIADH.

Question 18: Correct Answer: B) Physical appearance changes
Rationale: Physical appearance changes due to cancer treatment such as hair loss, weight fluctuations, or surgical scars can have a profound impact on a patient's self-esteem and body image, directly affecting their sense of intimacy. While financial burden, emotional support, and communication skills are important aspects of cancer care, they may not directly influence intimacy as significantly as physical changes do.

Question 19: Correct Answer: C) Unrelated donor's stem cells
Rationale: Allogeneic transplants involve using stem cells from a donor, which can be a family member, unrelated donor, or cord blood unit. The donor must be a close genetic match to the recipient to reduce the risk of complications.

Question 20: Correct Answer: B) Involves emotional preparation for an impending loss
Rationale: Anticipatory grief involves the process of mourning and emotional preparation for an anticipated loss, allowing individuals to gradually adjust to the idea of impending death. Options A, C, and D do not accurately describe anticipatory grief, making option B the correct answer.

Question 21: Correct Answer: D) Case Manager
Rationale: During the care continuum, a case manager plays a pivotal role in coordinating various aspects of a patient's care, including symptom management, emotional support, and resource allocation. While oncologists focus on medical treatments, psychologists address mental health, and dietitians provide nutritional guidance, the case manager ensures seamless transitions and comprehensive support for patients like John.

Question 22: Correct Answer: B) Offering respite care services
Rationale: Respite care services allow caregivers to take a break from their responsibilities, recharge, and attend to their own needs. This can prevent caregiver burnout and improve the quality of care provided to the patient. Options A, C, and D are counterproductive and can lead to increased stress and isolation for the caregiver, making them incorrect choices.

Question 23: Correct Answer: B) Hormonal changes
Rationale: Hormonal changes, such as those resulting from cancer treatment, can significantly impact libido and contribute to sexual dysfunction in male cancer survivors. Regular exercise, healthy diet, and adequate sleep may have positive effects but are not direct contributors to sexual dysfunction in this context.

Question 24: Correct Answer: C) Managing symptoms and improving quality of life
Rationale: Palliative care in cancer patients aims to manage symptoms such as pain, nausea, and fatigue, while also focusing on improving the patient's quality of life. It does not focus on curing the cancer itself but rather on providing holistic care that addresses physical, emotional, and spiritual needs.

Question 25: Correct Answer: C) Nebulized morphine
Rationale: In end-stage COPD, dyspnea can be severe and debilitating. Nebulized morphine is often used in palliative care to relieve dyspnea by acting as a respiratory depressant. Inhaled corticosteroids and long-acting beta-agonists are more commonly used for managing COPD exacerbations and maintenance therapy. Oral antibiotics are indicated for treating COPD exacerbations due to infections, not for dyspnea relief.

Question 26: Correct Answer: B) Consider switching to a different opioid
Rationale: In cases of inadequate pain control, switching to a different opioid with a different mechanism of action or adjusting the dose is recommended. Corticosteroids are not typically used for pain management in this context. Methotrexate is a chemotherapy drug and not indicated for pain relief in palliative care.

Question 27: Correct Answer: B) Offering empathy and compassion
Rationale: Offering empathy and compassion is essential in supporting bereaved individuals in end-of-life care settings. Disregarding cultural beliefs, avoiding discussions about the deceased, and providing generic responses can alienate the grieving individual and hinder the healing process.

Question 28: Correct Answer: B) Providing constructive feedback
Rationale: Prioritizing providing constructive feedback when mentoring novice nurses helps them develop skills, gain confidence, and improve their practice. Discouraging questions, limiting exposure to diverse cases, and avoiding sharing experiences can hinder the learning and growth of novice nurses under the mentorship of an OCN.

Question 29: Correct Answer: C) Engaging in continuous learning and skill development
Rationale: Continuous learning and skill development are essential components of maintaining quality of practice in oncology nursing. By staying updated on the latest evidence-based practices and participating in professional development opportunities, nurses can enhance their knowledge and skills to provide high-quality care. Options A, B, and D are incorrect as they do not align with the principles of quality practice, which emphasize the importance of ongoing learning and improvement.

Question 30: Correct Answer: B) Safety goggles
Rationale: Safety goggles are crucial in protecting the eyes from exposure to hazardous chemicals, bodily fluids, and other potentially harmful substances in the oncology setting. Stethoscope, penlight, and watch are not considered PPE and do not provide the necessary protection against environmental hazards in the oncology practice.

Question 31: Correct Answer: A) The Joint Commission
Rationale: The Joint Commission is a renowned accrediting body that evaluates and accredits healthcare organizations based on stringent quality and safety standards, including those specific to oncology care. The organization plays a crucial role in ensuring that healthcare facilities adhere to best practices in delivering oncology services, thus enhancing patient outcomes and safety.

Question 32: Correct Answer: D) Providing oral rehydration solutions
Rationale: Chemotherapy-induced diarrhea can lead to dehydration. Providing oral rehydration solutions helps maintain electrolyte balance and prevent complications. Encouraging a low-fiber diet, administering antiemetics, and monitoring for mucositis are not primary interventions for managing chemotherapy-induced diarrhea.

Question 33: Correct Answer: B) Providing a quiet space for prayer or meditation
Rationale: Acknowledging and accommodating diverse spiritual beliefs by offering a designated space for prayer or meditation demonstrates respect for patients' individual needs. Encouraging patients to embrace their own spiritual practices fosters a sense of comfort, support, and holistic care. Disregarding or imposing personal beliefs can alienate patients and hinder the therapeutic relationship.

Question 34: Correct Answer: D) The number of individuals diagnosed with prostate cancer at a specific point in time
Rationale: Prevalence refers to the total number of individuals diagnosed with a disease at a specific point in time in a given population. It provides insights into the burden of the disease. Options A, B, and C do not accurately define prevalence and are therefore incorrect.

Question 35: Correct Answer: A) Ageism
Rationale: Ageism is a prevalent form of discrimination where individuals are treated differently based on their age, impacting the care and support received by cancer survivors. Gender equality, socioeconomic parity, and religious tolerance, although

important, do not directly address the specific challenges faced by survivors due to age-related biases in the care continuum.

Question 36: Correct Answer: B) Setting boundaries between work and personal life
Rationale: Setting boundaries between work and personal life is essential for preventing burnout and compassion fatigue. By establishing clear limits on work-related activities and dedicating time for self-care and relaxation, oncology nurses can maintain a healthy work-life balance. Working overtime, avoiding breaks, and ignoring signs of stress can lead to increased fatigue, emotional exhaustion, and decreased job satisfaction.

Question 37: Correct Answer: D) Genetic mutations
Rationale: Genetic mutations play a crucial role in carcinogenesis by altering the normal functioning of genes involved in cell growth regulation. Options A, B, and C are incorrect as apoptosis promotion, DNA repair enhancement, and angiogenesis inhibition are mechanisms that typically counteract carcinogenesis rather than promote it.

Question 38: Correct Answer: B) Prescribe antidepressant medication
Rationale: Antidepressant medication is a common intervention used to manage depression in cancer patients, along with psychotherapy and supportive care. Avoiding discussions on emotions, ignoring signs of distress, and limiting access to support services can hinder the management of depression and overall patient well-being.

Question 39: Correct Answer: A) Psychological support and counseling services
Rationale: Psychological support and counseling services play a crucial role in addressing anxiety and concerns related to cancer recurrence in survivors. Options B, C, and D are not evidence-based strategies for addressing cancer recurrence concerns and may not be beneficial or appropriate for survivorship care.

Question 40: Correct Answer: C) Compression therapy
Rationale: Compression therapy is a cornerstone in managing lymphedema as it helps reduce swelling and improve lymphatic flow. Heat packs, avoiding limb movement, and massaging the affected area can exacerbate lymphedema and are not recommended interventions.

Question 41: Correct Answer: B) Provide resources on body image support groups for cancer survivors.
Rationale: Supporting patients' psychosocial needs is essential in cancer care. By offering resources on body image support groups, the nurse can help Taylor navigate post-surgery challenges and connect with others facing similar experiences. Options A, C, and D overlook the importance of addressing body image and intimacy concerns in a comprehensive and patient-centered manner.

Question 42: Correct Answer: B) By engaging in continuous learning and professional development
Rationale: Oncology nurses can advance evidence-based practice in cancer care by actively engaging in continuous learning, staying updated on the latest research, and participating in professional development activities. By enhancing their knowledge and skills, nurses can effectively integrate evidence-based interventions into practice, leading to improved patient outcomes. Relying on tradition, avoiding research involvement, or isolating from interdisciplinary collaboration can impede progress in evidence-based practice and limit the quality of care provided to cancer patients.

Question 43: Correct Answer: C) Connecting Sarah with a counselor for emotional support
Rationale: Connecting Sarah with a counselor for emotional support can provide her with a safe space to explore her feelings, develop coping strategies, and receive professional guidance. This intervention acknowledges the importance of addressing Sarah's psychosocial distress and offers her tailored support to navigate her emotional challenges. Options A, B, and D are not recommended as they neglect Sarah's emotional needs and may exacerbate her feelings of isolation.

Question 44: Correct Answer: D) Stop the infusion and administer epinephrine
Rationale: In the scenario described, the patient is exhibiting signs and symptoms of anaphylaxis. The priority nursing action is to stop the infusion and administer epinephrine to reverse the allergic reaction. Administering corticosteroids, normal saline, or placing the patient in Trendelenburg position are not the initial interventions for anaphylaxis and may delay appropriate treatment. Epinephrine is crucial in the management of anaphylaxis as it acts quickly to counteract the allergic response and stabilize the patient's condition.

Question 45: Correct Answer: B) Mammography
Rationale: Mammography is the recommended screening modality for breast cancer, especially in individuals with a family history of the disease. Colonoscopy is used for colorectal cancer screening, PSA test for prostate cancer, and Pap smear for cervical cancer.

Question 46: Correct Answer: B) HIPAA regulations
Rationale: HIPAA (Health Insurance Portability and Accountability Act) regulations are essential legal guidelines that oncology nurses must adhere to in order to protect patient information and maintain confidentiality. Breaching patient confidentiality, sharing information without consent, or ignoring privacy concerns are violations of ethical and legal standards, which can lead to legal consequences and jeopardize patient trust and safety.

Question 47: Correct Answer: C) Opioids
Rationale: Opioids are the mainstay for managing severe cancer-related bone pain. NSAIDs and acetaminophen may not provide adequate pain relief for severe bone pain. Corticosteroids are not typically used as first-line agents for cancer-related bone pain.

Question 48: Correct Answer: B) Providing clear information and involving them in decision-making
Rationale: Supporting patients experiencing 'Loss of personal control' involves providing clear information, involving them in decision-making processes, and empowering them to make informed choices. Options A, C, and D are counterproductive as they hinder patient autonomy and decision-making, exacerbating feelings of loss of control.

Question 49: Correct Answer: A) PD-1
Rationale: PD-1 (Programmed Cell Death Protein 1) is a common immune checkpoint protein targeted in immunotherapy for cancer. PD-1 inhibitors block the interaction between PD-1 on T cells and PD-L1 on cancer cells, allowing the immune system to recognize and attack the cancer cells. HER2, EGFR, and BCR-ABL are not immune checkpoint proteins targeted in immunotherapy for cancer, making A) PD-1 the correct answer.

Question 50: Correct Answer: B) The time after cancer treatment ends
Rationale: Cancer survivorship refers to the time after cancer treatment ends and focuses on the physical, emotional, and psychosocial aspects of recovery and well-being. It includes follow-up care, monitoring for recurrence, managing long-term side effects, and promoting overall health and quality of life. The other options do not fully capture the comprehensive nature of cancer survivorship.

Question 51: Correct Answer: D) High Deductible Health Plan (HDHP)
Rationale: High Deductible Health Plans (HDHPs) usually offer lower monthly premiums but come with higher deductibles and out-of-pocket costs. This option is the correct answer as it aligns with the characteristic of having lower premiums and higher costs when care is required. HMOs, PPOs, and EPOs generally have higher monthly premiums but lower out-of-pocket costs compared to HDHPs.

Question 52: Correct Answer: B) Respecting and embracing diversity
Rationale: Respecting and embracing diversity (option B) is fundamental in providing culturally competent care to sexual and gender minorities, fostering trust and understanding. Making assumptions based on stereotypes (option A) can lead to biased care. Using conversion therapy techniques (option C) is harmful and unethical. Excluding family involvement in care decisions (option D) can impact the support system crucial for patients' well-being.

Question 53: Correct Answer: C) Superior vena cava syndrome
Rationale: The symptoms described are classic for superior vena cava syndrome, often seen in patients with lymphomas. While congestive heart failure may present with similar symptoms, it typically does not cause dilated veins over the chest wall. COPD exacerbation would not explain the dilated veins and facial swelling. Pericarditis presents with chest pain that worsens with inspiration, not necessarily with facial swelling and dilated veins.

Question 54: Correct Answer: C) Increases risk of non-compliance with treatment
Rationale: Depression can significantly impact cancer treatment outcomes by increasing the risk of non-compliance with treatment regimens, leading to poorer prognosis and decreased quality of life. Improving response to treatment, having no effect on outcomes, and reducing side effects are not typical effects of depression on cancer treatment.

Question 55: Correct Answer: B) Smoking history
Rationale: Smoking history is a significant risk factor for the development of pneumonitis in oncology patients. Tobacco smoke can damage lung tissue, making individuals more susceptible to lung inflammation and injury. Hypertension, diabetes mellitus, and osteoarthritis are not directly linked to an increased risk of pneumonitis in this patient population.

Question 56: Correct Answer: B) Breaking down information into smaller segments
Rationale: Breaking down information into smaller segments can help James digest the content more effectively, reducing feelings of overwhelm. Providing additional reading materials (option A) may add to the information overload. Increasing the pace (option C) can further overwhelm him. Using technical terminology (option D) can complicate understanding, adding to his sense of being overwhelmed.

Question 57: Correct Answer: D) Renal failure
Rationale: SIADH is commonly associated with small cell lung cancer, head injury, and certain other malignancies. Renal failure is not a typical cause of SIADH. In SIADH, there is excessive release of antidiuretic hormone (ADH) leading to water retention and dilutional hyponatremia.

Question 58: Correct Answer: A) Disability Insurance
Rationale: Disability Insurance offers income replacement when a policyholder is unable to work due to illness or injury. Long-Term Care Insurance covers long-term services, not lost wages. Vision and dental insurance focus on eye and dental care, respectively, and do not address the financial concerns related to lost wages during treatment.

Question 59: Correct Answer: C) Stage III
Rationale: In colon cancer staging, Stage III indicates the cancer has spread to nearby lymph nodes but not to distant organs. Stage I is localized, Stage II may involve nearby tissues, and Stage IV signifies distant organ metastasis, making Stage III the appropriate choice for John's case.

Question 60: Correct Answer: C) Lactic acidosis
Rationale: Lactic acidosis is a common laboratory finding in septic shock, including in oncology patients. It results from tissue hypoperfusion and anaerobic metabolism due to the body's response to severe infection. Hypernatremia, hypokalemia, and hypoglycemia are not typically associated with septic shock and may indicate other conditions.

Question 61: Correct Answer: C) "Research involving human subjects must prioritize participant safety and well-being."
Rationale: Ethical considerations in oncology research emphasize the protection of participants' rights, safety, and well-being. Option C aligns with this principle by highlighting the importance of prioritizing participant safety in research studies. Options A, B, and D present unethical practices or inaccuracies regarding research ethics in oncology.

Question 62: Correct Answer: C) Encouraging patient involvement in decision-making
Rationale: In oncology nursing practice, it is essential to involve patients in treatment decisions to ensure patient-centered care. By encouraging patient involvement, OCNs empower patients, promote shared decision-making, and improve treatment adherence. Options A, B, and D are incorrect as limiting options may not consider patient preferences, complex language can confuse patients, and rushing discussions can lead to misunderstandings and anxiety.

Question 63: Correct Answer: B) Pneumonitis
Rationale: The patient's symptoms of dyspnea, dry cough, and bilateral lung infiltrates in the setting of radiation therapy to the chest are highly suggestive of radiation-induced pneumonitis. While pulmonary embolism can present with similar symptoms, the presence of lung infiltrates on imaging points towards pneumonitis as the primary diagnosis. Lung metastases and pleural effusion would typically present differently on imaging studies.

Question 64: Correct Answer: A) Administering antidiarrheal medication
Rationale: Administering antidiarrheal medication is essential in managing chemotherapy-induced diarrhea to improve patient comfort and prevent complications. Increasing fluid intake is important to prevent dehydration but may not directly address the diarrhea. A high-fiber diet can exacerbate diarrhea and is not recommended in this scenario. Encouraging bed rest may be necessary for some patients but does not target the primary symptom of diarrhea.

Question 65: Correct Answer: A) Thrombocytopenia
Rationale: Splenomegaly in CLL can lead to sequestration and destruction of platelets, resulting in thrombocytopenia. Hypertension, hyperglycemia, and hypokalemia are not typically associated with splenomegaly in CLL.

Question 66: Correct Answer: B) Psychologist
Rationale: The correct answer is B) Psychologist. Psychologists specialize in evaluating and treating the psychological and emotional aspects of cancer care, providing counseling and support to patients dealing with the emotional impact of their diagnosis and treatment. While occupational therapists focus on daily living activities, speech therapists address communication issues, and respiratory therapists manage breathing problems, psychologists are specifically trained to address the psychological needs of cancer patients.

Question 67: Correct Answer: B) Collaborating with interdisciplinary teams to optimize resource allocation
Rationale: Collaborating with interdisciplinary teams (Option B) is essential for effective resource utilization in oncology nursing practice. Prioritizing cost over patient outcomes (Option A) goes against the core principles of patient-centered care. Hoarding supplies (Option C) is unethical and impedes equitable resource distribution. Disregarding evidence-based practice guidelines (Option D) undermines quality care delivery. Therefore, the correct answer is B as it highlights the importance of teamwork in optimizing resource allocation.

Question 68: Correct Answer: C) Support groups
Rationale: Support groups play a crucial role in providing emotional support, sharing experiences, and coping strategies for cancer patients. While chemotherapy, radiation therapy, and surgery are essential medical treatments, they do not directly address the psychosocial needs of patients. Support groups offer a platform for individuals to connect with others facing similar challenges, reducing feelings of isolation and improving overall well-being.

Question 69: Correct Answer: C) Providing honest and clear information
Rationale: In end-of-life care discussions, honesty and clarity are essential for building trust, facilitating understanding, and supporting informed decision-making. OCNs should communicate openly, address concerns, and provide support during these sensitive conversations. Options A, B, and D are incorrect as avoiding the topic can lead to misunderstandings, euphemisms may obscure important information, and rushing through discussions can cause additional distress and hinder effective communication.

Question 70: Correct Answer: C) Breast cancer originates in the milk ducts or lobules of the breast.
Rationale: Breast cancer typically begins in the cells of the milk ducts or lobules of the breast. The abnormal cells can form a

tumor that may invade surrounding tissues. Options A, B, and D are incorrect as breast cancer is not caused by viral infections, non-cancerous lumps, or hormonal imbalances.

Question 71: Correct Answer: C) Cognitive-behavioral therapy
Rationale: Cognitive-behavioral therapy (CBT) is a recommended intervention for managing cancer-related fatigue. CBT helps patients identify and change negative thought patterns and behaviors that may contribute to fatigue. Limiting fluid intake, avoiding physical activity, and isolation can worsen fatigue by impacting hydration, muscle strength, and emotional well-being, respectively. Encouraging social interactions and maintaining a balanced level of physical activity are essential components of fatigue management.

Question 72: Correct Answer: B) Engaging in peer support groups and debriefing sessions
Rationale: Engaging in peer support groups and debriefing sessions allows oncology nurses to share their experiences, emotions, and coping strategies with colleagues who understand the challenges of caring for cancer patients. This promotes a sense of camaraderie, validation, and emotional support, which are essential for building resilience and preventing burnout. Suppressing emotions, taking on additional work responsibilities, and relying solely on medication are not effective long-term solutions and can contribute to increased stress and emotional strain.

Question 73: Correct Answer: A) Intensity-modulated radiation therapy (IMRT)
Rationale: IMRT is a sophisticated radiation therapy technique that allows for precise targeting of tumors with varying radiation intensities. MRI, PET, and CT scans are imaging modalities used for diagnosis and staging, not for delivering radiation therapy.

Question 74: Correct Answer: A) Encouraging regular exercise
Rationale: Encouraging regular exercise can help combat fatigue, improve energy levels, and enhance overall functioning in patients with cancer. Increasing caffeine intake may provide temporary alertness but does not address the underlying fatigue. Antidepressant medication may be considered for associated depression but is not the primary intervention for cancer-related fatigue. While naps can be beneficial, promoting physical activity has more long-term benefits.

Question 75: Correct Answer: A) Democratic leadership
Rationale: Democratic leadership involves involving team members in decision-making processes, fostering collaboration and open communication. Mark's emphasis on these aspects aligns with democratic leadership. Servant leadership focuses on serving others, Charismatic leadership involves inspiring others through charisma, and Situational leadership adapts to different situations and needs.

Question 76: Correct Answer: D) Initiate a turning schedule to prevent pressure ulcers
Rationale: Immobility in patients with bone metastases can lead to pressure ulcers. Initiating a turning schedule helps prevent skin breakdown and pressure ulcers. Options A, B, and C focus on other aspects of care but are not directly related to preventing complications of immobility.

Question 77: Correct Answer: D) Palliative Care Physician
Rationale: The correct answer is D) Palliative Care Physician. Palliative care physicians specialize in managing pain and symptoms, focusing on improving quality of life and providing comfort to patients with serious illnesses. While radiologists perform imaging studies, oncology nurses deliver direct patient care, and anesthesiologists administer anesthesia, palliative care physicians are specifically trained to address pain and symptom management in the context of palliative care, making them the most suitable choice in this scenario.

Question 78: Correct Answer: C) Educating patients about treatment options
Rationale: In the context of navigation and coordination of care, educating patients about treatment options is a crucial role of an Oncology Certified Nurse. This involves explaining different treatment modalities, potential side effects, and helping patients make informed decisions. Options A and B are typically performed by surgeons and oncologists, respectively, while option D falls under the purview of hospital administrators, not nurses.

Question 79: Correct Answer: D) Genetic mutations
Rationale: Genetic mutations play a crucial role in determining the prognosis of cancer patients. Certain genetic mutations can impact treatment response, disease progression, and overall survival outcomes. Family history of cancer, socioeconomic status, and emotional well-being are important considerations in cancer care but may not have as direct an impact on prognosis as specific genetic mutations that can influence the biological behavior of the cancer. Understanding the genetic profile of a patient's cancer can help oncology nurses tailor treatment plans and provide personalized care to improve prognosis.

Question 80: Correct Answer: C) Smoking cessation
Rationale: Smoking is a well-established risk factor for various cancers, including subsequent malignancies in cancer survivors. Therefore, smoking cessation is a crucial strategy to reduce the risk of developing secondary cancers. Regular screenings, physical activity, and sun protection are also important in cancer survivorship but do not directly address the risk of subsequent malignancies as effectively as smoking cessation.

Question 81: Correct Answer: C) Neutrophils
Rationale: Neutropenia is a condition characterized by a low level of neutrophils, which are a type of white blood cell important for fighting infections. Options A, B, and D are incorrect as they represent different types of white blood cells that are not primarily affected in neutropenia.

Question 82: Correct Answer: C) Leaning in attentively
Rationale: Leaning in attentively demonstrates active engagement and empathy, showing the patient that the OCN is present and attentive to their emotional needs. Options A, B, and D are incorrect as crossing arms can convey defensiveness, a neutral facial expression may be perceived as lack of interest, and checking the time frequently can signal impatience or disengagement, all of which hinder effective emotional support.

Question 83: Correct Answer: C) Respect John's dietary restrictions and work with the healthcare team to accommodate them.
Rationale: Respecting and accommodating a patient's cultural dietary practices is crucial in promoting adherence to treatment and overall well-being. Option C is the correct choice as it demonstrates cultural competence and patient-centered care. Options A, B, and D are incorrect as they do not consider the importance of cultural beliefs in patient care.

Question 84: Correct Answer: B) Respecting patient autonomy and preferences
Rationale: Patient advocacy in oncology nursing aims to respect patient autonomy and preferences, ensuring that patients are actively involved in decision-making regarding their care. Options A, C, and D are incorrect as they do not align with the core principle of patient advocacy, which is to support and respect the patient's right to self-determination.

Question 85: Correct Answer: C) Seeking continuing education opportunities
Rationale: Professional accountability in oncology nursing involves taking responsibility for one's actions, seeking opportunities for professional growth and development, and adhering to evidence-based practice guidelines. Blaming others, falsifying records, or disregarding evidence-based practice are unethical behaviors that can compromise patient safety and trust. By engaging in continuing education, oncology nurses demonstrate their commitment to providing high-quality care and staying updated on best practices in the field.

Question 86: Correct Answer: C) Sharing information openly and transparently
Rationale: Open and transparent communication among team members is crucial for effective collaboration in oncology care, leading to improved patient outcomes. Professional silos, limited communication, and avoidance of interprofessional discussions can hinder collaboration and impact the quality of care provided to oncology patients.

Question 87: Correct Answer: A) Secondary malignancy
Rationale: A secondary malignancy refers to a new cancer that

develops as a result of previous cancer treatment. In Sarah's case, the lung mass is not a recurrence of her breast cancer or a metastasis from the original tumor. It is crucial to differentiate between secondary malignancies and recurrent cancers to guide appropriate treatment decisions and follow-up care.

Question 88: Correct Answer: A) Initiate antiemetic therapy with a different mechanism of action
Rationale: In cases of intractable nausea and vomiting, switching to an antiemetic with a different mechanism of action or adding another antiemetic is recommended. Increasing the dose of the current antiemetic may not be effective. High-dose radiation therapy and surgical procedures are not first-line interventions for palliative care symptom management.

Question 89: Correct Answer: B) Case Manager
Rationale: The correct answer is B) Case Manager. Case managers are pivotal in the care continuum, coordinating care, advocating for patients, and ensuring smooth transitions between various healthcare settings. While nurse practitioners provide direct patient care, pharmacists focus on medication management, and radiology technologists perform imaging studies, the case manager's role is specifically centered around care coordination and continuity.

Question 90: Correct Answer: A) Lung Cancer
Rationale: Superior vena cava syndrome is most commonly caused due to the proximity of the superior vena cava to the lungs. Lung cancer can compress or invade the superior vena cava, leading to the syndrome. Breast, prostate, and colorectal cancers are less likely to directly cause this syndrome.

Question 91: Correct Answer: A) BRCA1
Rationale: BRCA1 gene mutation is frequently linked to hereditary breast and ovarian cancer syndrome, emphasizing the importance of genetic testing for individuals with a family history of these cancers. Options B, C, and D are unrelated to this syndrome and are not commonly associated with breast and ovarian cancers.

Question 92: Correct Answer: C) Sucralfate mouthwash
Rationale: Sucralfate mouthwash is often used to alleviate mucositis symptoms by forming a protective barrier over the mucosa. Nystatin oral suspension is an antifungal agent. Cetirizine is an antihistamine used for allergies. Dexamethasone may be used for inflammation but is not a primary choice for mucositis management.

Question 93: Correct Answer: C) Turning the patient to the side
Rationale: During a seizure episode, the appropriate nursing action is to turn the patient to the side to prevent aspiration and maintain a clear airway. Restraining the patient's movements can lead to injury. Placing a padded tongue blade in the mouth is contraindicated as it can cause oral injuries. Administering anticoagulants is not indicated during a seizure and can be harmful.

Question 94: Correct Answer: D) Occupational exposure to carcinogens
Rationale: John's occupational exposure to carcinogens is a significant modifiable risk factor for his colorectal cancer. While smoking, high intake of processed meats, and sedentary lifestyle are risk factors for various cancers, in John's case, occupational exposure plays a more direct role in his condition.

Question 95: Correct Answer: D) Excessive alcohol consumption
Rationale: Excessive alcohol consumption is not typically recommended to reduce the risk of cancer recurrence. In contrast, regular physical activity, a healthy diet rich in fruits and vegetables, and smoking cessation are commonly advised lifestyle modifications to lower the risk of cancer recurrence. Alcohol consumption, especially in excess, can have detrimental effects on overall health and may potentially increase the risk of cancer development or recurrence. Therefore, limiting alcohol intake is important in survivorship care to promote better outcomes and overall well-being.

Question 96: Correct Answer: B) Bloom-Richardson grade
Rationale: The correct answer is B) Bloom-Richardson grade, which is a histologic classification system used for breast cancer. Option A) Gleason score is used for prostate cancer, Option C) Ann Arbor staging is used for lymphomas, and Option D) Lugano classification is used for lymphoma staging. Therefore, the Bloom-Richardson grade is the appropriate choice for classifying breast cancer.

Question 97: Correct Answer: C) Wearing lead apron and thyroid shield when in the radiation therapy room
Rationale: The correct answer is C) Wearing a lead apron and thyroid shield when in the radiation therapy room. Oncology nurses must wear appropriate shielding equipment to minimize radiation exposure during therapy sessions. Options A, B, and D do not address radiation safety measures and may compromise environmental health and safety by increasing the risk of radiation exposure to healthcare providers and patients.

Question 98: Correct Answer: C) Melanoma
Rationale: Melanoma is one of the cancers that has shown significant responses to immunotherapy, particularly with checkpoint inhibitors. Immunotherapy has revolutionized the treatment of melanoma, leading to durable responses and improved survival rates. While immunotherapy is also used in other cancers like lung cancer and bladder cancer, melanoma has been a standout success. Breast cancer, prostate cancer, and leukemia have not shown as significant responses to immunotherapy as melanoma has. Hence, the correct answer is C) Melanoma.

Question 99: Correct Answer: C) CA-125 blood test
Rationale: CA-125 blood test can be considered for ovarian cancer screening, especially in individuals with a family history of the disease. Pap smear is for cervical cancer, mammography for breast cancer, and colonoscopy for colorectal cancer.

Question 100: Correct Answer: B) Sepsis
Rationale: Sepsis is a common trigger for DIC in oncology patients due to the release of pro-inflammatory cytokines and activation of the coagulation cascade. Hypocalcemia, hypernatremia, and hypoalbuminemia are not typically direct triggers for DIC.

Question 101: Correct Answer: B) Recognizing and respecting cultural differences
Rationale: Recognizing and respecting cultural differences is a fundamental aspect of providing culturally congruent care in oncology nursing. It involves acknowledging the uniqueness of each patient's cultural background and tailoring care to meet their specific needs. Imposing the nurse's values, avoiding cultural discussions, or assuming homogeneity among patients can lead to cultural insensitivity and impact the quality of care.

Question 102: Correct Answer: C) Morphine
Rationale: Morphine is an opioid analgesic that is widely recognized as the cornerstone of cancer pain management due to its effectiveness in treating moderate to severe pain. Acetaminophen and ibuprofen are more commonly used for mild pain and are not as potent as opioids like morphine in managing cancer-related pain. Gabapentin is primarily used for neuropathic pain and is not typically the first-line choice for moderate to severe cancer pain.

Question 103: Correct Answer: D) Healthcare providers, lawyers, or family members
Rationale: Individuals can seek assistance from healthcare providers, lawyers, or family members to help them complete an advance directive. These professionals can provide guidance and ensure that the document accurately reflects the individual's wishes. Options A, B, and C are incorrect as they limit the scope of who can assist in completing an advance directive.

Question 104: Correct Answer: C) "It is essential to assess the scientific evidence supporting the use of complementary therapies."
Rationale: Evidence-based practice in oncology requires evaluating the scientific evidence supporting complementary therapies before recommending their use. Option C emphasizes the importance of assessing evidence to ensure the safety and efficacy of complementary interventions. Options A, B, and D present inaccurate or incomplete views on integrating complementary therapies based on evidence.

Question 105: Correct Answer: D) Pap smear

Rationale: Pap smear, also known as Pap test, is the standard screening method for cervical cancer. It involves collecting cells from the cervix to detect any abnormalities or precancerous changes. Colonoscopy is for colorectal cancer, PSA test for prostate cancer, and mammography for breast cancer, not cervical cancer.

Question 106: Correct Answer: B) Offering resources and support
Rationale: The best way to support a patient disclosing a history of domestic violence is by offering resources and support. This can include providing information on shelters, hotlines, counseling services, and safety planning. Minimizing the impact of the abuse, dismissing the patient's experience, or avoiding the topic can make the patient feel unheard and isolated, hindering their ability to seek help.

Question 107: Correct Answer: D) To restore the body's ability to produce blood cells
Rationale: The main goal of a blood and marrow transplant in cancer treatment is to restore the body's ability to produce healthy blood cells, which may have been damaged by high-dose chemotherapy or radiation.

Question 108: Correct Answer: D) Advise pureed or soft foods
Rationale: Pureed or soft foods are easier to swallow for patients with dysphagia. Large food bites can pose a choking hazard, thin liquids may be difficult to swallow, and straws can increase the risk of aspiration in these patients.

Question 109: Correct Answer: D) Arranging for a visit from a hospital chaplain
Rationale: A visit from a hospital chaplain can help James explore his feelings of guilt, unworthiness, and disconnection from his faith. Chaplains are trained to provide spiritual support, guidance, and a compassionate presence to individuals facing spiritual distress. This intervention focuses on addressing James's spiritual well-being and can help him find comfort and healing in his beliefs. The other options do not directly address his spiritual distress and may not provide the same level of support and understanding.

Question 110: Correct Answer: B) Referring John to a mental health professional for counseling.
Rationale: Referring John to a mental health professional for counseling is crucial in addressing his depression as it allows for specialized support and interventions tailored to his emotional well-being. Encouraging emotional suppression can exacerbate his condition. Avoiding discussions about his emotions may lead to feelings of neglect. Providing self-help books alone may not offer the personalized support needed to manage his depression effectively.

Question 111: Correct Answer: A) Encouraging increased fluid intake
Rationale: Hypercalcemia is a common complication in multiple myeloma due to bone destruction. Encouraging increased fluid intake helps promote renal excretion of calcium. Administering furosemide can worsen dehydration. Limiting weight-bearing activities is not directly related to managing hypercalcemia. Providing a high-calcium diet would exacerbate hypercalcemia.

Question 112: Correct Answer: A) Methylphenidate
Rationale: Methylphenidate is often prescribed to address cancer-related fatigue by improving alertness and energy levels. Alprazolam is a benzodiazepine used for anxiety and not fatigue. Diphenhydramine is an antihistamine with sedative effects. Sertraline is an antidepressant and not typically used for cancer-related fatigue.

Question 113: Correct Answer: B) Furosemide
Rationale: Furosemide, a diuretic, is commonly used to reduce intracranial pressure in oncologic emergencies by decreasing cerebral edema. Insulin is used to manage blood sugar levels, aspirin for pain and inflammation, and morphine for pain relief, not specifically for reducing intracranial pressure.

Question 114: Correct Answer: B) Referring her to a support group for cancer survivors
Rationale: Referring Ms. Johnson to a support group for cancer survivors would provide her with a safe space to share her experiences, connect with others facing similar challenges, and receive emotional support. This intervention acknowledges the significance of her emotional state and offers her a supportive environment to cope with her feelings. Options A, C, and D are not appropriate as they neglect the importance of addressing Ms. Johnson's psychosocial distress and may hinder her emotional well-being.

Question 115: Correct Answer: D) Provide corticosteroids
Rationale: The immediate management priority for a patient with suspected spinal cord compression in oncology is to provide corticosteroids to reduce inflammation and swelling around the spinal cord. Administering pain medication, initiating radiation therapy, or performing surgery may be considered later in the treatment plan after stabilizing the patient with corticosteroids.

Question 116: Correct Answer: A) Administering beta-blockers
Rationale: The patient's symptoms and ECG findings are consistent with atrial fibrillation, a common complication of cancer treatment. Beta-blockers are the first-line therapy for rate control in atrial fibrillation. Anticoagulation therapy is indicated to reduce the risk of thromboembolism. Electrical cardioversion is reserved for hemodynamically unstable patients. Calcium channel blockers are contraindicated in the presence of reduced left ventricular function.

Question 117: Correct Answer: C) Wearing protective clothing and hats
Rationale: Wearing protective clothing and hats is a crucial preventive health practice for reducing the risk of skin cancer. Exposure to harmful UV rays from the sun is a significant risk factor for skin cancer, and wearing protective clothing and hats helps shield the skin from these damaging rays. Avoiding sunscreen, tanning bed use, and excessive sun exposure are high-risk behaviors that can increase the likelihood of developing skin cancer.

Question 118: Correct Answer: B) Developing individualized care plans for patients
Rationale: The correct answer is B because developing individualized care plans for patients is a key responsibility within the scope of practice for an Oncology Certified Nurse (OCN). Ordering diagnostic imaging tests, performing surgical procedures, and prescribing medications are typically outside the scope of practice for nurses and are usually performed by physicians or advanced practice providers. Developing care plans tailored to each patient's unique needs is essential in oncology nursing practice.

Question 119: Correct Answer: B) Provide education on managing fatigue and its impact on intimacy.
Rationale: Providing education on managing fatigue and its impact on intimacy is essential in addressing James's concerns. This empowers him to make informed decisions and adapt intimacy practices to accommodate his energy levels. Options A, C, and D are incorrect as they do not directly address the impact of fatigue on intimacy and may not be suitable interventions.

Question 120: Correct Answer: A) Fluid restriction
Rationale: Fluid restriction is a cornerstone in managing SIADH to decrease water intake and correct hyponatremia. Administering hypotonic fluids, increasing ADH levels, and encouraging free water intake can exacerbate hyponatremia in patients with SIADH.

Question 121: Correct Answer: B) Breslow Thickness Classification
Rationale: The Breslow Thickness Classification is specifically used for staging melanoma based on the thickness of the primary tumor and the presence of ulceration. It helps in determining the prognosis and treatment approach for melanoma patients. The other options mentioned, such as the Gleason Score, are used for grading prostate cancer, not melanoma.

Question 122: Correct Answer: B) Initiating palliative care services
Rationale: Initiating palliative care services is crucial in end-of-life care for terminally ill cancer patients as it focuses on improving quality of life, managing symptoms, and providing psychosocial support. Administering aggressive chemotherapy, scheduling additional radiation therapy sessions, or performing

major surgical procedures may not be appropriate at this stage as they can cause more harm than benefit, leading to unnecessary suffering and decreased quality of life.

Question 123: Correct Answer: D) Immune-related adverse events
Rationale: A common side effect of biotherapy is immune-related adverse events, which occur due to the activation of the immune system. These side effects can range from mild to severe and may affect various organs in the body. Hair loss, nausea and vomiting, and fatigue are more commonly associated with traditional cancer treatments like chemotherapy, rather than biotherapy.

Question 124: Correct Answer: B) Involving him in developing strategies to manage side effects
Rationale: Involving the patient in managing side effects empowers them and restores a sense of control. Options A, C, and D diminish the patient's autonomy and worsen feelings of overwhelm.

Question 125: Correct Answer: C) Suprapubic pain
Rationale: Suprapubic pain is a common clinical manifestation of urinary obstruction in oncology patients due to the distension of the bladder. Bradycardia, hemoptysis, and vision changes are not typically associated with urinary obstructions.

Question 126: Correct Answer: C) Chemotherapy side effects
Rationale: Chemotherapy side effects such as nausea, fatigue, and cognitive impairment can pose significant barriers to learning for oncology patients. These side effects can impact concentration, memory, and overall cognitive function, making it challenging for patients to engage in the learning process. While regular follow-up appointments (option A), adequate pain management (option B), and emotional support groups (option D) are important aspects of oncology care, addressing chemotherapy side effects is crucial to optimize patients' ability to learn and retain information during treatment.

Question 127: Correct Answer: B) Resistance training
Rationale: Resistance training is the most suitable intervention for addressing muscle weakness and fatigue in cancer survivors. It helps improve muscle strength, endurance, and overall physical function. Aerobic exercise can also be beneficial but may not specifically target muscle weakness. Yoga and meditation, as well as massage therapy, may help with relaxation and stress management but may not directly address the physical symptoms Mr. Johnson is experiencing.

Question 128: Correct Answer: C) Intravenous
Rationale: Intravenous administration is preferred for rapid pain relief in breakthrough cancer pain as it allows for the quickest onset of action compared to other routes. Oral and transdermal routes may have delayed onset times, while subcutaneous administration is generally slower than intravenous for achieving rapid pain relief in this context.

Question 129: Correct Answer: A) Colorectal cancer is characterized by the formation of polyps in the colon.
Rationale: Colorectal cancer often begins as a growth called a polyp in the inner lining of the colon or rectum. Over time, some polyps can develop into cancer. Options B, C, and D are incorrect as colorectal cancer is not primarily caused by vitamin deficiencies, skin cancer, or inflammation in the small intestine.

Question 130: Correct Answer: A) Phase I
Rationale: Phase I trials are designed to determine the safety, side effects, and dosage of a new treatment. This phase typically involves a small number of participants and aims to establish the maximum tolerated dose. Options B, C, and D are incorrect as they focus on different aspects of clinical trials such as efficacy, comparison with standard treatments, and post-marketing surveillance, respectively.

Question 131: Correct Answer: B) Offer supportive counseling and resources
Rationale: Offering supportive counseling and resources acknowledges Mr. Patel's emotional distress and provides him with tools to cope effectively. Discouraging mirror use, minimizing discussions, or solely focusing on physical recovery may neglect his psychosocial needs, exacerbating his self-esteem issues.

Question 132: Correct Answer: A) Providing information on disability insurance benefits
Rationale: It is crucial for the oncology nurse to prioritize providing information on disability insurance benefits to Sarah as it can help alleviate her financial concerns during her time off work. Disability insurance can provide financial support when individuals are unable to work due to illness or injury. This option addresses Sarah's specific worry about the impact of her treatment on her financial situation.

Question 133: Correct Answer: B) Neuropathy
Rationale: Ms. Johnson's symptoms of numbness and tingling in her fingers and toes are indicative of chemotherapy-induced peripheral neuropathy, a common chronic side effect of certain chemotherapeutic agents. Fatigue, lymphedema, and cognitive impairment are also potential chronic side effects of cancer treatment, but they do not typically present with these specific symptoms.

Question 134: Correct Answer: A) Gender
Rationale: Gender is a non-modifiable risk factor as males have a lower risk of developing breast cancer compared to females. Smoking history, physical activity level, and diet are modifiable risk factors and do not directly influence the predisposition to breast cancer based on gender.

Question 135: Correct Answer: B) Performing Kegel exercises
Rationale: Kegel exercises help strengthen the pelvic floor muscles, which can improve urinary incontinence in patients post-prostatectomy. Encouraging high fluid intake, administering laxatives, and recommending weight-bearing exercises are not directly related to managing urinary incontinence in prostate cancer patients.

Question 136: Correct Answer: B) Minimizing waste by accurately assessing patient needs
Rationale: As an OCN, it is crucial to optimize resource utilization by accurately assessing patient needs to minimize waste. Ordering excessive supplies (Option A) can lead to unnecessary expenses and potential waste. Using outdated equipment (Option C) compromises patient care and violates standards. Ignoring budget constraints (Option D) is not in line with responsible resource management. Therefore, the correct answer is B as it aligns with efficient resource allocation in oncology nursing practice.

Question 137: Correct Answer: A) Osteoporosis
Rationale: Prolonged use of corticosteroids in cancer patients can lead to osteoporosis, a chronic condition characterized by decreased bone density and increased fracture risk. While corticosteroids can cause fluid retention leading to peripheral edema, they are more commonly associated with hyperglycemia and may contribute to hypertension, but osteoporosis is a more direct and specific chronic side effect.

Question 138: Correct Answer: C) Carvedilol
Rationale: Carvedilol, a beta-blocker with antioxidant properties, has been shown to improve left ventricular function and reduce cardiac remodeling in patients with chemotherapy-induced cardiomyopathy. Digoxin is not recommended due to its potential toxicity in this population. Amiodarone is used for arrhythmias, and Furosemide is a diuretic for volume overload but does not address the underlying cardiomyopathy.'

Question 139: Correct Answer: D) Hormone Replacement Therapy
Rationale: Hormone replacement therapy is not a fertility preservation method but rather a treatment for menopausal symptoms. Egg freezing, ovarian transposition, and sperm banking are options to preserve fertility before cancer treatment that may impact reproductive function. These methods aim to safeguard fertility potential for future family planning post-treatment.

Question 140: Correct Answer: B) Haloperidol
Rationale: Haloperidol, an antipsychotic medication, is often used as an adjunct in managing refractory nausea and vomiting in palliative care patients. It helps by blocking dopamine receptors in the chemoreceptor trigger zone. Ondansetron, Diazepam, and Prochlorperazine are more commonly used as first-line antiemetics and may not be as effective in refractory

cases.

Question 141: Correct Answer: B) Acknowledge John's grief and validate his feelings of loss.
Rationale: Validating John's feelings of grief and loss is crucial in providing effective bereavement support. By acknowledging his emotions and offering empathy, the nurse can create a supportive environment for John to express his feelings openly. Options A, C, and D are incorrect as they involve minimizing discussions, discouraging help-seeking, and promoting distraction, which can invalidate John's grief experience and impede his healing process.

Question 142: Correct Answer: C) Administering medication
Rationale: Implementation is the phase where the nurse carries out the interventions as planned during the planning phase. Administering medication, providing treatments, and carrying out nursing actions are all part of the implementation phase. Setting patient goals is part of the planning phase, collecting patient data is part of the assessment phase, and evaluating patient outcomes is part of the evaluation phase.

Question 143: Correct Answer: A) Inducing apoptosis
Rationale: Chemotherapy exerts its anti-cancer effects by triggering apoptosis, which is programmed cell death in cancer cells. Options B, C, and D are incorrect as chemotherapy works by causing cell death rather than promoting division, enhancing repair, or suppressing the immune response. Apoptosis induction is a key mechanism through which chemotherapy eliminates cancer cells from the body.

Question 144: Correct Answer: C) Hyperphosphatemia
Rationale: Tumor lysis syndrome is characterized by the release of intracellular contents into the bloodstream due to rapid cell lysis, leading to elevated levels of potassium, phosphate, uric acid, and decreased calcium. Hyperphosphatemia is a hallmark feature of tumor lysis syndrome, as phosphate is released from the breakdown of nucleic acids. Hypercalcemia, hypokalemia, and hypouricemia are not typically seen in tumor lysis syndrome, making them incorrect choices.

Question 145: Correct Answer: B) Superior vena cava syndrome
Rationale: The symptoms described are indicative of superior vena cava syndrome, commonly seen in patients with malignancies such as testicular cancer. Aortic dissection presents with severe tearing chest pain, esophageal cancer may cause dysphagia but not facial plethora, and thyroid storm presents with hyperthyroid symptoms such as tachycardia and fever.

Question 146: Correct Answer: D) Elevating the head of the bed
Rationale: Elevating the head of the bed is a priority intervention in managing increased intracranial pressure as it helps reduce intracranial pressure by promoting venous drainage from the brain. Administering antibiotics, providing oxygen therapy, and initiating chemotherapy are not primary interventions for managing increased intracranial pressure.

Question 147: Correct Answer: C) Respecting the patient's cultural beliefs and practices
Rationale: Culturally congruent care in oncology nursing involves respecting the patient's cultural beliefs and practices. This approach acknowledges the importance of cultural diversity in healthcare and promotes patient-centered care. Providing materials in only English, using complex medical terms, or disregarding family preferences can hinder effective communication and understanding, leading to potential disparities in care.

Question 148: Correct Answer: A) Acupuncture
Rationale: Acupuncture involves the insertion of thin needles into specific points on the body to help alleviate various symptoms, including chemotherapy-induced nausea and vomiting. Reiki is a form of energy healing, Tai Chi is a mind-body practice involving gentle movements, and homeopathy uses highly diluted substances to stimulate the body's healing processes. While these modalities may offer benefits in other areas, acupuncture is specifically recognized for its antiemetic effects.

Question 149: Correct Answer: B) Providing resources for sexual counseling
Rationale: Offering resources for sexual counseling can empower patients to address sexual dysfunction, improve communication, and explore solutions. Dismissing sexual health, encouraging avoidance, or minimizing treatment impact are counterproductive approaches, making them incorrect choices.

Question 150: Correct Answer: D) Wearing a disposable gown when handling chemotherapy drugs
Rationale: The correct answer is D) Wearing a disposable gown when handling chemotherapy drugs. Oncology nurses should wear appropriate PPE, including gowns, when handling chemotherapy drugs to prevent skin contact and contamination. Options A, B, and C pose risks of exposure to the nurse and potential environmental contamination, emphasizing the importance of following safe handling practices.

OCN Exam Practice Questions [SET 4]

Question 1: Mr. Patel, a 65-year-old patient undergoing chemotherapy, develops a grade 2 radiation-induced skin reaction on his chest. Which nursing intervention is essential for managing his skin reaction?
A) Applying ice packs to the affected area
B) Using a mild soap for cleansing
C) Administering topical corticosteroids
D) Encouraging frequent scratching to relieve itching

Question 2: Which diagnostic measure is commonly employed to diagnose lung cancer?
A) Biopsy
B) Echocardiogram
C) Liver function test
D) Urinalysis

Question 3: Which type of immune cell is responsible for producing antibodies in response to cancer cells?
A) T cells
B) B cells
C) Natural killer cells
D) Macrophages

Question 4: Scenario: Sarah, an Oncology Nurse, is documenting a patient's chemotherapy administration. She notices a discrepancy in the dosage prescribed by the physician and the dosage administered by the nurse. What should Sarah do next?
A) Alter the documentation to match the administered dosage.
B) Inform the physician immediately about the discrepancy.
C) Ignore the error and continue with her duties.
D) Wait until the end of the shift to report the error.

Question 5: Which of the following best describes the scope of practice for an Oncology Certified Nurse (OCN)?
A) Performing surgical procedures
B) Administering chemotherapy and biotherapy
C) Conducting radiation therapy sessions
D) Prescribing medications

Question 6: Which statement is true regarding anxiety in oncology patients?
A) Anxiety has no impact on treatment adherence
B) Anxiety is always a sign of depression
C) Anxiety can manifest as physical symptoms
D) Anxiety does not affect quality of life

Question 7: Which of the following study designs is most appropriate for investigating the association between a risk factor and a disease outcome over time?
A) Case-control study
B) Cross-sectional study
C) Cohort study
D) Randomized controlled trial

Question 8: After receiving radiation therapy for prostate cancer, Mr. Brown develops a localized, painful, erythematous skin reaction at the treatment site. Which type of hypersensitivity reaction is most likely responsible for his skin changes?
A) Type I
B) Type II
C) Type III
D) Type IV

Question 9: Which site-specific cancer is associated with the Philadelphia chromosome?
A) Chronic myeloid leukemia
B) Skin melanoma
C) Thyroid
D) Bone

Question 10: James, a 55-year-old lung cancer patient, is experiencing significant caregiver burnout as his wife takes on the role of primary caregiver. Which support intervention would be most beneficial for addressing James' psychosocial needs as a caregiver?
A) Arranging respite care services for his wife
B) Providing him with relaxation techniques to manage stress
C) Connecting him with a caregiver support group
D) Recommending he take up a new hobby for distraction

Question 11: Which coping mechanism is characterized by an individual diverting their thoughts, feelings, or behaviors to something more neutral or acceptable?
A) Displacement
B) Rationalization
C) Sublimation
D) Repression

Question 12: Which of the following is a common trigger for anaphylaxis in oncology patients?
A) Chemotherapy
B) Radiation therapy
C) Surgery
D) Blood transfusion

Question 13: Scenario: Emily, a 55-year-old patient with lung cancer, is exploring biotherapy options. Which biotherapy modality involves the introduction of genetic material into cells to fight cancer?
A) Monoclonal Antibodies
B) Cytokine Therapy
C) Gene Therapy
D) Cancer Vaccines

Question 14: Mr. Lee, a 60-year-old patient, is diagnosed with colorectal cancer. Which staging system is commonly used to determine the extent of spread of colorectal cancer?
A) Lugano classification
B) Dukes staging
C) FIGO staging
D) TNM staging

Question 15: Scenario: John, a 60-year-old patient undergoing chemotherapy, is experiencing taste changes and mouth sores, making it challenging for him to eat. Which dietary recommendation would be most beneficial for John?
A) Increase intake of spicy foods to enhance taste perception
B) Encourage consumption of citrus fruits to stimulate saliva production
C) Suggest using plastic utensils to reduce metallic taste sensation
D) Recommend soft, bland foods at room temperature to ease discomfort

Question 16: Scenario: Emily, a 45-year-old female, is undergoing radiation therapy for lung cancer. She experiences difficulty swallowing and oral mucositis. Which nursing intervention is most appropriate for managing these side effects?
A) Encouraging spicy foods to stimulate saliva production
B) Providing ice chips for oral intake
C) Administering alcohol-based mouthwash
D) Recommending soft, bland foods and oral hygiene care

Question 17: What is the significance of maintaining a clean and organized work environment in oncology nursing practice?
A) Enhancing workplace aesthetics
B) Promoting efficient workflow
C) Minimizing the need for hand hygiene
D) Reducing patient satisfaction

Question 18: Mr. Lee, a 70-year-old patient with prostate cancer, is experiencing confusion and disorientation. Which assessment tool is most appropriate for evaluating his cognitive function?
A) Pain scale
B) Mini-Mental State Examination (MMSE)
C) Blood pressure cuff
D) Electrocardiogram (ECG)

Question 19: Scenario: Maria, a 55-year-old Latina patient, has been diagnosed with advanced breast cancer. She expresses a strong belief in the healing power of prayer and requests to have a religious leader visit her in the hospital. How should the oncology nurse best respond to Maria's request?
A) Allow the religious leader to visit Maria and facilitate spiritual support.
B) Explain to Maria that hospital policies do not allow religious leaders to visit.
C) Disregard Maria's request as it may interfere with medical treatment.
D) Suggest to Maria that she should focus on medical treatments only.

Question 20: Scenario: Emily, a 30-year-old patient with lymphoma, is undergoing chemotherapy that requires a continuous infusion of medication. Which vascular access device would be most appropriate for Emily's treatment?
A) Arteriovenous Graft
B) Peripherally Inserted Central Catheter (PICC)
C) Dialysis Catheter
D) Implantable Port

Question 21: Mr. Johnson, a 55-year-old male with newly diagnosed Burkitt's lymphoma, is admitted for chemotherapy. On the second day of treatment, he develops muscle weakness, nausea, and oliguria. Laboratory findings reveal hyperkalemia, hyperphosphatemia, hypocalcemia, and elevated serum uric acid levels. What is the most appropriate initial intervention for Mr. Johnson?
A) Administer intravenous furosemide
B) Initiate allopurinol therapy
C) Provide aggressive intravenous hydration
D) Administer calcium gluconate

Question 22: Sarah, a 30-year-old cervical cancer survivor, is struggling with body image issues post-treatment. Which of the following interventions can help address the psychological effects of sexual dysfunction in cancer survivors?
A) Cognitive-behavioral therapy
B) Chemotherapy
C) Radiation therapy
D) Surgery

Question 23: Scenario: Sarah, a 55-year-old patient with breast cancer, is admitted to the oncology unit for chemotherapy. During the assessment, the nurse notes that Sarah is experiencing nausea and vomiting. Which step of the nursing process should the nurse prioritize in this situation?
A) Planning
B) Evaluation
C) Assessment
D) Implementation

Question 24: Mr. Patel, a 60-year-old prostate cancer survivor, has been prescribed antidepressant medication for his depressive symptoms. Which class of antidepressants is commonly recommended for cancer patients due to their favorable side effect profile and potential for managing pain symptoms?
A) Tricyclic Antidepressants (TCAs)
B) Monoamine Oxidase Inhibitors (MAOIs)
C) Selective Serotonin Reuptake Inhibitors (SSRIs)
D) Serotonin-Norepinephrine Reuptake Inhibitors (SNRIs)

Question 25: Which cultural practice may impact a patient's decision-making process regarding cancer treatment?
A) Fasting during specific religious holidays
B) Regular exercise routine
C) Consumption of herbal supplements
D) Participation in support groups

Question 26: Which genitourinary intervention is commonly used for symptom management in advanced cervical cancer?
A) Nephrostomy tube placement
B) Suprapubic catheter insertion
C) Ureteral stent placement
D) Urinary diversion surgery

Question 27: Which non-pharmacologic comfort measure involves the use of guided imagery and relaxation techniques to help patients manage pain and anxiety?
A) Hypnosis
B) Surgery
C) Blood Transfusion
D) Physical Therapy

Question 28: Mr. Garcia, a 60-year-old patient with gastric cancer, is scheduled for a palliative gastrectomy to relieve symptoms and improve quality of life. Which of the following goals is most appropriate for this surgical intervention?
A) Complete eradication of cancer cells
B) Prolonging overall survival
C) Alleviating symptoms and improving comfort
D) Preventing cancer recurrence

Question 29: Scenario: Sarah, an oncology nurse, is reviewing the Scope and Standards of Practice for Oncology Nursing. Which of the following best describes the Scope of Practice for an Oncology Certified Nurse (OCN)?
A) Performing surgical procedures in the oncology setting
B) Administering chemotherapy and biotherapy agents
C) Conducting radiation therapy sessions
D) Providing physical therapy services to oncology patients

Question 30: Which hypersensitivity reaction is characterized by a delayed response involving sensitized T lymphocytes and macrophages, leading to tissue damage?
A) Type I
B) Type II
C) Type III
D) Type IV

Question 31: Which of the following best describes the role of OCNs in professional practice evaluation?
A) Conducting research studies
B) Implementing evidence-based practice
C) Participating in quality improvement initiatives
D) Managing hospital finances

Question 32: Which alteration in functioning is a common side effect of chemotherapy in oncology patients?
A) Hypertension

B) Peripheral neuropathy
C) Hyperthyroidism
D) Osteoporosis

Question 33: Which diagnostic measure is typically used to confirm a diagnosis of skin cancer?
A) MRI scan
B) Skin biopsy
C) Stool occult blood test
D) Renal function test

Question 34: What is the first-line treatment for anaphylaxis in oncology patients?
A) Intramuscular epinephrine
B) Oral antihistamines
C) Intravenous fluids
D) Oxygen therapy

Question 35: Scenario: Sarah, an Oncology Nurse, is reviewing the standards set by The Joint Commission for oncology care. Which of the following is a key focus area of The Joint Commission accreditation in oncology nursing practice?
A) Patient Education and Counseling
B) Staffing Ratios
C) Hospital Revenue Generation
D) Marketing Strategies

Question 36: Mrs. Smith, a 45-year-old patient with breast cancer, is scheduled for a lumpectomy. What is the primary goal of a lumpectomy in the treatment of breast cancer?
A) To remove the entire breast.
B) To remove the tumor and a margin of surrounding healthy tissue.
C) To perform reconstructive surgery.
D) To administer chemotherapy directly to the tumor site.

Question 37: Which leadership quality is essential for an OCN to promote a culture of safety and quality improvement in oncology nursing practice?
A) Authoritarianism
B) Open communication
C) Blaming individuals for errors
D) Resisting change

Question 38: Scenario: Sarah, a 55-year-old female with metastatic breast cancer, is being considered for targeted therapy. Which of the following is a characteristic of targeted therapies in cancer treatment?
A) Targeted therapies work by killing both cancerous and healthy cells.
B) Targeted therapies are effective for all types of cancer.
C) Targeted therapies aim to specifically target cancer cells while minimizing harm to normal cells.
D) Targeted therapies have severe side effects similar to traditional chemotherapy.

Question 39: Which phase of the nursing process involves the systematic collection of patient data?
A) Planning
B) Implementation
C) Assessment
D) Evaluation

Question 40: Mr. Johnson, a 58-year-old patient with metastatic lung cancer, is receiving his first cycle of chemotherapy with carboplatin and paclitaxel. During the infusion, he develops sudden onset of dyspnea, urticaria, and hypotension. What is the most appropriate initial intervention for suspected anaphylaxis in this patient?
A) Administer epinephrine intramuscularly
B) Stop the infusion and administer diphenhydramine
C) Increase the rate of the infusion to push through the reaction
D) Administer corticosteroids intravenously

Question 41: Mr. Roberts, a 65-year-old patient with lung cancer, is receiving radiation therapy. Which of the following interventions is essential for the nurse to implement to manage treatment-related side effects?
A) Encouraging the patient to increase caffeine intake
B) Providing education on the importance of sun exposure
C) Applying aloe vera gel to the radiation site
D) Monitoring the patient for signs of radiation dermatitis

Question 42: How can oncology nurses support cancer patients with depression?
A) Minimize communication with patients
B) Disregard emotional needs of patients
C) Encourage social isolation
D) Provide emotional support and empathy

Question 43: Mr. Smith, a 58-year-old patient, is diagnosed with non-small cell lung cancer. Which TNM classification system is commonly used to stage lung cancer?
A) AJCC
B) FIGO
C) SEER
D) Dukes

Question 44: What fertility preservation option is most suitable for a female patient diagnosed with leukemia who wishes to preserve her fertility before starting chemotherapy?
A) Ovarian transposition
B) Egg freezing
C) Tubal ligation
D) Hormonal therapy

Question 45: Ms. Johnson, a 45-year-old patient undergoing treatment for breast cancer, develops fever, joint pain, and a widespread rash following administration of a new chemotherapy drug. Which hypersensitivity reaction is most likely responsible for her symptoms?
A) Type I
B) Type II
C) Type III
D) Type IV

Question 46: Scenario: David, a 70-year-old male patient with non-small cell lung cancer, is being treated with monoclonal antibody therapy. Which of the following best describes the mechanism of action of monoclonal antibodies in cancer treatment?
A) Directly killing cancer cells
B) Blocking specific targets on cancer cells
C) Stimulating cancer cell growth
D) Inhibiting immune response

Question 47: Which of the following is a common symptom of spinal cord compression in oncology patients?
A) Headache
B) Abdominal pain
C) Weakness or numbness in extremities
D) Chest pain

Question 48: Which intervention can help address altered body image in cancer patients?
A) Meditation techniques
B) Cosmetic surgery
C) Group therapy
D) Avoiding discussions about body image

Question 49: How is pneumonitis managed in oncology patients?
A) Antibiotics
B) Corticosteroids

C) Antifungal medications
D) Chemotherapy

Question 50: Which of the following best describes the concept of quality of practice in oncology nursing?
A) Meeting the minimum requirements for patient care
B) Providing care that is cost-effective
C) Delivering evidence-based, patient-centered care
D) Completing tasks efficiently to save time

Question 51: Scenario: Sarah, a 45-year-old female patient with metastatic breast cancer, is receiving chemotherapy. She presents with a low white blood cell count, specifically neutropenia. Which of the following interventions is most appropriate for managing neutropenia in this patient?
A) Administering erythropoietin
B) Initiating prophylactic antibiotics
C) Encouraging consumption of raw fruits and vegetables
D) Avoiding hand hygiene

Question 52: Which of the following strategies can help address discrimination concerns in the care continuum for cancer survivors?
A) Implementing cultural competency training for healthcare staff
B) Ignoring patient feedback on discriminatory experiences
C) Limiting access to survivorship resources based on age
D) Excluding diverse perspectives in survivorship program development

Question 53: Mrs. Lee, a 55-year-old patient with end-stage breast cancer, is experiencing profound fatigue. Which of the following interventions is most appropriate for managing her symptom in palliative care?
A) Initiate physical therapy
B) Prescribe erythropoietin-stimulating agents
C) Recommend regular exercise regimen
D) Adjust medications to manage contributing factors

Question 54: A young adult cancer survivor expresses fears of facing discrimination in social settings due to changes in their physical appearance post-treatment. How can the Oncology Certified Nurse best assist this patient?
A) Recommend the patient to isolate themselves from social interactions
B) Provide strategies for building self-confidence and coping with stigma
C) Disregard the patient's concerns as part of normal post-treatment anxiety
D) Advise the patient to undergo further cosmetic procedures to fit in

Question 55: Which of the following actions by an oncology nurse best demonstrates adherence to environmental health standards?
A) Proper disposal of hazardous waste
B) Wearing jewelry during patient care
C) Using personal mobile phone in patient areas
D) Reusing disposable gloves

Question 56: Scenario: Emily, a 55-year-old female, presents with a suspicious skin lesion on her face. A biopsy reveals abnormal cells confined to the epidermis without invasion into the dermis. What is the most likely stage of this skin cancer?
A) Stage 0
B) Stage I
C) Stage II
D) Stage III

Question 57: Scenario: Emily, a 45-year-old lung cancer patient, is receiving radiation therapy. The nurse notices that the radiation machine is frequently left running idle between patient sessions, leading to energy wastage. What action should the nurse take to improve resource utilization?
A) Ignore the idle machine as it is common in radiation therapy units
B) Inform the radiation therapy team about the idle machine issue
C) Continue with the current practice of leaving the machine running
D) Implement a schedule to optimize machine usage

Question 58: Which delayed-onset side effect is a concern for patients who have undergone radiation therapy to the chest area?
A) Fatigue
B) Cardiotoxicity
C) Diarrhea
D) Hair loss

Question 59: Which alteration in functioning is a priority concern in the palliative care of oncology patients with advanced disease?
A) Improved mobility
B) Enhanced taste perception
C) Alleviation of dyspnea
D) Increased blood pressure

Question 60: Which imaging modality is commonly used to diagnose bowel obstruction in oncology patients?
A) Electrocardiogram (ECG)
B) Magnetic resonance imaging (MRI)
C) Bone scan
D) Abdominal X-ray

Question 61: Mr. Lee, a 70-year-old patient with lung cancer, is experiencing severe neuropathic pain that is not adequately controlled with opioids. Which pharmacologic intervention is the first-line treatment for neuropathic pain in cancer patients?
A) Gabapentin
B) Morphine
C) Acetaminophen
D) Ibuprofen

Question 62: Mr. Johnson, a 65-year-old patient with metastatic bone cancer, is experiencing severe bone pain that is not adequately controlled with current analgesics. Which intervention should the nurse prioritize to manage his pain effectively?
A) Initiate physical therapy for range of motion exercises
B) Administer a bisphosphonate to strengthen bone density
C) Implement regular repositioning schedule to prevent pressure ulcers
D) Start palliative radiation therapy to the painful bone site

Question 63: What is the recommended treatment for an extravasation caused by a vesicant chemotherapy agent?
A) Apply heat to the affected area
B) Elevate the affected limb
C) Infiltrate with hyaluronidase
D) Massage the area gently

Question 64: Scenario: Emily, an oncology nurse, is educating a group of nursing students about the Scope and Standards of Practice for Oncology Nursing. Which of the following activities is within the Scope of Practice for an OCN?
A) Performing diagnostic imaging procedures for oncology patients
B) Developing individualized care plans for oncology patients
C) Prescribing medications for oncology treatment
D) Performing surgical interventions for oncology patients

Question 65: What is the role of a radiation oncology nurse

in the care of patients undergoing radiation therapy?
A) Administering chemotherapy drugs
B) Monitoring and managing side effects
C) Performing radiation therapy procedures
D) Conducting surgical interventions

Question 66: Which of the following is a common symptom of cognitive dysfunction in cancer patients undergoing treatment?
A) Increased attention span
B) Enhanced memory recall
C) Impaired decision-making
D) Improved problem-solving skills

Question 67: Scenario: John, a 60-year-old male, is undergoing evaluation for suspected lung cancer. His oncologist recommends a procedure to obtain a tissue sample for further analysis. Which diagnostic measure involves the removal of a small piece of lung tissue for examination?
A) Bronchoscopy
B) MRI
C) Ultrasound
D) Echocardiogram

Question 68: Which of the following is a common barrier to learning for oncology patients?
A) Supportive family members
B) Positive reinforcement
C) Emotional distress
D) Clear communication

Question 69: What is a characteristic of chronic symptoms in oncology patients?
A) Sudden onset
B) Intensity decreases over time
C) Resolved with treatment completion
D) Insidious development

Question 70: Mrs. Lee, a 70-year-old patient receiving radiation therapy for head and neck cancer, is experiencing mucositis. Which intervention is most appropriate for managing her mucositis?
A) Alcohol-based mouthwash
B) Regular dental flossing
C) Ice-cold beverages
D) Oral cryotherapy

Question 71: Scenario: David, a 70-year-old patient with lung cancer, is experiencing dyspnea-related anxiety and distress due to his cancer diagnosis. Which non-pharmacological intervention would be most beneficial for addressing David's dyspnea-related anxiety?
A) Relaxation techniques
B) Benzodiazepines
C) Antidepressants
D) Cognitive-behavioral therapy (CBT)

Question 72: Which immune-related adverse event involves inflammation of the liver and may manifest as elevated liver enzymes and jaundice in patients undergoing immunotherapy?
A) Thyroiditis
B) Dermatitis
C) Hepatitis
D) Myositis

Question 73: What is a crucial aspect of the standards of practice for an Oncology Certified Nurse (OCN) regarding patient advocacy?
A) Making treatment decisions on behalf of the patient
B) Respecting patient autonomy and preferences
C) Withholding information from patients
D) Disregarding patient rights

Question 74: Which nursing intervention is essential for preventing lymphedema in patients following axillary lymph node dissection?
A) Encouraging vigorous arm exercises
B) Avoiding limb compression
C) Applying heat packs to the affected arm
D) Allowing blood pressure measurements on the affected arm

Question 75: Which treatment-related consideration is crucial for oncology patients undergoing surgery?
A) Pain management
B) Blood sugar monitoring
C) Lung function tests
D) Urine analysis

Question 76: Which of the following is a high-risk behavior that can contribute to the development of colorectal cancer?
A) Consuming a diet rich in fruits and vegetables
B) Regular colorectal cancer screening
C) Smoking tobacco
D) Maintaining a healthy weight

Question 77: Scenario: Sarah, a 55-year-old breast cancer patient, is undergoing chemotherapy. She asks the nurse about the benefits of using cold caps to prevent hair loss during treatment. Which of the following statements by the nurse best reflects evidence-based practice?
A) "Cold caps are not effective in preventing hair loss during chemotherapy."
B) "Using cold caps may reduce the risk of hair loss, but individual results vary."
C) "Cold caps are guaranteed to prevent hair loss in all chemotherapy patients."
D) "There is no research supporting the use of cold caps for hair preservation."

Question 78: Which factor influences the selection of targeted therapies in oncology?
A) Tumor histology
B) Patient's blood type
C) Smoking history
D) Body mass index (BMI)

Question 79: Which opioid side effect can be effectively managed with the use of laxatives and stool softeners in cancer patients?
A) Nausea
B) Constipation
C) Sedation
D) Respiratory depression

Question 80: Scenario: Emily, a 45-year-old cancer survivor, is mourning the loss of her close friend who passed away from cancer. She expresses feelings of guilt and regrets about not being able to save her friend. What is a suitable approach to address Emily's feelings of guilt in bereavement?
A) Reinforce Emily's sense of responsibility for her friend's death.
B) Encourage Emily to suppress her feelings of guilt to focus on her recovery.
C) Validate Emily's emotions and help her reframe her thoughts about guilt.
D) Advise Emily to avoid discussing her feelings of guilt with others.

Question 81: Mr. Patel, a 60-year-old prostate cancer patient, is experiencing erectile dysfunction following treatment. Which intervention would be most appropriate to support Mr. Patel's sexual health?
A) Recommend mindfulness meditation to reduce stress.
B) Encourage open communication with his partner about his

concerns.
C) Advise complete avoidance of any sexual activity.
D) Prescribe testosterone supplements without further assessment.

Question 82: What is the primary purpose of advance care planning?
A) To ensure that healthcare providers make decisions on behalf of the patient.
B) To provide guidance to family members on medical treatment options.
C) To empower individuals to make decisions about their future healthcare.
D) To limit access to medical care for individuals with chronic conditions.

Question 83: Scenario: Emily, a 50-year-old lung cancer survivor, is worried about the impact of her cancer history on her ability to secure health insurance. What should the oncology nurse educate Emily about regarding insurance coverage post-cancer treatment?
A) Advising Emily to avoid disclosing her cancer history to insurance providers
B) Informing Emily about the importance of maintaining continuous health insurance coverage
C) Suggesting Emily to forgo health insurance coverage due to pre-existing condition concerns
D) Recommending Emily to switch insurance providers frequently to avoid scrutiny

Question 84: Ms. Johnson, a 55-year-old breast cancer survivor, presents with swelling in her right arm following axillary lymph node dissection. Which intervention is most appropriate for managing her lymphedema?
A) Application of heat packs
B) Manual lymphatic drainage
C) High-impact weightlifting
D) Tight bandaging of the affected arm

Question 85: Which of the following interventions can help address sexual dysfunction in cancer patients?
A) Avoiding communication with healthcare providers
B) Ignoring the impact of cancer treatment on sexual function
C) Engaging in open dialogue with a healthcare team
D) Isolating oneself from partners

Question 86: Which treatment-related consideration is essential to monitor for oncology patients undergoing chemotherapy?
A) Blood pressure
B) Liver function
C) Bone density
D) Vision acuity

Question 87: How can a nurse promote cultural competence in caring for oncology patients?
A) Stereotyping patients based on cultural background
B) Avoiding discussions about cultural differences
C) Seeking education on diverse cultural practices
D) Imposing the nurse's cultural norms on patients

Question 88: Ms. Johnson, a 55-year-old breast cancer patient, has been experiencing persistent feelings of sadness, hopelessness, and loss of interest in activities she once enjoyed. She often feels fatigued and has trouble sleeping. Which of the following assessment tools is most appropriate for evaluating her symptoms of depression?
A) Pain Assessment
B) Karnofsky Performance Status Scale
C) Patient Health Questionnaire-9 (PHQ-9)
D) Edmonton Symptom Assessment System (ESAS)

Question 89: Scenario: Emily, an oncology nurse, is preparing to change the dressing on a patient's central line. She notices signs of infection around the insertion site. What should Emily do first?
A) Proceed with the dressing change as planned
B) Notify the physician about the signs of infection
C) Consult the patient about the discomfort
D) Apply an antibiotic ointment to the site

Question 90: Which term describes the process of providing comfort and support to cancer patients experiencing cognitive decline near the end of life?
A) Curative care
B) Hospice care
C) Respite care
D) Palliative care

Question 91: Which factor is NOT typically associated with an increased risk of cancer recurrence in survivors?
A) Age at diagnosis
B) Type of cancer
C) Gender of the patient
D) Stage of the cancer

Question 92: Mr. Patel, a 60-year-old patient undergoing chemotherapy for lung cancer, expresses anger and frustration about his diagnosis and treatment. He mentions feeling abandoned by his faith community. What action by the nurse is most appropriate to address Mr. Patel's spiritual distress?
A) Referring him to a support group for cancer patients
B) Encouraging him to ignore his feelings of anger
C) Suggesting he focuses on work to distract himself
D) Arranging for a visit from a hospital chaplain

Question 93: Which of the following symptoms is NOT commonly associated with hypercalcemia in oncologic emergencies?
A) Fatigue
B) Nausea and vomiting
C) Muscle weakness
D) Hypotension

Question 94: Which of the following is a type of biotherapy that involves using antibodies to target cancer cells?
A) Gene therapy
B) Cytokine therapy
C) Monoclonal antibody therapy
D) Stem cell transplant

Question 95: When is it appropriate to initiate palliative care for cancer patients?
A) Only in the terminal stage of cancer
B) At the time of cancer diagnosis
C) After all curative treatment options have failed
D) When the patient requests it

Question 96: Which of the following is a common mechanism of action for targeted therapies in oncology?
A) Inhibition of specific molecules involved in cancer growth
B) Non-specific activation of the immune system
C) Induction of general cell death in the body
D) Promotion of angiogenesis in tumor cells

Question 97: Which of the following is a common psychosocial distress symptom experienced by cancer patients?
A) Increased appetite
B) Decreased anxiety
C) Social withdrawal
D) Improved sleep quality

**Question 98: Scenario: Michael, a 50-year-old male patient with pancreatic cancer, is experiencing cancer-related

fatigue. Which of the following interventions is most appropriate for managing cancer-related fatigue in this patient?
A) Encouraging frequent napping during the day
B) Limiting physical activity
C) Implementing a structured exercise program
D) Consuming caffeine before bedtime

Question 99: What is the purpose of using radiation therapy in cancer treatment?
A) To directly target and kill cancer cells
B) To boost the immune system
C) To promote cancer cell growth
D) To reduce the size of tumors

Question 100: Scenario: Sarah, a 45-year-old female, has recently been diagnosed with lung cancer. She has a history of smoking for the past 20 years. Which modifiable risk factor is most likely associated with her diagnosis?
A) High-fat diet
B) Sedentary lifestyle
C) Smoking
D) Occupational exposure to asbestos

Question 101: Which of the following is a hallmark of cancer cells?
A) Increased apoptosis
B) Contact inhibition
C) Self-sufficiency in growth signals
D) Limited angiogenesis

Question 102: Mr. Patel, a 60-year-old male with metastatic lung cancer, is receiving chemotherapy. He presents with lethargy, muscle cramps, and ECG changes showing peaked T waves. Which electrolyte abnormality is most likely responsible for these findings in the context of tumor lysis syndrome (TLS)?
A) Hyperkalemia
B) Hypernatremia
C) Hypomagnesemia
D) Hypercalcemia

Question 103: Mrs. Patel, a 70-year-old female, is diagnosed with ovarian cancer. Which grading system is commonly used to classify the aggressiveness of ovarian tumors based on cellular features?
A) Gleason score
B) Bloom-Richardson grade
C) Fuhrman grade
D) FIGO grade

Question 104: Mr. Johnson, a 58-year-old male with metastatic lung cancer, presents with sudden onset bruising, petechiae, and mucosal bleeding. Laboratory findings reveal thrombocytopenia, prolonged PT and PTT, and decreased fibrinogen levels. What oncologic emergency is Mr. Johnson likely experiencing?
A) Tumor Lysis Syndrome
B) Superior Vena Cava Syndrome
C) Disseminated Intravascular Coagulation (DIC)
D) Hypercalcemia of Malignancy

Question 105: Which of the following best describes the concept of 'Loss of personal control' in the context of psychosocial distress for oncology patients?
A) Feeling empowered and confident in decision-making
B) Surrendering decision-making to healthcare providers
C) Actively participating in treatment planning
D) Seeking emotional support from family and friends

Question 106: Scenario: David, a 55-year-old male, is receiving chemotherapy for prostate cancer. The nurse discusses the role of genetic mutations in carcinogenesis. Which of the following best describes the impact of genetic mutations on carcinogenesis?
A) Genetic mutations have no role in carcinogenesis
B) Genetic mutations always lead to cancer development
C) Genetic mutations can increase the risk of cancer by altering cell function
D) Genetic mutations only occur in cancer cells

Question 107: Which of the following statements best describes an advance directive?
A) It is a legal document that specifies the type of medical care a person wishes to have in the event they are unable to communicate their preferences.
B) It is a document that only healthcare providers can access.
C) It is a document that is only applicable to individuals over the age of 75.
D) It is a document that can be changed by healthcare providers without patient consent.

Question 108: What role can oncology nurses play in addressing financial concerns of cancer patients?
A) Providing financial assistance directly
B) Offering emotional support only
C) Connecting patients with financial resources and support services
D) Ignoring financial concerns

Question 109: Mr. Johnson, a 58-year-old patient with metastatic melanoma, presents with diarrhea, colitis, and skin rash after receiving immunotherapy. Which immune-related adverse event is he most likely experiencing?
A) Pneumonitis
B) Hepatitis
C) Dermatitis
D) Enterocolitis

Question 110: Which surgical alteration may result in the development of lymphedema in oncology patients?
A) Mastectomy
B) Nephrectomy
C) Colectomy
D) Prostatectomy

Question 111: Which cognitive impairment is characterized by a decline in memory, language, problem-solving, and other thinking skills that affect a person's ability to perform everyday activities?
A) Delirium
B) Dementia
C) Amnesia
D) Aphasia

Question 112: Which accreditation program focuses specifically on oncology practices and aims to improve the quality of cancer care?
A) QOPI
B) ANCC Magnet Recognition Program
C) National Comprehensive Cancer Network (NCCN)
D) The Joint Commission

Question 113: What is a common palliative care intervention for managing nausea and vomiting in cancer patients with gastrointestinal issues?
A) Antibiotics
B) Chemotherapy
C) Antiemetics
D) Anticoagulants

Question 114: Which of the following is a common metastatic location for breast cancer?
A) Liver
B) Prostate
C) Colon

D) Thyroid

Question 115: Which statement best describes the impact of spiritual distress on cancer patients?
A) Spiritual distress has no effect on the overall well-being of cancer patients
B) Spiritual distress can lead to increased anxiety and depression
C) Spiritual distress only affects patients' religious practices
D) Spiritual distress is easily resolved with medical interventions

Question 116: Mr. Lee, a 60-year-old lung cancer patient, exhibits signs of depression and social withdrawal following his diagnosis. Which nursing action is most appropriate to assess and address Mr. Lee's psychosocial distress?
A) Encouraging Mr. Lee to isolate himself for self-reflection
B) Conducting a comprehensive psychosocial assessment
C) Prescribing antidepressant medication without evaluation
D) Dismissing his emotional concerns as a normal reaction to cancer

Question 117: What is the primary goal of managing skin alterations in cancer patients receiving palliative care?
A) Preventing infection
B) Promoting comfort
C) Enhancing wound healing
D) Minimizing scarring

Question 118: Scenario: Sarah, a 55-year-old female, is undergoing radiation therapy for breast cancer. She experiences skin redness and irritation in the treated area. Which of the following interventions is most appropriate for managing this side effect?
A) Applying heating pads to the affected area
B) Using harsh soaps to cleanse the skin
C) Wearing tight clothing over the treated area
D) Applying fragrance-free moisturizers

Question 119: Which of the following is a common barrier to effective care navigation for cancer patients?
A) Clear communication among healthcare providers
B) Limited access to transportation services
C) Timely and accurate diagnosis
D) Adequate financial resources

Question 120: Which intervention is commonly used to address psychosocial distress in cancer patients?
A) Chemotherapy
B) Radiation therapy
C) Support groups
D) Surgery

Question 121: Mr. Patel, a 55-year-old prostate cancer patient, is experiencing erectile dysfunction following his treatment. Which of the following psychological effects may exacerbate sexual dysfunction in cancer patients?
A) Increased self-esteem
B) Anxiety
C) Positive body image
D) Social support

Question 122: Scenario: Mark, an oncology nurse, is part of a quality improvement initiative to enhance patient safety in the oncology unit. Which approach best exemplifies effective collaboration in this initiative?
A) Mark implements changes based solely on his observations without consulting other team members.
B) Mark collaborates with the nursing staff but excludes input from patients and families.
C) Mark actively involves all stakeholders, including patients, families, and healthcare providers, in identifying and implementing safety improvements.
D) Mark disregards feedback from the hospital administration regarding safety protocols.

Question 123: Mr. Garcia, a 60-year-old patient with pancreatic cancer, develops jaundice, pruritus, and dark urine. Which of the following patterns of symptoms is indicative of late symptoms in cancer patients?
A) Acute dyspnea and chest pain
B) Chronic diarrhea and abdominal cramping
C) Late-onset jaundice and pruritus
D) Acute confusion and hallucinations

Question 124: Which of the following is a key characteristic of evidence-based practice in oncology nursing?
A) Relying solely on personal experience
B) Incorporating patient preferences and values
C) Disregarding current research findings
D) Following outdated protocols

Question 125: Which insurance type is commonly utilized by oncology patients to cover medical expenses related to cancer treatment?
A) Home insurance
B) Car insurance
C) Health insurance
D) Travel insurance

Question 126: How can healthcare providers address sexual concerns in cancer patients effectively?
A) Avoid discussing sexual issues to prevent discomfort
B) Provide resources and referrals to sexual health specialists
C) Minimize communication about sexuality to focus on medical treatment
D) Dismiss sexual concerns as non-essential during cancer care

Question 127: Scenario: Sarah, a 35-year-old female patient with a history of domestic violence, presents to the oncology clinic with signs of distress and anxiety. She confides in the nurse about her abusive relationship. What is the most appropriate initial action for the nurse to take?
A) Provide Sarah with resources for shelters and support groups.
B) Encourage Sarah to confront her abuser directly.
C) Advise Sarah to keep the abuse a secret to avoid further conflict.
D) Dismiss Sarah's concerns as unrelated to her oncology treatment.

Question 128: Which hypersensitivity reaction involves the formation of immune complexes that deposit in tissues, leading to complement activation and tissue damage?
A) Type I
B) Type II
C) Type III
D) Type IV

Question 129: Which of the following is a common psychosocial challenge faced by caregivers of oncology patients?
A) Financial burden
B) Physical therapy techniques
C) Medical terminology
D) Surgical procedures

Question 130: How can financial concerns impact the psychosocial well-being of cancer patients?
A) Decreased stress levels
B) Improved quality of life
C) Increased anxiety and depression
D) Enhanced social support

Question 131: Scenario: John, a 55-year-old prostate cancer survivor, is experiencing emotional distress due to financial concerns related to his ongoing care. Which insurance benefit can help John manage the psychosocial dimensions

of his care?
A) Copayment
B) Coinsurance
C) Mental Health Parity
D) Out-of-Pocket Maximum

Question 132: Which of the following best describes the impact of a cancer diagnosis on social relationships and family dynamics?
A) Strengthening of existing relationships
B) Decreased communication within the family
C) Increased conflict due to stress
D) Improved financial stability

Question 133: Which skin manifestation is commonly associated with radiation therapy in cancer patients?
A) Petechiae
B) Erythema
C) Purpura
D) Xerosis

Question 134: Scenario: Emily, a 30-year-old patient undergoing chemotherapy, is struggling with feelings of sadness and hopelessness. Which coping mechanism should the nurse discourage Emily from using?
A) Engaging in creative activities
B) Seeking professional counseling
C) Self-isolation
D) Physical exercise

Question 135: What is the role of the oncology nurse in ensuring legal and ethical practice?
A) Disregarding patient rights
B) Advocating for patient autonomy
C) Engaging in fraudulent activities
D) Neglecting informed consent process

Question 136: What is a crucial aspect to consider when assessing a patient experiencing domestic violence?
A) Blaming the victim for the situation
B) Assuming the abuser's behavior is justified
C) Maintaining confidentiality
D) Reporting the abuse without consent

Question 137: Which of the following is a characteristic of malignant tumors?
A) Well-differentiated cells
B) Slow growth rate
C) Invasive growth
D) Encapsulated structure

Question 138: Ms. Patel, a 45-year-old female undergoing chemotherapy for breast cancer, complains of sharp chest pain that worsens with inspiration. She appears restless and diaphoretic. On examination, you note muffled heart sounds and pulsus paradoxus. What is the likely diagnosis?
A) Myocardial infarction
B) Cardiac tamponade
C) Aortic dissection
D) Pericarditis

Question 139: Sarah, a 30-year-old leukemia patient, is struggling with feelings of isolation and loneliness during her hospital stay. Which intervention would best address Sarah's psychosocial needs?
A) Limiting visitors to prevent overwhelming Sarah.
B) Arranging for a therapy dog to visit Sarah in the hospital.
C) Discouraging Sarah from expressing her emotions to avoid negativity.
D) Keeping Sarah's room devoid of personal items to maintain cleanliness.

Question 140: Which surgical procedure involves the removal of the entire breast, including the nipple, areola, and overlying skin?
A) Lumpectomy
B) Mastectomy
C) Sentinel lymph node biopsy
D) Breast-conserving surgery

Question 141: Which musculoskeletal symptom is commonly associated with bone metastases in cancer patients?
A) Muscle weakness
B) Joint stiffness
C) Pathologic fractures
D) Numbness and tingling

Question 142: Ms. Smith, a 40-year-old patient with multiple myeloma, is undergoing an autologous stem cell transplant. What is the source of stem cells in this type of transplant?
A) Bone marrow
B) Peripheral blood
C) Umbilical cord blood
D) Adipose tissue

Question 143: Scenario: Michael, a 50-year-old patient receiving radiation therapy, is experiencing nausea and vomiting as side effects. Which dietary recommendation would be most suitable for Michael?
A) Avoid all fruits and vegetables to reduce fiber intake
B) Opt for high-fat meals to prevent stomach irritation
C) Consume small, frequent meals and snacks throughout the day
D) Increase intake of spicy foods to stimulate appetite

Question 144: Mrs. Patel, a 60-year-old female, was diagnosed with stage I ovarian cancer. She underwent surgery and completed chemotherapy. Follow-up tests reveal no signs of cancer. What can be inferred about Mrs. Patel's prognosis?
A) Excellent prognosis
B) Poor prognosis
C) Moderate prognosis
D) Uncertain prognosis

Question 145: Mrs. Lee, a 70-year-old lung cancer patient, completed immunotherapy treatment four months ago. She now presents with new-onset diarrhea and abdominal cramping. Which delayed-onset side effect of immunotherapy is she most likely experiencing?
A) Thyroid dysfunction
B) Hepatitis
C) Colitis
D) Pneumonitis

Question 146: Which imaging modality is commonly used to diagnose Superior vena cava syndrome?
A) MRI
B) CT Scan
C) X-ray
D) Ultrasound

Question 147: What imaging modality is typically used to assess increased intracranial pressure in oncologic emergencies?
A) Echocardiogram
B) MRI
C) Colonoscopy
D) Electroencephalogram

Question 148: Where do colorectal cancers commonly metastasize?
A) Liver
B) Lungs
C) Spleen

D) Bladder

Question 149: How can healthcare providers support the maintenance of social relationships during cancer treatment?
A) Encouraging isolation to focus on treatment
B) Providing resources for family counseling
C) Discouraging involvement of friends and extended family
D) Suggesting complete independence from family support

Question 150: Which integrative modality focuses on promoting relaxation, reducing stress, and enhancing overall well-being through gentle touch or manipulation?
A) Qigong
B) Ayurveda
C) Therapeutic touch
D) Naturopathy

ANSWER WITH DETAILED EXPLANATION SET [4]

Question 1: Correct Answer: B) Using a mild soap for cleansing
Rationale: Using a mild soap for cleansing helps maintain skin integrity and prevents further irritation. Ice packs can worsen skin damage. Topical corticosteroids are reserved for severe reactions. Scratching can lead to skin breakdown and infection.

Question 2: Correct Answer: A) Biopsy
Rationale: A biopsy involves the removal of a small tissue sample for examination under a microscope to confirm the presence of cancer cells. An echocardiogram assesses heart function, a liver function test evaluates liver health, and a urinalysis examines urine composition. Therefore, the correct option is A.

Question 3: Correct Answer: B) B cells
Rationale: B cells are responsible for producing antibodies, which can target cancer cells for destruction. T cells are involved in directly killing infected or abnormal cells, while natural killer cells and macrophages are primarily responsible for identifying and destroying abnormal cells through different mechanisms.

Question 4: Correct Answer: B) Inform the physician immediately about the discrepancy.
Rationale: In oncology nursing practice, it is crucial to address any medication errors promptly. Informing the physician immediately ensures patient safety and allows for timely intervention. Altering documentation or ignoring the error can lead to serious consequences for the patient and legal implications for the nurse. Waiting to report the error at the end of the shift delays necessary actions that could prevent harm to the patient.

Question 5: Correct Answer: B) Administering chemotherapy and biotherapy
Rationale: The correct answer is B because as an Oncology Certified Nurse (OCN), administering chemotherapy and biotherapy falls within the scope of practice. Surgical procedures, radiation therapy, and prescribing medications are typically outside the scope of practice for nurses and are usually performed by physicians or advanced practice providers. Administering chemotherapy and biotherapy is a crucial aspect of oncology nursing practice, requiring specialized knowledge and skills.

Question 6: Correct Answer: C) Anxiety can manifest as physical symptoms
Rationale: Anxiety in oncology patients can manifest as physical symptoms such as headaches, muscle tension, fatigue, and gastrointestinal disturbances. These physical symptoms can impact the patient's overall well-being and quality of life. Anxiety can also affect treatment adherence, is not always a sign of depression, and can significantly impact the patient's emotional and psychological state.

Question 7: Correct Answer: C) Cohort study
Rationale: Cohort studies follow a group of individuals over time to observe how their exposure to certain risk factors influences the development of specific outcomes. Case-control studies are retrospective and compare individuals with a disease to those without the disease. Cross-sectional studies assess exposure and outcome at a single point in time, while randomized controlled trials involve random allocation of participants to different interventions.

Question 8: Correct Answer: D) Type IV
Rationale: Mr. Brown is experiencing a Type IV hypersensitivity reaction, also known as delayed-type hypersensitivity. This reaction typically occurs 48-72 hours after exposure to an antigen and is characterized by a localized inflammatory response. Type I involves immediate allergic reactions, Type II involves cytotoxic reactions, and Type III involves immune complex deposition, none of which match Mr. Brown's presentation of localized skin changes post-radiation therapy.

Question 9: Correct Answer: A) Chronic myeloid leukemia
Rationale: The Philadelphia chromosome is a genetic abnormality found in chronic myeloid leukemia, aiding in its diagnosis and targeted treatment. Skin melanoma, thyroid, and bone cancers do not exhibit this specific chromosomal abnormality, distinguishing them from chronic myeloid leukemia.

Question 10: Correct Answer: C) Connecting him with a caregiver support group
Rationale: Connecting James with a caregiver support group would be the most beneficial intervention to address his psychosocial needs as a caregiver experiencing burnout. Caregiver support groups offer emotional support, coping strategies, and a sense of community with others facing similar challenges, which can help alleviate feelings of isolation and stress. While respite care, relaxation techniques, and hobbies are important for self-care, a caregiver support group would provide James with targeted support and understanding from peers in similar situations.

Question 11: Correct Answer: C) Sublimation
Rationale: Sublimation involves channeling negative emotions or impulses into positive and socially acceptable behaviors. This differs from displacement (A), which involves transferring emotions from one target to another, rationalization (B), which involves justifying behaviors with logical reasoning, and repression (D), which involves unconsciously blocking out thoughts or feelings.

Question 12: Correct Answer: A) Chemotherapy
Rationale: Chemotherapy is a common trigger for anaphylaxis in oncology patients due to the potential for hypersensitivity reactions to the medications used. While radiation therapy and surgery may have their own associated complications, they are not typically direct triggers for anaphylaxis. Blood transfusions can lead to transfusion reactions but are not as commonly associated with anaphylaxis in oncology patients.

Question 13: Correct Answer: C) Gene Therapy
Rationale: Gene therapy aims to modify genetic material within cells to enhance their ability to combat cancer. Monoclonal antibodies target specific antigens, cytokine therapy boosts immune responses, and cancer vaccines prevent cancer development.

Question 14: Correct Answer: D) TNM staging
Rationale: The correct answer is D) TNM staging, which is the most commonly used staging system for colorectal cancer. Option A) Lugano classification is used for lymphomas, Option B) Dukes staging is used for colorectal cancer, and Option C) FIGO staging is used for gynecological cancers. Therefore, TNM staging is the appropriate choice for determining the extent of spread in colorectal cancer.

Question 15: Correct Answer: D) Recommend soft, bland foods at room temperature to ease discomfort
Rationale: Patients experiencing taste changes and mouth sores benefit from consuming soft, bland foods at room temperature as they are gentle on the mouth and easier to tolerate. Spicy foods can exacerbate mouth sores, citrus fruits may be irritating, and plastic utensils do not alter taste perception significantly.

Question 16: Correct Answer: D) Recommending soft, bland foods and oral hygiene care
Rationale: Soft, bland foods and oral hygiene care help alleviate difficulty swallowing and oral mucositis during radiation therapy. Spicy foods can further irritate the mucosa, ice chips may be too harsh on the sensitive tissues, and alcohol-based mouthwash can exacerbate mucositis.

Question 17: Correct Answer: B) Promoting efficient workflow
Rationale: A clean and organized work environment in oncology nursing promotes efficient workflow, reduces errors, and enhances patient care delivery. While workplace aesthetics are important, the primary focus is on optimizing workflow. Maintaining cleanliness also plays a crucial role in infection control, contrary to minimizing the need for hand hygiene. Patient satisfaction is influenced by various factors beyond just the cleanliness of the environment.

Question 18: Correct Answer: B) Mini-Mental State Examination (MMSE)
Rationale: The Mini-Mental State Examination (MMSE) is a widely used tool for assessing cognitive function, including

orientation, memory, and attention. It helps healthcare providers evaluate the severity of cognitive impairment and monitor changes over time. A pain scale, blood pressure cuff, and electrocardiogram are not specific tools for assessing cognitive function and would not provide relevant information in this case.

Question 19: Correct Answer: A) Allow the religious leader to visit Maria and facilitate spiritual support.
Rationale: Acknowledging and respecting a patient's cultural and spiritual beliefs is essential in providing holistic care. Allowing the religious leader to visit Maria will provide her with the spiritual support she needs during this challenging time. Options B, C, and D are incorrect as they do not address Maria's cultural and spiritual needs, which are crucial aspects of psychosocial care in oncology.

Question 20: Correct Answer: B) Peripherally Inserted Central Catheter (PICC)
Rationale: A PICC line is suitable for continuous infusions of chemotherapy as it provides long-term access with fewer complications. Options A and C are specific to dialysis needs, while option D is more commonly used for intermittent infusions.

Question 21: Correct Answer: C) Provide aggressive intravenous hydration
Rationale: The initial management of tumor lysis syndrome (TLS) involves aggressive intravenous hydration to prevent renal damage from uric acid, phosphate, and potassium crystal deposition. Furosemide may exacerbate electrolyte imbalances, allopurinol is used for prophylaxis, and calcium gluconate is indicated for symptomatic hypocalcemia.

Question 22: Correct Answer: A) Cognitive-behavioral therapy
Rationale: Cognitive-behavioral therapy is an effective intervention for addressing the psychological effects of sexual dysfunction in cancer survivors by helping them cope with body image issues and anxiety. Chemotherapy, radiation therapy, and surgery are not specifically targeted at addressing psychological effects.

Question 23: Correct Answer: C) Assessment
Rationale: In this scenario, the nurse should prioritize the assessment step of the nursing process to gather data about Sarah's nausea and vomiting. Assessment involves collecting and analyzing information to identify the patient's problems and needs. Planning (option A) comes after assessment and involves setting goals and outcomes. Evaluation (option B) is the final step to determine if the goals were met. Implementation (option D) is the step where the nurse carries out the plan of care.

Question 24: Correct Answer: D) Serotonin-Norepinephrine Reuptake Inhibitors (SNRIs)
Rationale: SNRIs, such as duloxetine and venlafaxine, are often preferred in cancer patients for managing depression due to their dual mechanism of action targeting both serotonin and norepinephrine. They are also effective in managing pain symptoms commonly experienced by cancer patients. TCAs and MAOIs have more side effects and drug interactions, while SSRIs primarily target serotonin levels.

Question 25: Correct Answer: A) Fasting during specific religious holidays
Rationale: Cultural practices such as fasting during religious holidays can significantly influence a patient's adherence to treatment plans, including medication schedules and dietary restrictions. This practice may affect the timing and administration of cancer treatments, potentially leading to complications or suboptimal outcomes. Understanding and respecting these cultural beliefs are crucial for providing patient-centered care.

Question 26: Correct Answer: C) Ureteral stent placement
Rationale: Ureteral stent placement is often utilized in advanced cervical cancer to relieve urinary obstruction caused by tumor growth. Nephrostomy tubes are more for kidney drainage. Suprapubic catheters are used for bladder drainage. Urinary diversion surgery is considered for more extensive genitourinary issues beyond simple obstruction.

Question 27: Correct Answer: A) Hypnosis
Rationale: Hypnosis is a non-pharmacologic comfort measure that utilizes guided imagery and relaxation techniques to help patients manage pain, anxiety, and other symptoms. This approach can be beneficial in improving the patient's overall well-being. Surgery, blood transfusion, and physical therapy are not primarily focused on utilizing guided imagery and relaxation techniques for comfort measures in cancer care.

Question 28: Correct Answer: C) Alleviating symptoms and improving comfort
Rationale: In palliative gastrectomy, the primary goal is to alleviate symptoms such as pain, bleeding, or obstruction, and to improve the patient's quality of life. This procedure is not aimed at complete cancer eradication, prolonging survival, or preventing recurrence, making option C the most appropriate goal for Mr. Garcia's palliative surgical intervention.

Question 29: Correct Answer: B) Administering chemotherapy and biotherapy agents
Rationale: The correct answer is B because administering chemotherapy and biotherapy agents falls within the Scope of Practice for an Oncology Certified Nurse (OCN). Options A, C, and D are incorrect as they involve tasks that are typically performed by other healthcare professionals in the oncology setting, such as surgeons, radiation therapists, and physical therapists.

Question 30: Correct Answer: D) Type IV
Rationale: Type IV hypersensitivity reactions are delayed hypersensitivity reactions mediated by sensitized T lymphocytes and macrophages. This type of reaction is involved in conditions like contact dermatitis, graft rejection, and some autoimmune diseases. Unlike Type I, II, and III hypersensitivity reactions, Type IV does not involve antibodies but rather cell-mediated immune responses causing tissue damage over time.

Question 31: Correct Answer: C) Participating in quality improvement initiatives
Rationale: OCNs play a crucial role in professional practice evaluation by actively engaging in quality improvement initiatives within oncology settings. They contribute to enhancing patient care standards, implementing evidence-based practices, and ensuring adherence to professional guidelines. While research and financial management are important aspects of nursing practice, the focus of professional practice evaluation for OCNs is on quality improvement and patient-centered care.

Question 32: Correct Answer: B) Peripheral neuropathy
Rationale: Chemotherapy often leads to peripheral neuropathy in oncology patients, causing symptoms such as numbness, tingling, and pain in the extremities. Hypertension (option A), hyperthyroidism (option C), and osteoporosis (option D) are not typically direct side effects of chemotherapy.

Question 33: Correct Answer: B) Skin biopsy
Rationale: A skin biopsy involves the removal of a suspicious skin lesion for examination to determine if cancerous cells are present. An MRI scan is used for detailed imaging, a stool occult blood test screens for colorectal cancer, and a renal function test assesses kidney health. Therefore, the correct option is B.

Question 34: Correct Answer: A) Intramuscular epinephrine
Rationale: Intramuscular epinephrine is the first-line treatment for anaphylaxis in oncology patients as it helps reverse the systemic effects of the allergic reaction. While antihistamines, fluids, and oxygen therapy may be used as adjunct treatments, epinephrine is the most critical intervention.

Question 35: Correct Answer: A) Patient Education and Counseling
Rationale: The Joint Commission emphasizes patient education and counseling as essential components of oncology care to ensure patients receive comprehensive information about their diagnosis, treatment options, and supportive care services. Staffing ratios, hospital revenue generation, and marketing strategies are not primary areas of focus for The Joint Commission in oncology accreditation.

Question 36: Correct Answer: B) To remove the tumor and a margin of surrounding healthy tissue.
Rationale: A lumpectomy, also known as breast-conserving surgery, aims to remove the tumor along with a margin of healthy tissue around it while preserving the breast. This approach helps in achieving local control of the disease while maintaining

cosmesis. Options A, C, and D are incorrect as a lumpectomy does not involve removing the entire breast, performing reconstructive surgery, or administering chemotherapy directly to the tumor site.

Question 37: Correct Answer: B) Open communication
Rationale: Open communication fosters transparency, encourages reporting of errors, and facilitates continuous quality improvement efforts in oncology nursing practice. Authoritarianism, blaming individuals for errors, and resisting change can create barriers to a culture of safety and quality improvement.

Question 38: Correct Answer: C) Targeted therapies aim to specifically target cancer cells while minimizing harm to normal cells.
Rationale: Targeted therapies are designed to interfere with specific molecules involved in cancer cell growth and survival. Unlike traditional chemotherapy, they are intended to target cancer cells with precision, minimizing damage to normal, healthy cells. This specificity is a key advantage of targeted therapies, reducing the likelihood of severe side effects compared to non-targeted treatments.

Question 39: Correct Answer: C) Assessment
Rationale: Assessment is the first phase of the nursing process where the nurse collects data about the patient's health status. This data includes physical, emotional, social, and spiritual aspects. Planning involves setting goals and outcomes, implementation is the phase where interventions are carried out, and evaluation is the final phase where the nurse determines the effectiveness of the care provided.

Question 40: Correct Answer: A) Administer epinephrine intramuscularly
Rationale: In the scenario described, the patient is experiencing signs and symptoms of anaphylaxis, which is a life-threatening emergency. The immediate and most effective treatment for anaphylaxis is the administration of epinephrine. Epinephrine acts quickly to reverse the symptoms of anaphylaxis by constricting blood vessels, improving breathing, and increasing heart function. Stopping the infusion, administering diphenhydramine, or increasing the infusion rate are not the first-line interventions for anaphylaxis and may delay appropriate treatment, potentially leading to a worsening of the patient's condition.

Question 41: Correct Answer: D) Monitoring the patient for signs of radiation dermatitis
Rationale: Monitoring the patient for signs of radiation dermatitis is crucial during radiation therapy to assess skin reactions and provide appropriate interventions. Encouraging increased caffeine intake, promoting sun exposure, and applying aloe vera gel are not recommended interventions and may exacerbate side effects.

Question 42: Correct Answer: D) Provide emotional support and empathy
Rationale: Oncology nurses play a crucial role in supporting cancer patients with depression by providing emotional support, empathy, and a caring presence. Minimizing communication, disregarding emotional needs, and encouraging social isolation can exacerbate feelings of depression and isolation in patients.

Question 43: Correct Answer: A) AJCC
Rationale: The correct answer is A) AJCC, which stands for the American Joint Committee on Cancer. The AJCC TNM staging system is widely used for lung cancer staging. Option B) FIGO is used for gynecological cancers, Option C) SEER is a database, and Option D) Dukes is used for colorectal cancer staging. Therefore, the AJCC system is the appropriate choice for staging lung cancer.

Question 44: Correct Answer: B) Egg freezing
Rationale: Egg freezing is the most effective method for fertility preservation in female cancer patients. Options A, C, and D are not typically used for fertility preservation and may not be suitable or effective in this scenario.

Question 45: Correct Answer: C) Type III
Rationale: Ms. Johnson is experiencing a Type III hypersensitivity reaction, characterized by immune complex deposition in tissues leading to inflammation. Symptoms such as fever, joint pain, and rash are typical of this reaction. Type I involves immediate allergic responses, Type II involves cytotoxic reactions, and Type IV involves delayed hypersensitivity, none of which match Ms. Johnson's presentation.

Question 46: Correct Answer: B) Blocking specific targets on cancer cells
Rationale: Monoclonal antibodies work by blocking specific targets on cancer cells, leading to their destruction. Options A, C, and D are incorrect as monoclonal antibodies do not directly kill cancer cells, stimulate cancer cell growth, or inhibit the immune response.

Question 47: Correct Answer: C) Weakness or numbness in extremities
Rationale: Weakness or numbness in extremities is a common symptom of spinal cord compression in oncology patients due to the pressure on the spinal cord. Headache, abdominal pain, and chest pain are not typically associated with spinal cord compression but may indicate other conditions.

Question 48: Correct Answer: C) Group therapy
Rationale: Group therapy can be an effective intervention to address altered body image in cancer patients by providing a supportive environment where individuals can share their experiences, receive feedback, and learn coping strategies. Meditation techniques can help with relaxation but may not directly target body image concerns. Cosmetic surgery is not always recommended or feasible for all patients. Avoiding discussions about body image can lead to increased distress and isolation.

Question 49: Correct Answer: B) Corticosteroids
Rationale: The mainstay of treatment for pneumonitis in oncology patients is corticosteroids. These medications help reduce inflammation in the lungs and alleviate symptoms. Antibiotics and antifungal medications are not typically used unless there is an underlying infection. Chemotherapy may exacerbate pneumonitis and should be carefully evaluated in these patients to prevent further lung damage.

Question 50: Correct Answer: C) Delivering evidence-based, patient-centered care
Rationale: Quality of practice in oncology nursing involves delivering care that is evidence-based, ensuring that interventions are supported by research and tailored to individual patient needs. This approach emphasizes patient-centered care, where the focus is on the patient's preferences, values, and goals. Options A and D do not encompass the comprehensive nature of quality care, while option B, although important, does not capture the essence of patient-centeredness and evidence-based practice which are crucial in oncology nursing.

Question 51: Correct Answer: B) Initiating prophylactic antibiotics
Rationale: Neutropenia puts the patient at high risk for infections. Initiating prophylactic antibiotics helps prevent bacterial infections in neutropenic patients. Administering erythropoietin is used to treat anemia, not neutropenia. Encouraging consumption of raw fruits and vegetables can increase the risk of infections due to bacteria present on them. Avoiding hand hygiene is detrimental as proper hand hygiene is crucial in preventing infections in immunocompromised patients.

Question 52: Correct Answer: A) Implementing cultural competency training for healthcare staff
Rationale: Implementing cultural competency training can help healthcare staff better understand and address the diverse needs of cancer survivors, reducing instances of discrimination and promoting inclusive care practices. Ignoring patient feedback, limiting access based on age, and excluding diverse perspectives can exacerbate discrimination concerns, hindering the delivery of equitable and patient-centered survivorship care.

Question 53: Correct Answer: D) Adjust medications to manage contributing factors
Rationale: Fatigue in palliative care is often multifactorial. Adjusting medications, addressing anemia, optimizing pain control, and managing depression or anxiety can help alleviate fatigue. Physical therapy and exercise may not be suitable for

patients with profound fatigue.

Question 54: Correct Answer: B) Provide strategies for building self-confidence and coping with stigma
Rationale: Supporting the patient in developing self-confidence and resilience against societal stigma is crucial in promoting mental well-being. Encouraging isolation or unnecessary cosmetic procedures may worsen the patient's self-image and perpetuate feelings of discrimination. Acknowledging and addressing these concerns can help the patient navigate social challenges effectively.

Question 55: Correct Answer: A) Proper disposal of hazardous waste
Rationale: Proper disposal of hazardous waste is essential to maintain environmental health standards in oncology settings. Wearing jewelry, using personal mobile phones in patient areas, and reusing disposable gloves can introduce contaminants and compromise environmental safety.

Question 56: Correct Answer: A) Stage 0
Rationale: Stage 0, also known as carcinoma in situ, indicates abnormal cells confined to the original site without invasion into deeper layers. Stages I, II, and III involve increasing degrees of invasion and spread, making Stage 0 the appropriate choice for Emily's case.

Question 57: Correct Answer: D) Implement a schedule to optimize machine usage
Rationale: Implementing a schedule to optimize machine usage will help reduce energy wastage and improve resource utilization in radiation therapy. Informing the radiation therapy team about the idle machine issue is crucial for addressing the inefficiency. Ignoring the idle machine or continuing with the current practice will not address the resource utilization problem effectively.

Question 58: Correct Answer: B) Cardiotoxicity
Rationale: Radiation therapy to the chest area can lead to delayed-onset cardiotoxicity, which may manifest years after treatment. This condition increases the risk of heart disease. Fatigue, diarrhea, and hair loss are more immediate side effects of radiation therapy and are not typically classified as delayed-onset.

Question 59: Correct Answer: C) Alleviation of dyspnea
Rationale: Alleviation of dyspnea (difficulty breathing) is a priority concern in the palliative care of oncology patients with advanced disease, as it significantly impacts quality of life. Improved mobility (option A), enhanced taste perception (option B), and increased blood pressure (option D) are not typically primary concerns in this context.

Question 60: Correct Answer: D) Abdominal X-ray
Rationale: Abdominal X-ray is frequently utilized to diagnose bowel obstruction in oncology patients due to its ability to visualize air-fluid levels and distended loops of bowel. ECG, MRI, and bone scans are not typically used for diagnosing bowel obstructions.

Question 61: Correct Answer: A) Gabapentin
Rationale: Gabapentin is a first-line treatment for neuropathic pain in cancer patients due to its efficacy in managing nerve-related pain. Morphine is an opioid and may not target neuropathic pain specifically. Acetaminophen and ibuprofen are not typically used as first-line agents for neuropathic pain.

Question 62: Correct Answer: D) Start palliative radiation therapy to the painful bone site
Rationale: Palliative radiation therapy is a common intervention for managing bone pain in patients with metastatic bone cancer. It helps reduce pain by targeting the tumor and surrounding tissues. Options A, B, and C are not the first-line interventions for managing severe bone pain in this scenario.

Question 63: Correct Answer: C) Infiltrate with hyaluronidase
Rationale: Infiltrating the affected area with hyaluronidase (Option C) is the recommended treatment for an extravasation caused by a vesicant chemotherapy agent to help disperse the medication and reduce tissue damage. Applying heat (Option A) can worsen the injury. Elevating the limb (Option B) is beneficial for non-vesicant extravasations. Massaging the area (Option D) can increase tissue damage.

Question 64: Correct Answer: B) Developing individualized care plans for oncology patients
Rationale: The correct answer is B because developing individualized care plans for oncology patients is a core responsibility within the Scope of Practice for an OCN. Options A, C, and D are incorrect as they involve tasks that are typically performed by other healthcare professionals in the oncology setting.

Question 65: Correct Answer: B) Monitoring and managing side effects
Rationale: Radiation oncology nurses play a crucial role in assessing, educating, and supporting patients throughout their radiation therapy treatment. They focus on monitoring and managing side effects, providing emotional support, and ensuring patient safety. Administering chemotherapy, performing radiation therapy, and conducting surgeries are tasks typically carried out by other healthcare professionals in their respective specialties.

Question 66: Correct Answer: C) Impaired decision-making
Rationale: Cognitive dysfunction in cancer patients often manifests as impaired decision-making abilities rather than improved cognitive functions like increased attention span, enhanced memory recall, or improved problem-solving skills. Impaired decision-making can significantly impact a patient's ability to make informed choices about their treatment and care.

Question 67: Correct Answer: A) Bronchoscopy
Rationale: Bronchoscopy is a procedure where a thin, flexible tube with a camera is inserted through the nose or mouth into the lungs to visualize the airways and collect tissue samples for biopsy. MRI, ultrasound, and echocardiogram are imaging tests that do not involve tissue sampling from the lungs.

Question 68: Correct Answer: C) Emotional distress
Rationale: Emotional distress can significantly hinder the learning process for oncology patients. When individuals are overwhelmed by emotions such as fear, anxiety, or sadness, their ability to focus, retain information, and engage in the learning process is compromised. Supportive family members (option A) and positive reinforcement (option B) can actually facilitate learning by providing encouragement and a conducive environment. Clear communication (option D) is essential for effective learning but may not be as impactful as addressing emotional distress, which is a common barrier in oncology care.

Question 69: Correct Answer: D) Insidious development
Rationale: Chronic symptoms in oncology patients often have an insidious onset, gradually worsening over time. Unlike acute symptoms, chronic symptoms persist beyond the initial phase of treatment and may require long-term management. Sudden onset, decreasing intensity, and resolution with treatment completion are not typical of chronic symptoms.

Question 70: Correct Answer: D) Oral cryotherapy
Rationale: Oral cryotherapy, or ice chips, can help reduce the severity of mucositis by constricting blood vessels and decreasing blood flow to the mouth. Alcohol-based mouthwash can exacerbate mucositis. Regular dental flossing can irritate the mucosa. Ice-cold beverages can worsen mucositis by causing vasoconstriction.

Question 71: Correct Answer: A) Relaxation techniques
Rationale: Relaxation techniques, such as deep breathing exercises and guided imagery, can help alleviate anxiety associated with dyspnea in cancer patients. Benzodiazepines may cause respiratory depression and are not recommended as first-line treatment for dyspnea-related anxiety. Antidepressants are more suitable for managing depression symptoms. CBT may be beneficial for addressing underlying psychological distress but may not provide immediate relief for acute dyspnea-related anxiety.

Question 72: Correct Answer: C) Hepatitis
Rationale: Hepatitis is an immune-related adverse event characterized by liver inflammation, leading to symptoms such as elevated liver enzymes, jaundice, and abdominal pain. Thyroiditis (A) involves inflammation of the thyroid gland, dermatitis (B) is skin inflammation, and myositis (D) is muscle inflammation, all distinct from hepatitis in terms of affected organs and clinical presentation.

Question 73: Correct Answer: B) Respecting patient autonomy and preferences
Rationale: The correct answer is B because respecting patient autonomy and preferences is a crucial aspect of patient advocacy within the standards of practice for an Oncology Certified Nurse (OCN). Making treatment decisions on behalf of the patient, withholding information, and disregarding patient rights are contrary to the principles of patient advocacy and ethical nursing practice. Oncology nurses play a vital role in advocating for patients by honoring their autonomy, preferences, and rights throughout the care process.

Question 74: Correct Answer: B) Avoiding limb compression
Rationale: Avoiding limb compression is crucial for preventing lymphedema in patients following axillary lymph node dissection to reduce the risk of impaired lymphatic flow. Encouraging vigorous arm exercises (Option A) can exacerbate lymphedema. Applying heat packs (Option C) may increase blood flow but does not prevent lymphedema. Allowing blood pressure measurements (Option D) on the affected arm can increase the risk of lymphedema development.

Question 75: Correct Answer: A) Pain management
Rationale: Effective pain management is essential for oncology patients post-surgery to enhance recovery, improve quality of life, and facilitate early mobilization. Monitoring blood sugar levels is more relevant for diabetic patients, lung function tests are typically done for respiratory conditions, and urine analysis is not directly linked to surgical outcomes in oncology patients.

Question 76: Correct Answer: C) Smoking tobacco
Rationale: Smoking tobacco is a high-risk behavior that can contribute to the development of colorectal cancer. Tobacco smoke contains carcinogens that can enter the bloodstream and affect the colon cells, increasing the risk of colorectal cancer. Consuming a diet rich in fruits and vegetables, regular colorectal cancer screening, and maintaining a healthy weight are preventive health practices that can help reduce the risk of colorectal cancer by promoting overall colon health and early detection of any abnormalities.

Question 77: Correct Answer: B) "Using cold caps may reduce the risk of hair loss, but individual results vary."
Rationale: Evidence-based practice involves integrating clinical expertise with the best available evidence. Option B reflects this principle by acknowledging the potential benefit of cold caps while highlighting the variability in outcomes based on individual factors. Options A, C, and D present extreme or unsupported statements, which do not align with evidence-based practice.

Question 78: Correct Answer: A) Tumor histology
Rationale: The selection of targeted therapies in oncology is heavily influenced by the specific characteristics of the tumor, including its histology, genetic mutations, and protein expression patterns. These factors help oncologists determine the most appropriate targeted therapy for a particular patient. Options B, C, and D are not directly related to the selection of targeted therapies and are therefore incorrect choices in this context.

Question 79: Correct Answer: B) Constipation
Rationale: Constipation is a common side effect of opioid medications in cancer patients due to decreased gastrointestinal motility. It can be effectively managed with the use of laxatives and stool softeners to prevent complications such as bowel obstruction. Nausea is often managed with antiemetics, sedation may improve with dose adjustments, and respiratory depression is a serious but less common side effect that requires close monitoring and intervention.

Question 80: Correct Answer: C) Validate Emily's emotions and help her reframe her thoughts about guilt.
Rationale: Validating Emily's feelings of guilt and assisting her in reframing negative thoughts can promote healing and self-forgiveness. By offering support and guidance, the nurse can help Emily navigate through complex emotions associated with survivor's guilt. Options A, B, and D are incorrect as they involve reinforcing guilt, suppressing emotions, and avoiding discussions, which can exacerbate Emily's distress and hinder her bereavement process.

Question 81: Correct Answer: B) Encourage open communication with his partner about his concerns.
Rationale: Encouraging open communication with his partner about his concerns is essential in addressing Mr. Patel's sexual health. This fosters understanding, support, and exploration of alternative intimate activities. Options A, C, and D are incorrect as they do not directly address the issue of erectile dysfunction and may not be suitable or effective interventions.

Question 82: Correct Answer: C) To empower individuals to make decisions about their future healthcare.
Rationale: The primary purpose of advance care planning is to empower individuals to make informed decisions about their future healthcare, particularly in situations where they may not be able to communicate their preferences. Options A, B, and D do not accurately reflect the main goal of advance care planning and are therefore incorrect.

Question 83: Correct Answer: B) Informing Emily about the importance of maintaining continuous health insurance coverage
Rationale: The oncology nurse should educate Emily about the importance of maintaining continuous health insurance coverage post-cancer treatment. Continuous coverage ensures that Emily has access to necessary healthcare services and treatments without facing coverage gaps or pre-existing condition exclusions. This option addresses Emily's concern about securing health insurance post-cancer and emphasizes the significance of maintaining coverage for ongoing care.

Question 84: Correct Answer: B) Manual lymphatic drainage
Rationale: Manual lymphatic drainage is a gentle massage technique that helps reduce swelling in lymphedema by promoting lymph flow. Heat packs can worsen lymphedema by dilating blood vessels. High-impact weightlifting can exacerbate lymphedema by increasing fluid accumulation. Tight bandaging can impede lymphatic flow and should be avoided.

Question 85: Correct Answer: C) Engaging in open dialogue with a healthcare team
Rationale: Open communication with healthcare providers is crucial in addressing sexual dysfunction in cancer patients, allowing for tailored interventions and support. Avoiding communication, ignoring treatment impact, and isolating oneself can exacerbate issues, making them incorrect options.

Question 86: Correct Answer: B) Liver function
Rationale: Monitoring liver function is critical during chemotherapy as many chemotherapeutic agents are metabolized by the liver. Changes in liver function tests can indicate drug toxicity or potential liver damage. While monitoring blood pressure is important for overall health, bone density is more relevant in conditions like osteoporosis, and vision acuity is not directly impacted by chemotherapy in most cases.

Question 87: Correct Answer: C) Seeking education on diverse cultural practices
Rationale: Cultivating cultural competence involves actively seeking knowledge about various cultural beliefs, values, and practices to provide culturally sensitive care. Stereotyping, avoiding discussions, or imposing one's cultural norms can lead to misunderstandings, conflicts, and compromised patient outcomes. Continuous learning and respect for cultural diversity are essential in delivering quality oncology care.

Question 88: Correct Answer: C) Patient Health Questionnaire-9 (PHQ-9)
Rationale: The Patient Health Questionnaire-9 (PHQ-9) is a validated tool specifically designed to screen for and monitor the severity of depression symptoms in cancer patients. It assesses various symptoms such as depressed mood, anhedonia, sleep disturbances, fatigue, and changes in appetite. The other options, Pain Assessment, Karnofsky Performance Status Scale, and Edmonton Symptom Assessment System, focus on different aspects of patient assessment and symptom management, but they are not specific tools for evaluating depression symptoms.

Question 89: Correct Answer: B) Notify the physician about the signs of infection
Rationale: In oncology nursing practice, prompt recognition and management of infections are crucial. Notifying the physician about the signs of infection allows for timely intervention and appropriate treatment. Proceeding with the dressing change or

applying antibiotic ointment without physician consultation can worsen the condition.
Question 90: Correct Answer: D) Palliative care
Rationale: Palliative care focuses on providing relief from the symptoms and stress of a serious illness like cancer, including cognitive decline, to improve the quality of life for both the patient and their family. Unlike curative care, which aims to cure the disease, palliative care is designed to provide comfort and support, making it the most appropriate option for patients experiencing cognitive decline near the end of life.
Question 91: Correct Answer: C) Gender of the patient
Rationale: The risk of cancer recurrence is usually not significantly influenced by the gender of the patient. Factors such as age at diagnosis, type of cancer, and stage of the cancer play crucial roles in determining the likelihood of recurrence. Age at diagnosis can impact the body's ability to recover, the type of cancer affects its aggressiveness, and the stage of cancer indicates how far it has spread, all contributing to the recurrence risk. Therefore, gender alone is not a primary determinant of cancer recurrence.
Question 92: Correct Answer: D) Arranging for a visit from a hospital chaplain
Rationale: A hospital chaplain can provide Mr. Patel with spiritual support, guidance, and a listening ear to address his feelings of abandonment and distress. Chaplains are trained to help individuals navigate spiritual struggles and find comfort in their faith. Referring him to a support group may help, but addressing his immediate spiritual needs through a chaplain visit is more direct and beneficial.
Question 93: Correct Answer: D) Hypotension
Rationale: While fatigue, nausea and vomiting, and muscle weakness are common symptoms of hypercalcemia in oncologic emergencies, hypotension is not a typical symptom. Hypercalcemia often presents with dehydration, which can lead to hypotension, but hypotension itself is not a direct symptom of hypercalcemia.
Question 94: Correct Answer: C) Monoclonal antibody therapy
Rationale: Monoclonal antibody therapy is a type of biotherapy that uses antibodies designed to target specific antigens on cancer cells. These antibodies can either directly kill cancer cells or help the immune system recognize and destroy them. Gene therapy, cytokine therapy, and stem cell transplant are other biotherapy approaches but do not specifically involve the use of antibodies to target cancer cells.
Question 95: Correct Answer: B) At the time of cancer diagnosis
Rationale: Palliative care can be initiated at the time of cancer diagnosis and can be provided alongside curative treatments. It focuses on symptom management, emotional support, and improving quality of life throughout the cancer journey, not just in the terminal stage. Early integration of palliative care has been shown to improve patient outcomes and quality of life.
Question 96: Correct Answer: A) Inhibition of specific molecules involved in cancer growth
Rationale: Targeted therapies in oncology work by specifically targeting and inhibiting molecules or pathways that are crucial for cancer cell growth and survival. This approach differs from traditional chemotherapy, which affects both cancerous and healthy cells. Options B, C, and D are incorrect as they do not accurately describe the mechanism of action of targeted therapies. Option B is more aligned with immunotherapy, while options C and D are not reflective of the targeted nature of these therapies.
Question 97: Correct Answer: C) Social withdrawal
Rationale: Social withdrawal is a common psychosocial distress symptom in cancer patients due to factors such as fear, stigma, and coping mechanisms. Increased appetite and improved sleep quality are not typically associated with psychosocial distress in this context. Decreased anxiety would actually be a positive outcome rather than a distress symptom.
Question 98: Correct Answer: C) Implementing a structured exercise program
Rationale: Implementing a structured exercise program has been shown to reduce cancer-related fatigue and improve overall quality of life. Encouraging frequent napping can disrupt nighttime sleep patterns. Limiting physical activity can lead to deconditioning and worsen fatigue. Consuming caffeine before bedtime can interfere with sleep quality, exacerbating fatigue.
Question 99: Correct Answer: A) To directly target and kill cancer cells
Rationale: Radiation therapy aims to destroy cancer cells by damaging their DNA, preventing them from multiplying. It does not boost the immune system but works as a localized treatment. The goal is to shrink tumors, not promote cancer cell growth, and ultimately eliminate or control the cancer.
Question 100: Correct Answer: C) Smoking
Rationale: Smoking is a well-established modifiable risk factor for lung cancer. Sarah's long history of smoking significantly increases her risk of developing lung cancer. High-fat diet and sedentary lifestyle are important factors in overall health but are not directly linked to lung cancer. Occupational exposure to asbestos is associated with mesothelioma, not lung cancer.
Question 101: Correct Answer: C) Self-sufficiency in growth signals
Rationale: Cancer cells exhibit self-sufficiency in growth signals, meaning they can proliferate independently of external growth factors. This characteristic distinguishes them from normal cells. Increased apoptosis (Option A) is not a hallmark of cancer; instead, cancer cells often evade apoptosis. Contact inhibition (Option B) is a property of normal cells, where they stop dividing when they come into contact with other cells. Limited angiogenesis (Option D) is not a hallmark of cancer; in fact, cancer cells promote angiogenesis to ensure blood supply for tumor growth.
Question 102: Correct Answer: A) Hyperkalemia
Rationale: Peaked T waves on ECG are indicative of hyperkalemia, a common electrolyte abnormality in tumor lysis syndrome. Hypernatremia, hypomagnesemia, and hypercalcemia are not typically associated with TLS.
Question 103: Correct Answer: D) FIGO grade
Rationale: The correct answer is D) FIGO grade, which is used to grade ovarian tumors based on cellular features. Option A) Gleason score is used for prostate cancer, Option B) Bloom-Richardson grade is used for breast cancer, and Option C) Fuhrman grade is used for kidney cancer. Therefore, the FIGO grade is the appropriate choice for classifying ovarian tumors based on cellular features.
Question 104: Correct Answer: C) Disseminated Intravascular Coagulation (DIC)
Rationale: The scenario describes a classic presentation of DIC, a serious condition where widespread activation of coagulation leads to both thrombosis and bleeding. The combination of thrombocytopenia, prolonged clotting times, and low fibrinogen levels is indicative of DIC. Tumor Lysis Syndrome presents with metabolic abnormalities, Superior Vena Cava Syndrome with obstruction of the SVC, and Hypercalcemia of Malignancy with elevated calcium levels.
Question 105: Correct Answer: B) Surrendering decision-making to healthcare providers
Rationale: 'Loss of personal control' in psychosocial distress often manifests as patients feeling overwhelmed and relinquishing decision-making to healthcare providers due to the complex nature of cancer treatment. This can lead to increased anxiety and a sense of helplessness. Options A, C, and D focus on aspects of empowerment, active participation, and seeking support, which are not indicative of 'Loss of personal control' in this context.
Question 106: Correct Answer: C) Genetic mutations can increase the risk of cancer by altering cell function
Rationale: Genetic mutations play a significant role in carcinogenesis by altering the normal function of cells and promoting uncontrolled growth. While not all genetic mutations lead to cancer, they can increase the risk of cancer development. Options A, B, and D are incorrect as they do not accurately describe the impact of genetic mutations on carcinogenesis.
Question 107: Correct Answer: A) It is a legal document that

specifies the type of medical care a person wishes to have in the event they are unable to communicate their preferences.
Rationale: An advance directive is a legal document that allows individuals to express their preferences for medical treatment in the event they are unable to communicate their wishes. It provides guidance to healthcare providers and family members regarding the individual's healthcare decisions. Options B, C, and D are incorrect as they do not accurately describe what an advance directive is and its purpose.

Question 108: Correct Answer: C) Connecting patients with financial resources and support services
Rationale: Oncology nurses can play a crucial role in helping patients by connecting them with financial resources and support services that can assist with their financial concerns. Providing direct financial assistance is usually beyond the scope of nursing practice. Ignoring financial concerns or offering emotional support alone may not effectively address the root of the issue.

Question 109: Correct Answer: D) Enterocolitis
Rationale: Enterocolitis is a common immune-related adverse event associated with immunotherapy, presenting with symptoms such as diarrhea and colitis. Pneumonitis involves lung inflammation, hepatitis involves liver inflammation, and dermatitis involves skin inflammation, which are less likely in this scenario.

Question 110: Correct Answer: A) Mastectomy
Rationale: Lymphedema is a common complication following mastectomy, especially when lymph nodes are removed or damaged during the surgery. Nephrectomy, colectomy, and prostatectomy are not typically associated with the development of lymphedema.

Question 111: Correct Answer: B) Dementia
Rationale: Dementia is a broad term used to describe a decline in cognitive function severe enough to interfere with daily life. Delirium is a sudden state of confusion and disorientation that often has a reversible cause. Amnesia refers to memory loss, while aphasia is a language disorder. Therefore, among the options provided, dementia best fits the description of a decline in memory, language, problem-solving, and thinking skills affecting daily activities.

Question 112: Correct Answer: A) QOPI
Rationale: The Quality Oncology Practice Initiative (QOPI) is a program designed to assess and improve the quality of oncology practices. It focuses on various aspects of cancer care delivery, including adherence to evidence-based guidelines, patient safety, and quality improvement initiatives. QOPI accreditation signifies a commitment to providing high-quality cancer care.

Question 113: Correct Answer: C) Antiemetics
Rationale: Antiemetics are commonly used in palliative care to alleviate nausea and vomiting in cancer patients with gastrointestinal issues. These medications help control symptoms and improve the patient's comfort. Antibiotics, chemotherapy, and anticoagulants are not primarily indicated for managing nausea and vomiting in this context, making them incorrect choices.

Question 114: Correct Answer: A) Liver
Rationale: Breast cancer commonly metastasizes to the liver due to its rich blood supply and the presence of estrogen receptors. The liver provides a favorable environment for breast cancer cells to settle and grow. Prostate, colon, and thyroid are not typical sites for breast cancer metastasis, making them incorrect options.

Question 115: Correct Answer: B) Spiritual distress can lead to increased anxiety and depression
Rationale: Spiritual distress in cancer patients can significantly impact their emotional well-being, leading to increased anxiety and depression (option B). It goes beyond religious practices (option C) and cannot be easily resolved with medical interventions (option D). Ignoring the impact of spiritual distress (option A) can worsen the patient's overall quality of life.

Question 116: Correct Answer: B) Conducting a comprehensive psychosocial assessment
Rationale: Conducting a comprehensive psychosocial assessment allows the nurse to identify the underlying causes of Mr. Lee's distress, develop a tailored care plan, and refer him to appropriate support services. Encouraging isolation, prescribing medication without evaluation, or dismissing emotional concerns can exacerbate his condition and hinder effective management of psychosocial distress.

Question 117: Correct Answer: B) Promoting comfort
Rationale: In palliative care, the primary goal of managing skin alterations is to promote comfort and quality of life rather than aggressive wound healing or scar prevention. While preventing infection is important, comfort takes precedence in palliative care settings.

Question 118: Correct Answer: D) Applying fragrance-free moisturizers
Rationale: Applying fragrance-free moisturizers helps soothe and hydrate the irritated skin during radiation therapy. Heating pads can exacerbate skin irritation, harsh soaps can further dry out the skin, and tight clothing can cause friction and discomfort, worsening the condition.

Question 119: Correct Answer: B) Limited access to transportation services
Rationale: Limited access to transportation services can hinder a cancer patient's ability to attend appointments, receive treatments, and access supportive care services, impacting their overall care navigation. Options A, C, and D are facilitators rather than barriers to effective care navigation.

Question 120: Correct Answer: C) Support groups
Rationale: Support groups are a common intervention to address psychosocial distress in cancer patients by providing a platform for sharing experiences, coping strategies, and emotional support. Chemotherapy, radiation therapy, and surgery are treatment modalities for cancer itself and do not directly target psychosocial distress.

Question 121: Correct Answer: B) Anxiety
Rationale: Anxiety is a psychological effect commonly experienced by cancer patients that can exacerbate sexual dysfunction. Increased self-esteem and positive body image are more likely to have a positive impact on sexual function.

Question 122: Correct Answer: C) Mark actively involves all stakeholders, including patients, families, and healthcare providers, in identifying and implementing safety improvements.
Rationale: Effective collaboration in quality improvement initiatives in oncology nursing involves actively involving all stakeholders, including patients, families, healthcare providers, and administrators, in the process of identifying and implementing safety improvements. This inclusive approach ensures that diverse perspectives are considered, leading to more effective and sustainable changes. Options A, B, and D represent actions that do not reflect effective collaboration as they involve working in isolation, excluding key stakeholders, or disregarding valuable input from the administration.

Question 123: Correct Answer: C) Late-onset jaundice and pruritus
Rationale: Late symptoms in cancer patients may include manifestations such as late-onset jaundice and pruritus, which can indicate liver involvement or obstruction of the bile ducts. Acute dyspnea and chest pain are more suggestive of acute cardiac or pulmonary issues. Chronic diarrhea and abdominal cramping are characteristic of chronic gastrointestinal problems. Acute confusion and hallucinations are more likely related to metabolic disturbances or central nervous system issues.

Question 124: Correct Answer: B) Incorporating patient preferences and values
Rationale: Evidence-based practice in oncology nursing involves integrating the best available research evidence with clinical expertise and patient values. By considering patient preferences and values, nurses can provide individualized care that aligns with the patient's needs and goals, leading to improved outcomes. Relying only on personal experience, disregarding research findings, or following outdated protocols can compromise the quality of care and patient safety.

Question 125: Correct Answer: C) Health insurance
Rationale: Health insurance is essential for oncology patients to cover the costs of cancer treatment, including surgeries,

chemotherapy, and radiation therapy. Home, car, and travel insurance do not typically provide coverage for medical expenses related to cancer care.

Question 126: Correct Answer: B) Provide resources and referrals to sexual health specialists
Rationale: Addressing sexual concerns in cancer patients is crucial for their overall well-being. Healthcare providers should offer resources and referrals to sexual health specialists who can provide appropriate support and interventions. Avoiding discussions on sexual issues, minimizing communication, or dismissing concerns can lead to increased distress and hinder the patient's quality of life during and after cancer treatment.

Question 127: Correct Answer: A) Provide Sarah with resources for shelters and support groups.
Rationale: In cases of domestic violence, the priority is to ensure the safety of the patient. Providing resources for shelters and support groups can help Sarah access the help she needs. Encouraging confrontation or advising secrecy can escalate the situation and put Sarah at further risk.

Question 128: Correct Answer: C) Type III
Rationale: Type III hypersensitivity reactions result from the deposition of immune complexes in tissues, leading to complement activation, inflammation, and tissue damage. This process can contribute to conditions like serum sickness, Arthus reaction, and certain autoimmune diseases. Type I involves IgE-mediated immediate responses, Type II involves antibody-mediated cell destruction, and Type IV involves delayed cell-mediated responses.

Question 129: Correct Answer: A) Financial burden
Rationale: Caregivers often face financial challenges due to the costs associated with cancer treatment, transportation, and caregiving responsibilities. This can lead to increased stress and impact the caregiver's overall well-being. Options B, C, and D are not directly related to the psychosocial challenges faced by caregivers, making them incorrect choices.

Question 130: Correct Answer: C) Increased anxiety and depression
Rationale: Financial concerns can lead to increased anxiety and depression among cancer patients due to worries about medical bills, treatment costs, and financial stability. These concerns can significantly impact the psychosocial well-being of patients. The other options are incorrect as financial concerns typically do not decrease stress levels, improve quality of life, or enhance social support.

Question 131: Correct Answer: C) Mental Health Parity
Rationale: Mental Health Parity ensures that mental health services are covered at the same level as medical/surgical benefits. Copayments and coinsurance are cost-sharing methods, while the out-of-pocket maximum limits the total expenses a patient must pay. However, Mental Health Parity specifically addresses the psychosocial aspects of care, offering support for patients like John.

Question 132: Correct Answer: C) Increased conflict due to stress
Rationale: A cancer diagnosis can often lead to increased stress within the family, which may result in heightened conflict due to emotional strain, financial burdens, and changes in roles and responsibilities. This can challenge the family dynamics and communication patterns. While some relationships may strengthen through adversity, the overall impact tends to involve increased tension and conflict as the family navigates the challenges associated with cancer.

Question 133: Correct Answer: B) Erythema
Rationale: Erythema, or skin redness, is a common side effect of radiation therapy due to inflammation of the skin. It is characterized by redness, warmth, and sometimes itching. Petechiae and purpura are more commonly associated with blood disorders or certain infections. Xerosis refers to dry skin and is not specifically linked to radiation therapy.

Question 134: Correct Answer: C) Self-isolation
Rationale: Self-isolation is a maladaptive coping mechanism that can intensify feelings of sadness and hopelessness by limiting social interactions and support. Encouraging Emily to engage in creative activities, seek professional counseling, and participate in physical exercise can provide her with healthy outlets to express emotions, gain insights, and improve her overall well-being. These coping mechanisms promote emotional processing, resilience, and a sense of empowerment, unlike self-isolation, which can exacerbate feelings of loneliness and despair.

Question 135: Correct Answer: B) Advocating for patient autonomy
Rationale: Oncology nurses play a vital role in advocating for patient autonomy, respecting patient rights, and upholding ethical standards in practice. Engaging in fraudulent activities, neglecting informed consent, or disregarding patient rights are unethical behaviors that can compromise patient care quality and trust. By promoting patient autonomy, oncology nurses empower patients to make informed decisions about their care and treatment options.

Question 136: Correct Answer: C) Maintaining confidentiality
Rationale: When assessing a patient experiencing domestic violence, maintaining confidentiality is crucial to build trust and ensure the patient's safety. Blaming the victim or assuming the abuser's behavior is justified can further traumatize the individual. Reporting the abuse without consent may put the patient at risk of further harm and violate their autonomy.

Question 137: Correct Answer: C) Invasive growth
Rationale: Malignant tumors exhibit invasive growth, where they infiltrate surrounding tissues and can metastasize to distant sites. Well-differentiated cells (Option A) resemble normal cells and are characteristic of benign tumors. Malignant tumors typically have a rapid growth rate (Option B) compared to benign tumors. Encapsulated structure (Option D) is a feature of benign tumors, providing a clear boundary separating them from surrounding tissues.

Question 138: Correct Answer: B) Cardiac tamponade
Rationale: The clinical presentation of sharp chest pain worsening with inspiration, along with muffled heart sounds and pulsus paradoxus, is highly suggestive of cardiac tamponade. In this oncologic emergency, fluid accumulation in the pericardial sac impairs cardiac function. Myocardial infarction, aortic dissection, and pericarditis may present with chest pain but typically do not exhibit muffled heart sounds and pulsus paradoxus as seen in cardiac tamponade.

Question 139: Correct Answer: B) Arranging for a therapy dog to visit Sarah in the hospital.
Rationale: Arranging for a therapy dog to visit Sarah in the hospital can provide her with companionship, emotional support, and a sense of connection, thereby alleviating feelings of isolation and loneliness. Limiting visitors may further isolate Sarah. Discouraging emotional expression can hinder her coping mechanisms. Keeping her room devoid of personal items may contribute to a sterile environment that lacks warmth and comfort.

Question 140: Correct Answer: B) Mastectomy
Rationale: Mastectomy is the surgical procedure that involves the complete removal of the breast tissue. This procedure is indicated in cases of extensive breast cancer or as a preventive measure in high-risk individuals. Lumpectomy involves removing only the tumor and a small margin of surrounding tissue, while sentinel lymph node biopsy is done to determine if cancer has spread to the lymph nodes. Breast-conserving surgery aims to remove the tumor while preserving the breast.

Question 141: Correct Answer: C) Pathologic fractures
Rationale: Pathologic fractures are a common musculoskeletal symptom in cancer patients with bone metastases. These fractures occur due to weakened bones from cancer cells replacing normal bone cells. Muscle weakness (Option A) and joint stiffness (Option B) are less commonly associated with bone metastases compared to pathologic fractures. Numbness and tingling (Option D) are more indicative of neurological issues rather than musculoskeletal complications in this context.

Question 142: Correct Answer: B) Peripheral blood
Rationale: In an autologous stem cell transplant, the patient's own stem cells are collected from the peripheral blood. Bone

marrow, umbilical cord blood, and adipose tissue are not typically used as a source of stem cells in autologous transplants.

Question 143: Correct Answer: C) Consume small, frequent meals and snacks throughout the day
Rationale: Patients experiencing nausea and vomiting benefit from consuming small, frequent meals and snacks throughout the day to prevent an empty stomach, which can worsen symptoms. Avoiding fruits and vegetables can lead to nutrient deficiencies, high-fat meals may exacerbate stomach irritation, and spicy foods can further irritate the stomach lining.

Question 144: Correct Answer: A) Excellent prognosis
Rationale: Mrs. Patel's prognosis is excellent as there are no signs of cancer on follow-up tests post-treatment. Stage I ovarian cancer with no evidence of disease after treatment indicates a high likelihood of long-term survival and favorable prognosis.

Question 145: Correct Answer: C) Colitis
Rationale: Mrs. Lee's symptoms of diarrhea and abdominal cramping four months post-immunotherapy are suggestive of colitis, a delayed-onset side effect affecting the colon. Thyroid dysfunction, hepatitis, and pneumonitis are potential side effects of immunotherapy but are less likely to present with these gastrointestinal symptoms.

Question 146: Correct Answer: B) CT Scan
Rationale: CT scan is the preferred imaging modality for diagnosing Superior vena cava syndrome as it provides detailed images of the chest area, including the superior vena cava. MRI, X-ray, and ultrasound may also be used but are not as effective in visualizing the obstruction.

Question 147: Correct Answer: B) MRI
Rationale: MRI (Magnetic Resonance Imaging) is the preferred imaging modality to assess increased intracranial pressure in oncologic emergencies as it provides detailed images of the brain structures. Echocardiogram is used to assess heart function, colonoscopy for the colon, and electroencephalogram for brain electrical activity, not for imaging intracranial pressure.

Question 148: Correct Answer: A) Liver
Rationale: Colorectal cancer often spreads to the liver through the portal vein system. The liver's role in filtering blood makes it susceptible to metastatic deposits from colorectal tumors. Lungs, spleen, and bladder are not typical sites for colorectal cancer metastasis, making them incorrect choices.

Question 149: Correct Answer: B) Providing resources for family counseling
Rationale: Healthcare providers play a crucial role in supporting social relationships by offering resources for family counseling. This can help families navigate the emotional challenges, communication issues, and changes in roles that often arise during cancer treatment. Encouraging isolation or discouraging involvement of support networks can be detrimental to the patient's well-being and may lead to increased stress and feelings of loneliness.

Question 150: Correct Answer: C) Therapeutic touch
Rationale: Therapeutic touch involves practitioners using their hands to promote relaxation, reduce pain, and improve overall well-being by working with the body's energy field. Qigong and Ayurveda encompass broader traditional healing systems, while naturopathy emphasizes natural remedies and the body's ability to heal itself through lifestyle modifications and supplements. Therapeutic touch specifically emphasizes the power of touch and energy flow to benefit patients' health and well-being.

Made in United States
Troutdale, OR
04/04/2024